HETEROSEXUAL TRANSMISSION OF AIDS

CONRAD WORKSHOP SERIES EDITORS

Gary D. Hodgen, Ph.D.
Director
CONRAD Program

Henry L. Gabelnick, Ph.D.
Deputy Director
CONRAD Program

Nancy J. Alexander, Ph.D.
Director, Applied Fundamental Research
CONRAD Program

David F. Archer, M.D.
Director, Clinical Research
CONRAD Program

Anibal A. Acosta, M.D.
Director, Fellowships and Andrology
CONRAD Program

Jeffrey M. Spieler, M.Sc.
Senior Biomedical Research Advisor
Research Division, Office of Population
Agency for International Development

Marilyn A. Mendelson, Ph.D.
Technical Editor

Rose-Marie Bradley Jones
Production Editor

HETEROSEXUAL TRANSMISSION OF AIDS

Proceedings of the Second Contraceptive Research and Development (CONRAD) Program International Workshop, Held in Norfolk, Virginia, February 1–3, 1989

EDITORS

NANCY J. ALEXANDER
Contraceptive Research and Development Program
Eastern Virginia Medical School
Norfolk, Virginia

HENRY L. GABELNICK
Contraceptive Research and Development Program
Eastern Virginia Medical School
Arlington, Virginia

JEFFREY M. SPIELER
Office of Population
Agency for International Development
Washington, D.C.

WILEY-LISS, NEW YORK

Address all Inquiries to the Publisher
Alan R. Liss, Inc., 41 East 11th Street, New York, NY 10003

Printed in United States of America

Library of Congress Cataloging-in-Publication Data

Contraceptive Research and Development Program. International Workshop (2nd : 1989 : Norfolk, Va.)
Heterosexual transmission of AIDS: Proceedings of the Second Contraceptive Research and Development (CONRAD) Program International Workshop, held in Norfolk, Virginia, February 1–3, 1989 / editors, Nancy J. Alexander, Henry L. Gabelnick, Jeffrey M. Spieler.
p. cm.
ISBN 0-471-56208-4
1. AIDS (Disease)—Transmission—Congresses. I. Alexander, Nancy J. II. Gabelnick, Henry L. III. Spieler, Jeffrey M. IV. Title.
[DNLM: 1. Acquired Immunodeficiency Syndrome—prevention & control—congresses. 2. Acquired Immunodeficiency—transmission—congresses. 3. Contraceptive Devices, Male—congresses. 4. Disease Models, Animal—congresses. 5. Sex Behavior—congresses. WD C764h 1989]
RA644.A25C66 1989
616.97'9205—dc20
DNLM/DLC
for Library of Congress 89-22625
CIP

Cover and interior design by Virginia M. Rodgers.

Contents

PART II: ANIMAL MODELS FOR THE STUDY OF SEXUAL TRANSMISSION

PART III: MECHANICS OF HETEROSEXUAL TRANSMISSION

Contributors

NANCY J. ALEXANDER, Contraceptive Research and Development Program, Eastern Virginia Medical School, Norfolk, VA 23510 **[xiii,123]**

DEBORAH J. ANDERSON, Fearing Research Laboratory, Harvard Medical School, Boston, MA 02115 **[167]**

OMAR BAGASRA, Department of Microbiology, New Jersey School of Osteopathic Medicine, Camden, NJ 08109 **[155]**

GERALD S. BERNSTEIN, Department of Obstetrics and Gynecology, Women's Hospital, Los Angeles County, University of Southern California, Los Angeles, CA 90033 **[213]**

MARIANO E. BUSSO, Mount Sinai Medical Center, Miami Beach, FL 33140 **[311]**

BILL CAMERON, Ottawa General Hospital, Ottawa, Ontario K1H 8L6, Canada **[239]**

DIANE N. CATOTTI, Family Health International, Research Triangle Park, Durham, NC 27709 **[291]**

ERIC N. CHANTLER, Department of Obstetrics and Gynecology, University Hospital of South Manchester, West Didsbury, Manchester M2O 8LR, England **[303]**

JAMES CHIN, Global Programme on AIDS, World Health Organization, 1211 Geneva 27, Switzerland **[1]**

RICHARD A. CONE, The Thomas C. Jenkins Department of Biophysics, The Johns Hopkins University, Baltimore, MD 21218 **[115]**

ROBERT C. DUNCAN, University of Miami School of Medicine, Miami, FL 33124 **[311]**

MARTIN DYM, Georgetown University School of Medicine, Washington, DC 20007 **[181]**

TIMOTHY M.M. FARLEY, Special Programme of Research, Development and Research Training in Human Reproduction, World Health Organization, 1211 Geneva 27, Switzerland **[247]**

M. GASTON FARR, Family Health International, Research Triangle Park, Durham, NC 27709 **[291]**

M.F. FATHALLA, World Health Organization, 1211 Geneva 27, Switzerland **[225]**

PAUL J. FELDBLUM, Department of Reproductive Immunology and Sexually Transmitted Diseases, Family Health International, Research Triangle Park, Durham, NC 27709 **[69]**

ROBIN G. FOLDESY, Family Health International, Research Triangle Park, Durham, NC 27709 **[291]**

MICHAEL J. FREE, Program for Appropriate Technology in Health, Seattle, WA 98109 **[379]**

The numbers in brackets are the opening page numbers of the contributors' articles.

MATTHEW FREUND, New Jersey School of Osteopathic Medicine, Camden, NJ 08109 **[155]**

HENRY L. GABELNICK, Contraceptive Research and Development Program, Eastern Virginia Medical School, Arlington, VA 22209 **[xiii]**

MURRAY B. GARDNER, Department of Pathology, University of California, Davis, CA 95616 **[93,137,267]**

AGEGNEHU GETTIE, California Primate Research Center, University of California, Davis, CA 95616 **[123]**

JEFFREY R. HARRIS, Agency for International Development, Washington, DC 20523 **[327,399]**

STANLEY F. HAYES, Laboratory of Pathobiology, Public Health Service, NIAID, Rocky Mountain Labs, Hamilton, MT 59840 **[107]**

ANDREW G. HENDRICKX, California Primate Research Center, University of California, Davis, CA 95616 **[123]**

DAVID L. HEYMANN, Global Programme on AIDS, World Health Organization, 1211 Geneva 27, Switzerland **[1]**

GARY D. HODGEN, Contraceptive Research and Development Program, Eastern Virginia Medical School, Norfolk, VA 23510 **[415]**

ROBERT C. HOLMAN, Statistical Activities, Division of Immunologic, Oncologic and Hematologic Diseases, Center for Infectious Diseases, Centers for Disease Control, Atlanta, GA 30333 **[35]**

JANE HUTCHINGS, Program for Appropriate Technology in Health, Seattle, WA 98109 **[379]**

JANINE M. JASON, Applied Communications, Research Branch, National AIDS Information and Education Program, Centers for Disease Control, Atlanta, GA 30333 **[35]**

MYRA JENNINGS, Medical Pathology Department, University of Califonia, Davis, CA 95616 **[123]**

ANNE M. JOHNSON, Academic Department of Genito-Urinary Medicine, University College and Middlesex School of Medicine, London W1N 8AA, England **[9]**

FRANKLYN N. JUDSON, Denver Public Health Department; Department of Infectious Diseases, Denver General Hospital and Medical Center; and Departments of Medicine and Preventive Medicine, University of Colorado Health Sciences Center, Denver, CO 80220 **[355]**

LENNI W. KANGAS, Consultant, Agency for International Development, Washington, DC 20523 **[399]**

ANDREW A. LACKNER, California Primate Research Center, University of California, Davis, CA 95616 **[123]**

MARIE LAGA, Centers for Disease Control, Atlanta, GA 30333 **[9]**

PETER LAMPTEY, Family Health International, Research Triangle Park, Durham, NC 27709 **[255]**

DALE N. LAWRENCE, Epidemiologic Studies Branch, Division of Reproductive Health, Centers for Disease Control, Atlanta, GA 30333; present address: Clinical Development Section, Vaccine Research and Development Branch, Basic Research and Development Program, Division of AIDS, NIAID, National Institutes of Health, Rockville, MD 20852 **[35]**

JONATHAN M. MANN, Global Programme on AIDS, World Health Organization, 1211 Geneva 27, Switzerland **[1]**

ADRIANA MARTINEZ, Fearing Research Laboratory, Harvard Medical School, Boston, MA 02115 **[167]**

PRESTON A. MARX, Virology and Immunology Unit, California Primate Research Center, University of California, Davis, CA 95616 **[123]**

KENNETH MAYER, Infectious Diseases Division, Memorial Hospital, Pawtucket, RI 02860 **[167]**

FRANK J. McATEE, Public Health Service, NIAID, Rocky Mountain Labs, Hamilton, MT 59840 **[107]**

OLAV MEIRIK, Special Programme of Research, Development and Research Training in Human Reproduction, World Health Organization, 1211 Geneva 27, Switzerland **[247]**

CHRISTOPHER J. MILLER, California Primate Research Center, University of California, Davis, CA 95616 **[123]**

VERONICA E. MILLER, Department of Microbiology and Immunology, UCLA School of Medicine, Los Angeles, CA 90024 **[147]**

THOMAS R. MOENCH, The Johns Hopkins University, Baltimore, MD 21218 **[115]**

JOHN J. MURPHY, Epidemiology Studies, Center for Infectious Diseases, Centers for Disease Control, Atlanta, GA 30333 **[35]**

BARBARA B. NORTH, Healthworks Medical Group, Laguna Niguel, CA 92677 **[273]**

JAN ORENSTEIN, Department of Pathology, George Washington University School of Medicine, Washington, DC 20037 **[181]**

NANCY PADIAN, Department of Epidemiology, San Francisco General Hospital, San Francisco, CA 94110 **[25]**

THOMAS A. PETERMAN, Division of Sexually Transmitted Diseases, Centers for Disease Control, Atlanta, GA 30333 **[55]**

JOHN L. PORTIS, Laboratory of Persistent Viral Diseases, Public Health Service, NIAID, Rocky Mountain Labs, Hamilton, MT 59840 **[107]**

MALCOM POTTS, Family Health International, Research Triangle Park, Durham, NC 27709 **[69]**

JEFFREY PUDNEY, Fearing Research Laboratory, Harvard Medical School, Boston, MA 02115 **[167,197]**

LIONEL RESNICK, Mount Sinai Medical Center, Miami Beach, FL 33140 **[311]**

CORNELIS A.M. RIETMEIJER, Department of Dermatology and Venerology, Dijkzigt University Hospital, 3015 GD Rotterdam, The Netherlands; present address: Denver Disease Control Service, Denver, CO 80204-4507 **[355]**

VIRGINIA L. SCOFIELD, Department of Microbiology and Immunology, UCLA School of Medicine, Los Angeles, CA 90024 **[147]**

JAMES D. SHELTON, Research Division, Office of Population, Agency for International Development, Washington, DC 20523 **[327,399]**

KENNETH D. SOMMERS, Deparement of Microbiology and Immunology, Eastern Virginia Medical School, Norfolk, VA 23507 **[81]**

JEFFREY M. SPIELER, Research Division, Office of Population, Agency for International Development, Washington, DC 20523 **[xiii,419]**

SUGANTO SUTJIPTO, California Primate Research Center, University of California, Davis, CA 95616 **[123]**

A. CHARLES TANQUARY, Family Health International, Research Triangle Park, Durham, NC 27709 **[339]**

DEBORAH C. THOMPSON, Family Health International, Research Triangle Park, Durham, NC 27709 **[291]**

BRUCE VOELLER, Education and Research, The Mariposa Foundation, Topanga, CA 90290 **[365]**

ZHANG WENHAO, Fearing Research Laboratory, Harvard Medical School, Boston, MA 02115 **[167]**

KEVIN J. WHALEY, The Johns Hopkins University School of Medicine, Baltimore, MD 21218 **[115]**

STEVEN S. WITKIN, Department of Obstetrics and Gynecology, Cornell University Medical College, The New York Hospital, New York, NY 10021 **[205]**

JULIE HULL WITTE, Family Health International, Research Triangle Park, Durham, NC 27709 **[339]**

HANS WOLFF, Fearing Research Laboratory, Harvard Medical School, Boston, MA 02115 **[167]**

Preface

The Contraceptive Research and Development Program (CONRAD), funded by the Agency for International Development (A.I.D.), has as its primary mission the development of new and improved methods of fertility regulation suitable for use in developing countries. CONRAD supports research and development projects within its own laboratories and clinics at the Jones Institute for Reproductive Medicine at Eastern Virginia Medical School in Norfolk as well as in universities, research institutions, and private companies worldwide under subproject agreements administered through its Extramural Program.

Since the discovery in 1983 of the human immunodeficiency virus (HIV), which is responsible for AIDS, its has become apparent, perhaps too slowly, that research in contraceptive development needs to be concerned with the possible interaction between existing and new methods of family planning and the spread of sexually transmitted diseases (STDs), including AIDS. For this reason, the CONRAD Program has developed a focused basic and applied research effort, funded in part by the Center for Population Research, National Institute of Child Health and Human Development, aimed at understanding the mechanism and preventing the heterosexual transmission of HIV.

In order to facilitate research efforts, a workshop was held February 1–3, 1989, the aims of which were to:

— Assess the principal risk factors in the heterosexual transmission of HIV

— Understand how sexual behavior changes the risk of heterosexual HIV transmission

— Review the biology and pathogenic mechanisms of retroviruses

— Discuss the use of different animal models for investigating the mechanisms and prevention of heterosexual transmission of HIV

— Focus on the impact of specific contraceptive methods available today and under development in terms of their potential for preventing or enhancing the transmission of HIV

— Establish priorities for research to reduce the spread of AIDS through new contraceptive technology

The workshop brought together over 250 researchers, clinicians, and health care providers from academia, industry, government, and public and private sector organizations and foundations in 15 countries. The proceedings are being published so that an even wider audience may benefit from the information presented by, and the discussion held among, the leading investigators in this field.

Nancy J. Alexander
Henry L. Gabelnick
Jeffrey M. Spieler

1

A Global Overview of AIDS

David L. Heymann, James Chin, and Jonathan M. Mann

The acquired immune deficiency syndrome (AIDS) was recognized as a global emergency by the World Health Assembly and The United Nations General Assembly in 1987 and by Ministers of Health at a summit meeting in London in January, 1988. The World Health Organization (WHO) responded by developing the global AIDS strategy, which has three objectives: to prevent human immunodeficiency virus (HIV) infection, to reduce the personal and social impact of HIV infection, and to unify international and national efforts.

The WHO Global Programme on AIDS regularly receives reports of the number of AIDS cases in member countries and reports of studies of seroprevalence of HIV-1 and HIV-2. Of the 177 countries and territories regularly reporting to WHO, 143 (81%) have reported at least one case of AIDS, demonstrating the global importance of the disease [1].

As of January 1, 1989, these 143 countries reported a cumulative total of approximately 133,000 AIDS cases. Of these cases, approximately 21,000 (16%) were reported from pattern II countries, in which heterosexual transmission is the predominant mode of transmission. Pattern II countries are concentrated in sub-Saharan Africa. Pattern I countries, in which the predominant mode of transmission is among homosexual or bisexual males and intravenous drug users, are concentrated in North America and western Europe but include Australia and New Zealand. Latin America and the Caribbean countries have a combination of pattern I and pattern II transmission and appear to be evolving to pattern II. The remaining countries have pattern III transmission, a small number of cases, many of which are imported (Fig. 1).

Reporting of AIDS cases from pattern II countries is thought to be

Heterosexual Transmission of AIDS, pages 1–8

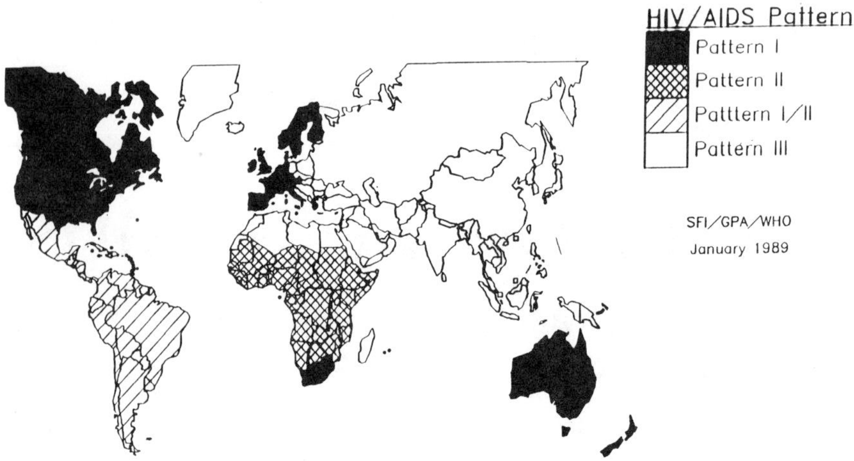

Fig. 1. Global patterns of HIV/AIDS.

incomplete. Based on serological data, the actual cumulative total of AIDS cases by January 1, 1989, was estimated to be more than 377,000, making pattern II, or heterosexual transmission, the dominant global pattern [2], accounting for about 200,000 cases. Pattern I transmission was estimated to have accounted for approximately 175,000 cases by the end of 1988; pattern III transmission is thought to have accounted for less than 1% of all AIDS cases (Table 1). Based on serological study data, the numbers of HIV-infected persons at present are estimated at approximately 2.5 million in sub-Saharan Africa, 2.0 million in the Americas, 0.5 million in Europe, and 0.1 million in Asia and the Pacific, for a global total of at least 5 million HIV-infected individuals [2]. Projections of AIDS have generally been accurate in countries where reporting is high. Projections have corresponded closely with reports from Europe and the United States through 1987; whereas globally, and in Africa, the low percentage of reporting is evident (Fig. 2). Once they are all received, 1988 reports from Europe and the U.S. are expected to correspond to projections.

Other than sexual transmission of the virus, two confirmed means of spread exist: through contaminated blood and blood products and from infected mother to infant during the perinatal period. Transmission due to blood transfusion and blood products in pattern I countries has decreased essentially to zero. The extent of transmission by blood is not known in pattern II countries, although it is thought to be much less important than sexual transmission. One study of children who received blood transfusions in a pattern II

TABLE 1. Reported and Estimated AIDS Cases: Global Data as of January 1, 1989

Region	Reported AIDS	Estimated AIDS	Percent reported
Africa	20,905	200,000	10.5
Americas	93,723	150,000	62.5
Asia	285	500	57.0
Europe	16,883	25,000	67.5
Oceania	1,180	1,500	78.7
Total	132,976	377,000	35.3

country, however, showed a strong relationship between blood transfusion and HIV seropositivity [3], and blood bank screening in certain pattern II cities, where 5% to 20% of blood samples are HIV seropositive, has demonstrated a potential for spread of HIV [4].

Perinatal transmission is thought to occur either in utero or during the birth process. Transmission rates from infected mother to child vary from 25% to 50% and appear to be associated with the state of immunosuppression of the mother; children born to women with low T4 cell counts or to women with clinical AIDS are thought to be at greatest risk of HIV infection [5]. The extent to which transmission from breast milk to infant contributes to perinatal infection has not been established, but transmission has occurred in isolated instances when women received HIV-infected blood transfusions after delivery [10]. Perinatal transmission of HIV-1 will increase in the immediate future as the AIDS pandemic continues to evolve.

Intravenous drug use generally is classified as a separate mode of transmission related to blood, and it accounts for up to 25% of AIDS cases in pattern I countries. Puncture wounds from blood-contaminated needles, transmission through mucous membrane, or transmission through nonvenereal skin lesions account for less than 1% of transmission in pattern I countries. Their importance and rates of transmission in pattern II countries are not yet fully defined.

Estimated rates of transmission by each route vary. Blood transfusion is the most efficient means of transmission, with a risk of over 90% after an infected transfusion, followed by perinatal transmission, with rates of 25% to 50%. The probability of transmission in heterosexual penovaginal intercourse appears to range from 1 in 100 to 1 in 1,000 for a single contact. Rates of transmission for single needle sharing or accidental needle puncture wounds are in the same range (approximately 0.5% to 1.0%).

Recent studies have shown an association between genital ulcerative disease (GUD) and HIV seropositivity. Experts who convened

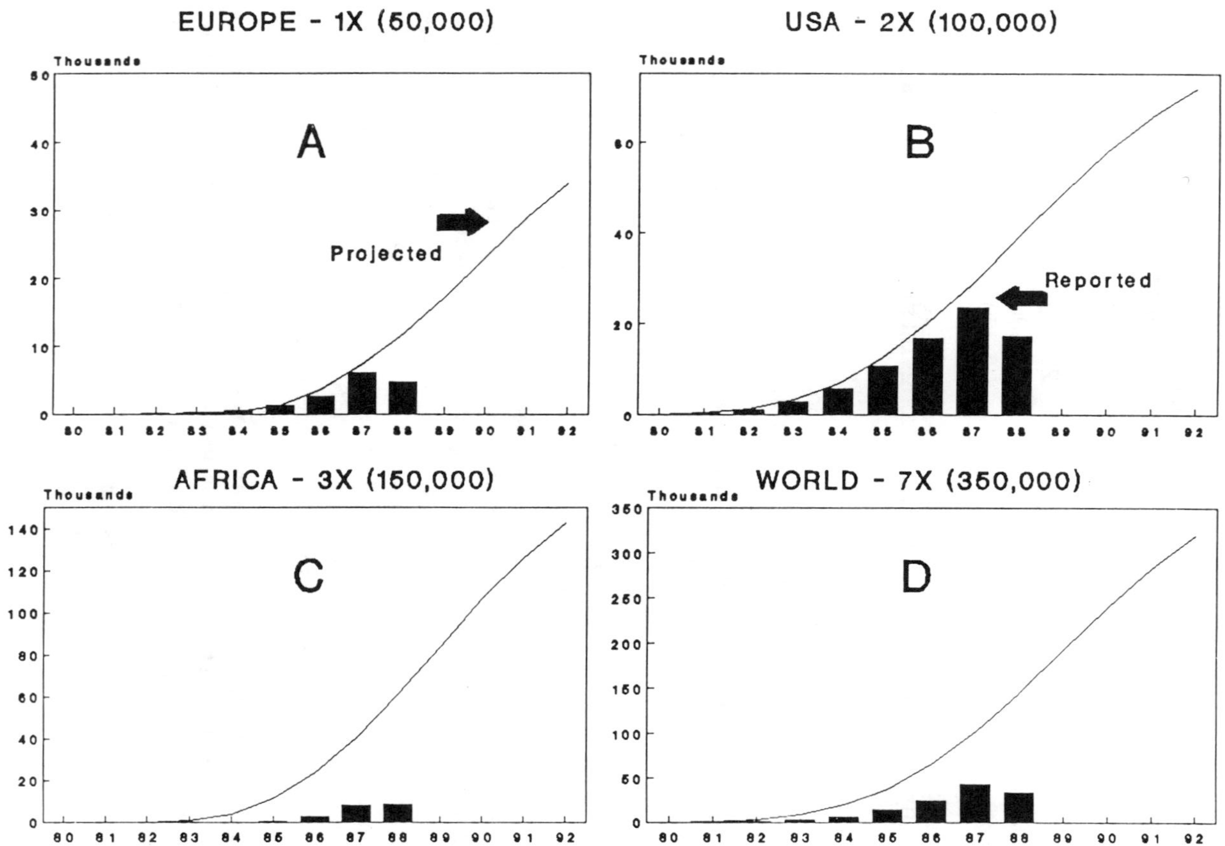
EUROPE - 1X (50,000)
A
Projected
USA - 2X (100,000)
B
Reported
AFRICA - 3X (150,000)
C
WORLD - 7X (350,000)
D
Thousands
80 81 82 83 84 85 86 87 88 89 90 91 92

at WHO in January, 1989, and reviewed all pertinent studies concluded that the association between HIV infection and GUD is sufficiently strong to recommend that GUD treatment may help prevent sexual transmission of HIV-1 [11]. Cohort studies, indicate that progression from infection to AIDS occurs at a rate of 2% to 5% per year in all three patterns of transmission, so that by 10 years after initial infection approximately 50% of individuals have progressed to AIDS [2]. More than 80% of those infected 10 years previously will, however, demonstrate some symptoms of infection.

The rate of tuberculosis is increasing in pattern I countries as the HIV epidemic evolves, and reports suggest that tuberculosis is increasing in several pattern II countries as well. Studies of adults with newly diagnosed tuberculosis in some pattern II countries have demonstrated 20–40% HIV seroprevalence [4]. Tuberculosis rates globally may increase as a direct result of immunosuppression in HIV-infected individuals and indirectly as a result of increased exposure to the tubercle bacillus among family members of HIV-infected individuals with tuberculosis. Relationships between HIV infection and other infectious diseases endemic in pattern II countries are less well defined. However, finding as many as one of five patients on infectious disease wards in pattern II countries infected with HIV-1 is not uncommon [4].

Much less is known about infection with HIV-2. A few epidemiologic studies suggest that modes of transmission for HIV-2 are the same as for HIV-1. It has also been suggested that HIV-2 has a longer latent period. To date, HIV-2 has been reported mainly from West Africa, Angola, and Mozambique (see Fig. 3). However, sporadic HIV-2 infections have been reported from the Americas, the Caribbean, and Europe [12]. Preliminary observations on the epidemiology of HIV-2 are based on small cohorts of HIV-2-infected individuals and on surveys and are complicated by difficulties in interpreting laboratory results for HIV-2 antibody.

AIDS and HIV infection pose a public health problem to all countries, regardless of the pattern of transmission or current prevalence of infection. AIDS appears to be one of the most severe human infectious diseases documented to date. Persons at risk are those having unprotected sex with infected partners, infants born to infected women, persons sharing unsterilized injection equipment with an infected person, persons receiving blood that has not been

Fig. 2. Reported and projected AIDS cases.

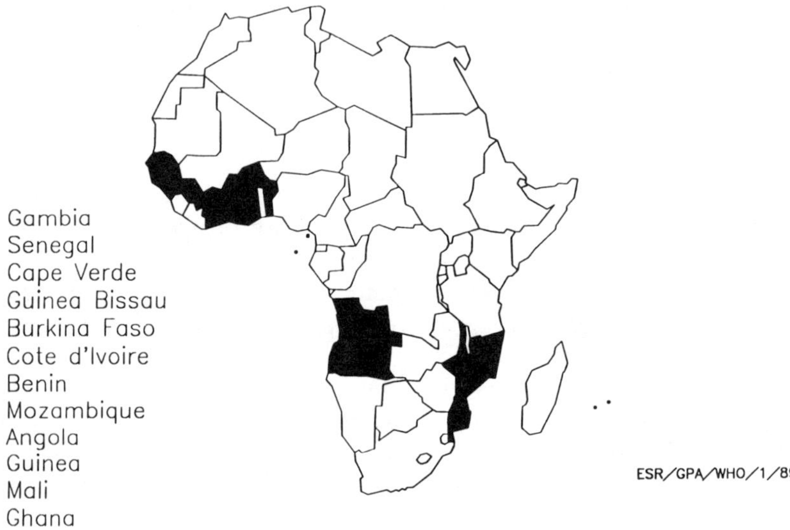

Fig. 3. Reported HIV-2 infection in Africa, December 31, 1988.

screened for antibody to HIV, and, occasionally, persons who are infected through accidents involving blood. Persons without these risks will remain at no measurable threat of HIV infection or AIDS. Mandatory testing as a requirement for entry to a country, or isolation of infected individuals within a country, will not stop the transmission of the HIV virus. In the absence of a vaccine and a curative antiviral medication, the effective control of AIDS will depend on the ability of countries to define the epidemiology of HIV infection and to apply these findings in developing interventions that decrease the risk of HIV transmission.

REFERENCES

1. **World Health Organization Global Programme on AIDS:** Update: AIDS Cases Reported to the Surveillance Forecasting, and Impact Assessment Unit, 4 January, 1989. Geneva: WHO, 1989.

2. **Mann JM, Chin J, Piot P:** The International Epidemiology of AIDS. Sci Am 259(4): 60–69, 1988.

3. **Greenberg AE, Nguyen-Dinh P, Mann JM, et al.:** The association between malaria, blood transfusion and HIV seropositivity in a pediatric population in Kinshasa, Zaire. JAMA 259:545–549, 1988.

4. **World Health Organization Global Programme on AIDS:** Unpublished data, 1988.

5. **Ryder RW, Rayfield M, Quinn T, et al.:** Transplacental HIV transmission in African newborns. Abstract 5123: IV International Conference on AIDS, Stockholm, June, 1988.

6. **Ziegler JB, Cooper DA, Johnson RO, Gold J:** Postnatal Transmission of AIDS-associated retroviruses from mother to infant. Lancet 1:896–897, 1985.

7. **Lepage P, Van de Perre P, Carael M, et al.:** Postnatal transmission of HIV from mother to child. Lancet 2:400, 1987.

8. **Weinbreck P, Lonstaud V, Denis F, Vidal B, Mounier M, de Lumley L:** Postnatal transmission of HIV infection. Lancet 1:482, 1988.

9. **Ziegler JB, Steward GJ, Penny R, Stuckey M, Good S:** Breast feeding and transmission of HIV from mother to infant. Abstract 5100: IV International Conference on AIDS, Stockholm, June, 1988.

10. **Colebunders R, Kapita B, Nekwei W, et al.:** Breast-feeding and transmission of human immunodeficiency. Abstract 5103: IV International Conference on AIDS, Stockholm, June, 1988.

11. **World Health Organization:** Consenses Statement From Consultation on Sexually Transmitted Diseases as a Risk Factor for HIV Transmission. Geneva: WHO, 1989.

12. **Essex M, Kanki PJ:** The origins of the AIDS virus. Sci Am 259(4):44–51, 1988.

DISCUSSION

DR. BIALY: What is the current budget of the WHO Global Programme on AIDS?

DR. HEYMANN: The budget last year was approximately 60 million dollars. Of this, almost 80% was spent in member countries for developing AIDS control programs.

DR. HARRIS: Many of us go to a lot of talks on AIDS, and I think at some point I began to not hear the numbers anymore. We also see reports, like that in the *Washington Post* a year or so ago, that say disease progression is slowing in Africa, that things have leveled off. Do you have a perspective on this, or do you have any data that will give us an idea of how quickly infection is or is not spreading? I am talking about HIV-1.

DR. HEYMANN: I think the article you are referring to was the one about Kinshasa, where it was stated that the prevalence of HIV due to blood transfusions was not increasing. All these quotations of seroprevalence in various populations are very difficult to interpret. They are certainly biased by selection of the individuals. Many times individuals who believe they are infected will not go for screening or to give blood. And, if they think they are going to be tested, they may stay away. So we are really not basing our ideas on the true incidence, but rather on reported seroprevalence and what we know about the epidemiology to come.

I think from all expert opinions, that the problem in pattern II countries is increasing each year. And, I think the estimate of 2–2.5 million HIV-infected people in pattern II countries will increase. I do not think it has yet stopped.

As you know, in pattern II counties, the disease in mainly limited to the urban areas. There is no evidence that in some countries it has spread into rural areas to any great extent. In countries with other patterns, it is spreading into the rural areas. So I think the problem is more dramatic than that portrayed in the papers.

DR. JOHN: I would suggest that pattern III sort of makes you feel comfortable, but many countries in the pattern III regions are currently experiencing a lot of heterosexual transmission. The numbers at this point do not give any comfort. For example, in the Asian region, you said there may be half a million people infected, but I think India alone probably has by now 500,000 people infected, based on a rough extrapolation from large-scale surveys.

DR. HEYMANN: Thank you. I might just add that in certain countries in Asia there are problems among drug users. And, in these populations, the seroprevalence has tripled in the past year. So, as you say, the problem is certainly increasing in Asia in the pattern III countries.

2

Heterosexual Transmission of HIV

Anne M. Johnson and Marie Laga

Heterosexual transmission from men to women and from women to men is a major mode of spread of the human immunodeficiency virus type 1 (HIV-1), particularly in urban centers of sub-Saharan Africa [1–5]. This chapter reviews the biological and epidemiological evidence for heterosexual transmission of HIV and considers research and prevention issues.

The epidemiology of heterosexually acquired HIV reflects major geographical differences [5]. In Europe, North America, much of Latin America, and Australia, transmission of HIV has occurred predominantly among homosexual men and injecting drug users (IDUs); in sub-Saharan Africa, the Carribean, and some parts of Latin America, HIV infection is mainly heterosexually acquired; in Asia, the Pacific region, the Middle East, and eastern Europe, HIV infection has been recently introduced and infection rates are very low. These different epidemiologic patterns are largely determined by the date the virus is introduced into a given community, the pattern of sexual and needle-sharing behavior, and population movements and their subsequent effect on sexual behavior.

THE UNITED STATES AND EUROPE

By the end of December 1988, 3,570 cases of acquired immune deficiency syndrome (AIDS) attributed to heterosexual transmission had been reported to the U.S. Centers for Disease Control (CDC). These cases accounted for 4% of all reported cases of AIDS. Just over one-third of the patients (1,248) were born in countries where heterosexual transmission is the major mode of spread; the remaining

Heterosexual Transmission of AIDS, pages 9–24

two-thirds (2,322) had heterosexual contact with a person with AIDS or at risk for AIDS. The U.S.-born cases increased from 1.1% of all AIDS cases before 1983 to 3.6% in 1988 [6,7] (Chamberland M, personal communication). Heterosexual spread of HIV in the United States occurs largely by transmission from IDUs. Approximately 70% of U.S.-born persons with heterosexually acquired AIDS have been partners of IDUs, and 13% have been partners of bisexual men. Following the pattern of infection among drug users, over 70% of these cases have occurred among black and Hispanic people [7].

Similar patterns are seen in Europe, where 7% of cases have been acquired through heterosexual transmission. Whereas in countries in southern Europe, such as Spain and Italy, heterosexual transmission occurs through IDUs, in countries such as the United Kingdom and Belgium sexual contact with persons from central Africa is also an important source of infection [8–10].

In contrast with their counterparts in Africa, female prostitutes in Europe without a history of injecting drug use show very low HIV infection rates (<1%) [3,11]. In the United States higher prevalence has been found [12]. A large multicenter collaborative study [13] found that 5% of nondrug-using prostitutes were seropositive. Seropositivity was associated with large numbers of nonpaying partners. The current low prevalence among nondrug-using Western prostitutes may reflect the low prevalence of HIV among their clients and the high rates of condom use. Although recruiting a representative group of prostitutes is a difficult task, prostitutes and their clients remain important groups to study for both surveillance and prevention of heterosexually transmitted HIV.

AIDS surveillance gives no estimate of current incidence rates of infection or of the prevalence of asymptomatic infection. The numbers of persons infected currently can only be estimated from studies in selected samples because of the absence of prevalence studies in representative population samples. These estimates rely on data from studies of groups such as blood donors, military recruits, pregnant women, and sexually transmitted diseases (STD) clinic attendees. In 1987, CDC [14] reviewed work in the United States. Aggregated prevalence studies were used, with estimates of the proportion of the population falling into different risk categories, to calculate the approximate numbers infected. An estimated 30,000 heterosexuals in the United States without specific identified risks and 45,000–127,000 heterosexuals born in Haiti and central Africa or with heterosexual partners at high risk had been infected by 1987. Added to these are an estimated 245,000 infected drug users and hemophiliacs, who may contribute to future heterosexual spread [14]. A similar exercise in the United Kingdom estimated that between 2,000 and 5,500 had become infected by heterosexual contact by the end of 1987 [15].

The difficulties of estimating the true incidence and prevalence of HIV infection have led to programs of HIV surveillance in more representative population samples. During 1988, a number of countries developed surveillance schemes for pregnant women through antenatal screening, testing cord blood, or using blood samples on filter paper from infants [14–21]. In the United States, prevalence has ranged from less than 1% in most areas to a high of 2.6% in the New York City area, with major potential for perinatal transmission. Studies in northern Europe [18,19] have found a lower prevalence of infection in antenatal clinic attendees (0.01–0.09%). Although they achieve accurate prevalence estimates, some of the blinded studies have the disadvantage of giving no information on risk factors. Named studies have the advantage that risk factor information can be collected. However, they may underestimate prevalence since persons declining testing may be most likely to be infected. Furthermore, self-reported risk behavior may not be accurate because individuals are reluctant to admit high-risk behaviors [22].

Infection among women attending antenatal clinics represents both transmission by drug use and heterosexual transmission. However, blinded studies with a well defined sampling frame and adequate sample size repeated over time can provide valuable data to monitor changes in prevalence. Attempts to improve serosurveillance in the general population are being made in a number of countries. However, these attempts have been hampered by legal and ethical issues. In the United Kingdom, for example, the government has only recently accepted the legality of blinded testing.

AFRICA

As of August, 1988, 14,818 cases of AIDS have been reported from the African region to the World Health Organization (WHO), but this number is believed to underestimate considerably the actual situation because of the lack of formal reporting systems. As much as 80% of HIV infection in Africa may be acquired heterosexually [23]. The most important risk factors for HIV infection in Africa are number of heterosexual sex partners, sex with prostitutes, being a prostitute, being a sex partner of an infected individual, and having a history of other STDs (especially genital ulceration) [23–28]. The prevalence of HIV antibody ranges from 1% to 20% in urban centers in sub-Saharan Africa. The highest rates are found among young adults, with slightly higher rates among women (male-to-female ratio 1:1.3) [23–33].

HIV infection is most severe in urban centers in Africa, with some evidence from rural Zaire of relatively low and stable levels of HIV infection [34]. Together with evidence of rapid spread in urban centers, this finding indicates that the HIV epidemic in part may result from recent social and economic changes and disruption of traditional lifestyles.

Longitudinal data [1,35] from Nairobi, Kenya, and Zaire show a rapidly rising prevalence of HIV antibody in cohorts of female prostitutes (from 4% in 1981 to 90% in 1987 in Kenya, and from 27% in 1985 to 50% in 1988 in Zaire). This demonstrates that HIV can spread as rapidly among heterosexuals with many partners as among homosexuals with similarly high rates of partner change in the United States. In contrast to the United States and Europe, in the African cities cited, clients of prostitutes appear to make limited use of condoms, further contributing to rapid dissemination of infection [35,36].

MECHANISMS OF HETEROSEXUAL TRANSMISSION

The isolation of HIV from semen and from cervical secretions of infected women provides biological plausibility for bidirectional heterosexual transmission of HIV [37–39]. Experimental vaginal infection of a chimpanzee and case reports of infection through artificial insemination indicate that infection can occur through nontraumatic vaginal exposure to virus and semen [40,41]. Early case reports and epidemiological evidence indicate that male-to-female and female-to-male sexual transmission can occur following only one or two episodes of vaginal intercourse [42–47]. Case cluster reports indicate that some individuals are infectious to successive partners for a number of years [48,49].

However, among many couples, the partner of an infected individual has remained uninfected despite unprotected sexual intercourse for several years following infection. The absence of simple quantitative measurements of levels of infectious virus in blood, semen, and cervical secretions contributes to our incomplete understanding of the biological variables that determine both infectivity of the index case and susceptibility of the contact case.

PROBABILITY OF HETEROSEXUAL TRANSMISSION

Studies in progress that examine the probability of and risk factors for transmission from an infected individual to a heterosexual part-

TABLE 1. Studies of Sexual Transmission of Human Immunodeficiency Virus (HIV)

Reference	Major risk factor in index case	No. of partners studied	Percent partners with antibodies to HIV
A. From men to women			
50	Hemophiliacs	56	9
51	Hemophiliacs	164	10
52	Hemophiliacs	124	14
45	Bisexual/injecting drug user	60	17
46	Blood transfusion	55	18
53	Not stated	60	21
54,55	Bisexual/injecting drug user	132	24
56	Mixed	104	28
57	Mixed (50% with African connections)	60	33
58	Bisexual men	75	35
59	Injecting drug user (AIDS/ARC)	114	45
60	African connections Heterosexuals	62	53
B. From women to men			
54,55	Injecting drug users	20	0
56	Mixed	27	4
46	Transfusion associated	25	8
45	Injecting drug users	13	8
57	Mixed (50% with African connections)	30	9
60	50% African heterosexuals	16	13
53	Not stated	Not stated	21
59	Injecting drug users (AIDS/ARC)	14	50

ner without other risk factors for infection are described in Table 1 [45,46,50–62]. These studies vary in methodology: in case ascertainment, risk group studied, clinical status of the index case, and definition of the contact case. Some studies examine only long-term partners. These methodological differences may, in part, explain the varying proportions of infected partners. Strikingly, a majority of recent studies found no relationship between the risk of transmission and length of relationship or number of acts of sexual intercourse (see references in Table 1). These studies seem to indicate that there is marked heterogeneity in infectivity and possibly in susceptibility between individuals and that infectivity may vary over the long incubation period from HIV infection to AIDS.

Studies from areas where HIV is primarily heterosexually transmitted show higher infection rates in heterosexual partners than the European and U.S. studies cited in Table 1 [61,62]. However, these results are difficult to interpret. In areas where seroprevalence in the general heterosexual population is high, infection from previous heterosexual partners cannot be excluded in couples among whom both partners are infected.

U.S. and European studies of transmission from an infected woman to a man without other risk factors for infection (Table 1) are few. Therefore, whether male-to-female and female-to-male transmissions differ in efficiency is difficult to determine. The studies cited suggest that transmission from women to men may be less efficient than from men to women, although larger numbers are required to draw firm conclusions. A difference in transmission risk is both biologically plausible and has been observed for other STDs such as gonorrhea [63].

COFACTORS FOR HETEROSEXUAL TRANSMISSION

Partner studies have examined factors that may influence the probability of heterosexual transmission, including clinical status of the index case, presence of concurrent STDs, anal intercourse, and circumcision. Evidence that infectivity increases as individuals progress towards advanced disease (CDC stage IV) was suggested in a study of 24 women who were partners of infected hemophiliacs [64]. Three women seroconverted more than 4 years after the date of their partners' infection despite repeated unprotected vaginal intercourse during that time. This coincided with a fall in T-helper lymphocyte counts in the men. Several ongoing studies [53,56,57,60] support this hypothesis by showing a higher risk of infection in women partners of men with CDC stage IV disease or low T-helper counts after controlling for sexual exposure. Two studies [52,53] also suggest an increase of transmission associated with antigenemia in the index case. Interpreting these findings is difficult since most are not based on observed seroconversions, so that biological variables are retrospectively correlated with the transmission events. Nevertheless, the hypothesis that declining immune function enhances infectivity is plausible, if it is associated with increased virus replication and levels of infectious virus in body fluids.

Evidence is accumulating that concomitant STDs, particularly genital ulceration, may enhance heterosexual transmission of HIV by increasing both infectivity and susceptibility [27,53,65–68]. (Implicated STDs include chancroid, syphilis, herpes simplex 2, gonorrhea, and chlamydia.) However, some of the evidence is unpublished and must be interpreted with caution because STDs are a marker for number of sexual partners, an important risk factor for HIV infection. Nevertheless, some intriguing data have emerged.

Cameron and coauthors [66] estimated that the incidence of female-to-male HIV transmission after a single exposure to a woman in the Nairobi prostitute cohort (nearly 90% of whom are infected) was 8%. Acquisition of genital ulcer disease following prostitute contact was a highly significant risk factor for HIV seroconversion in the men, suggesting that genital ulcer disease in the women enhanced transmission.

Although the precise role of other STDs in HIV transmission is not understood, that they might act as cofactors is biologically plausible. Genital ulcers, chlamydial infection, and other STDs could enhance penetration of HIV by causing epithelial disruption. They could increase infectivity in a seropositive individual by increasing lymphocyte populations.

Lack of circumcision may increase susceptibility to HIV infection [52,62]. Oral contraceptive use was found to be associated with an increased risk of HIV infection in a selected group of prostitutes at particularly high risk of HIV [67]. This finding should be examined in other populations before recommendations about contraceptive use in women at risk for HIV are made.

Different sexual practices may also influence HIV transmission. Padian and coauthors [54] reported a relative risk of 2.3 of HIV infection in the partners for those engaging in anal intercourse compared with those having only vaginal intercourse but emphasized that anal intercourse was not necessary for transmission. Four of nine studies [54–56,58,59] reporting on anal intercourse and included in Table 1 found a significantly increased risk of transmission in couples who report anal as well as vaginal intercourse.

All these risk factors are a measure of relative risk. The more important measure, in terms of prevention, is the degree to which these partly preventable cofactors contribute to the spread of disease in a population, that is, population attributable risk. This measure depends on the prevalence of these cofactors in a population. Thus, for example, where anal intercourse is infrequently practiced, the majority of infection can be attributed to vaginal intercourse. Conversely, where STDs are highly prevalent, the control of STDs per se may help to control HIV infection. Perhaps more importantly, treatment of STDs provides an educational opportunity to advise on reduction of partner numbers and on condom use to prevent transmission [53,71].

PREVENTION, SURVEILLANCE, AND FUTURE SPREAD

Predicting the potential extent of heterosexual spread is severely hampered by the absence of population measures of incidence of infection and patterns of behavior. Further viral spread will depend on rates of sexual partner change and on mixing between groups with high-risk and low-risk behavior patterns as well as on the probability of HIV transmission from men to women and from women to men. Quantitative information on rates of sexual partner change in different societies, and on the prevalence of high-risk behavior, is urgently needed. Such studies are being attempted in a number of countries using probability sample surveys [72,73]. In the United Kingdom, two pilot studies of 1,000 randomly selected individuals recently tested the feasibility of a major national survey, and similar work is being developed in the United States.

A rapidly growing heterosexual epidemic is being maintained in certain cities of sub-Saharan Africa [74]. Whether a widely disseminated self-sustaining heterosexual epidemic will occur in developed countries depends on the magnitude of the basic reproductive rate (Ro) for HIV. Ro measures the number of infections produced, on average, by an infected individual in a susceptible population. Using U.K. data on rates of partner change, Anderson and May [75] suggested that Ro may be just above or below one. If just above one, viral spread may increase very slowly and, at the low prevalence outside high-risk populations, require large seroprevalence surveys to detect changes of a small magnitude.

Support for blinded and repeated serosurveillance surveys to monitor trends in infection rates is increasing [75,76]. In the United States, a family of surveys in different clinical and nonclinical populations is being conducted through the CDC. In the United Kingdom, a similar family of surveys is being developed by the Medical Research Council.

Further understanding of heterosexual transmission probabilities requires greater emphasis on the biological determinants of transmission. This involves, in particular, the ability to develop quantitative assays of viral abundance in blood, semen, and vaginal secretions. Linking biological markers with transmission events will remain a difficult task, not least because of an ethical responsibility to counsel couples to prevent transmission from occurring. Many of the ethical, legal, and human rights issues that have made unbiased epidemiological studies difficult to conduct may diminish considerably if an effective and safe treatment for asymptomatic HIV infection becomes available. In such an event, another research issue may be whether treatment can reduce infectivity and itself act as a control measure.

For the foreseeable future, prevention demands sustained reduction in risk behaviors, which may be difficult to achieve in Western heterosexual populations, among whom the risk of infection is low. This demands continued publicity campaigns and intensive efforts targeted to persons at high risk, such as IDUs and prostitutes and their clients. Such targeted programs may include the introduction of contact tracing in low-prevalence communities [77–79]. In addition, educational and counselling programs should be evaluated if resources are to be used most effectively for prevention campaigns. A more difficult challenge is to address the sensitive policy issues relating to the treatment and prevention of drug injecting and to HIV control among prostitutes and their clients.

Although control will continue to depend on encouraging condom use and reducing partner numbers, the identification of modifiable cofactors for HIV transmission may have practical implications for HIV-control programs. Control of HIV must therefore depend on adequate STD treatment and control programs, particularly in areas of high incidence of STDs. Such programs offer an opportunity for effective care of other STDs and for individual education among persons at highest risk of HIV infection.

ACKNOWLEDGMENTS

This chapter is substantially based on a review article prepared after the IVth International Conference on AIDS and published by Gower Press (Johnson AM, Laga M: Heterosexual transmission of HIV. AIDS 2[Suppl 1]:S49–S56, 1988).

REFERENCES

1. **Piot P, Kreiss JK, Ndinya-Achola JO, et al.:** Editorial review. Heterosexual transmission of HIV. AIDS 1:199–206, 1987.

2. **Padian N:** Heterosexual transmission of acquired immunodeficiency syndrome: International perspectives and national projections. Rev Infect Dis 9:947–960, 1987.

3. **Johnson AM:** Heterosexual transmission of human immunodeficiency virus. Br Med J 296:1017–1020, 1988.

4. **Friedland GH, Klein RS:** Transmission of the human immunodeficiency virus. N Engl J Med 317:1125–1135, 1987.

5. **Piot P, Plummer FA, Mhalu FS, Lamboray JL, Chin J, Mann JM:** AIDS: An international perspective. Science 239:573–579, 1988.

6. **Curran JW, Jaffe HW, Hardy AM, Morgan WM, Selik RM, Dondero TJ:** Epidemiology of HIV infection and AIDS in the United States. Science 239:610–616, 1988.

7. **Chamberland M, Conley L, Dondero T:** Epidemiology and evolution of heterosexually acquired AIDS—United States. Abstract 4017: IV International Conference on AIDS, Stockholm, June, 1988.

8. **Anonymous:** AIDS update. Br Med J 297:244, 1988.

9. **Clumeck N, Magrez P, Roth D, De Wit S, Hermans SP, Schoumacher M:** Pattern of HIV heterosexual infection in Brussels. Abstract 4013: IV International Conference on AIDS, Stockholm, June, 1988.

10. **Bonneux L, Taelman H, Cornet J, et al.:** Case control study of HIV-seropositive versus HIV-seronegative European expatriates in Africa. Br Med J 297:581–584, 1988.

11. **Day S, Ward H, Harris JRW:** HIV and London prostitutes. Abstract 4052: IV International Conference on AIDS, Stockholm, June, 1988.

12. **Rosenberg MJ, Werner JM:** Prostitutes and AIDS: A health department priority? Am J Public Health 78:418–423, 1988.

13. **Darrow WW, Bigler W, Deppe D, et al.:** HIV antibody in 640 US prostitutes with no evidence of intravenous (IV) drug abuse. Abstract 4054: IV International Conference on AIDS, Stockholm, June, 1988.

14. **Centers for Disease Control:** Human immunodeficiency virus in the United States: A review of current knowledge. MMWR 36:(S-6):1–48, 1987.

15. **Report of a Working Group:** Short-Term Prediction of HIV Infection and AIDS in England and Wales. Department of Health, Welsh Office, London: HMSO, 1988.

16. **Landesman S, Minkoff H, Holam S, McCalla S, Sijin O:** Serosurvey of human immunodeficiency virus infection in parturients. Implications for human immunodeficiency virus testing programs of pregnant women. JAMA 258:2701–2703, 1987.

17. **Hoff R, Berardi VP, Weiblin BJ, Mahoney-Trout L, Mitchell ML, Grady GF:** Seroprevalence of human immunodeficiency virus among childbearing women. N Engl J Med 318:525–530, 1988.

18. **Brattebo G, Wiseberg T:** HIV monitoring of pregnant women. Lancet 1:713, 1988.

19. **Howard L, Hawkins D, Marwood R, Lawrence A, Gazzard BG:** The frequency of human immunodeficiency virus (HIV) infection in heterosexual women in central London. Abstract 4010: IV International Conference on AIDS, Stockholm, June, 1988.

20. **Goudeau A, Brossard Y, Larsen M, Huchet J, Barin F, Schwartz D:** A sero-epidemiological study of HIV in 15,465 pregnant women screened in Paris area between February 1987 and October 1987. Abstract 4632: IV International Conference on AIDS, Stockholm, June, 1988.

21. **Novick LF, Berns D, Stricof R, Stevens R:** HIV seroprevalence in newborn infants in New York state. Abstract 7221: IV International Conference on AIDS, Stockholm, June, 1988.

22. **Handsfield HH:** Heterosexual transmission of human immunodeficiency virus. JAMA 260:1943–1944, 1988.

23. **Ngaly B, Ryder RW:** Epidemiology of HIV in Africa. J Acquired Immune Deficiency Syndrome (in press).

24. **Quinn T, Mann JM, Curran JW, Piot P:** AIDS in Africa: An epidemiological paradigm. Science 234:955–963, 1986.

25. **Mhalu F, Bredberg-Raden V, Mbena E, et al.:** Prevalence of HIV infection in healthy subjects and groups of patients in Tanzania. AIDS 1:217–221, 1987.

26. **Van de Perre P, Carael M, Nzaramba O, Zissis G, Kayihigi J, Butzler JP:** Risk factors for HIV seropositivity in selected urban based Rwandese adults. AIDS, 1:207–211, 1987.

27. **Van de Perre P, Le Polain B, Carael M, Nzaramba D, Zissis G, Butzler JP:** HIV antibodies in a remote rural area in Rwanda, central Africa: An analysis of potential risk factors for HIV seropositivity. AIDS 1:213–215, 1987.

28. **Greenblatt RM, Lukehart SA, Plummer FA, et al.:** Genital ulceration as a risk factor for human immunodeficiency virus infection. AIDS 2:47–50, 1988.

29. **Carswell JW:** HIV infection in healthy persons in Uganda. AIDS 1:223–227, 1987.

30. **Gresenguel G, Somse P, Georges MC, et al.:** Sero-prevalence of HIV infection in Central Africa over a three year period (1985–1987). Abstract 5032: IV International Conference on AIDS, Stockholm, June, 1988.

31. **Josse R, Delaporte E, Kouka-Bemba D, et al.:** Continuing studies on seroepidemiological surveys of HIV infection in Central Africa: about 35 sample surveys. Abstract 5033: IV International Conference on AIDS, Stockholm, June, 1988.

32. **Melbye M, Mjelesani EK, Bayley A, et al.:** Evidence for heterosexual transmission and clinical manifestations of human immunodeficiency virus infection and related conditions in Lusaka, Zambia. Lancet 2:1113–1115, 1986.

33. **Clumeck N, Robert-Guroff M, Van de Perre P, et al.:** Seroepidemiological studies of HTLV III antibody prevalence among selected groups of heterosexual Africans. JAMA 254:2599–2602, 1985.

34. **Nzilambi N, De Cock KM, Fortha LDN, et al.:** The prevalence of infection with human immunodeficiency virus over a 10 year period in rural Zaire. N Engl J Med 318: 276–279, 1988.

35. **Piot P, Plummer FA, Rey MA, et al.:** Retrospective epidemiology of HIV infection in Nairobi populations. J Infect Dis 155:1108–1112, 1987.

36. **Mann J, Quinn TC, Piot P, et al.:** Condom use and HIV infection among prostitutes in Zaire. N Engl J Med 36:345, 1987.

37. **Zagury D, Bernard J, Leibowitch J, et al.:** HTLV III in cells cultured from semen of two patients with AIDS. Science 226:449–451, 1984.

38. **Wofsy CB, Cohen JB, Hauer LB, et al.:** Isolation of AIDS-associated retrovirus from genital secretions of women with antibodies to the virus. Lancet 1:527–529, 1986.

39. **Vogt MW, Witt DJ, Craven DE, et al.:** Isolation patterns of the human immunodeficiency virus from cervical secretions during the menstrual cycle of women at risk from the acquired immunodeficiency syndrome. Ann Intern Med 106:380–382, 1987.

40. **Fultz PN, McClure HM, Daugharty H, et al.:** Vaginal transmission of human immunodeficiency virus (HIV) to a chimpanzee. J Infect Dis 154:896–900, 1986.

41. **Stewart GJ, Tyler JPP, Cunningham AL, et al.:** Transmission of human T-cell lymphotropic virus type III (HTLV III) by artificial insemination by donor. Lancet 2:581–584, 1985.

42. **Cabane J, Thibierge E, Godeau P, Moreau A, Wattiaux MJ:** AIDS in an apparently risk-free woman. Lancet 2:105, 1984.

43. **Calabrese LH, Gopalakrishna KV:** Transmission of HTLV III infection from man to woman and woman to man. N Engl J Med 314:987, 1986.

44. **L'Age-Stehr J, Schwarz A, Offerman G, et al.:** HTLV III infection in kidney transplant recipients. Lancet 2:1361–1362, 1985.

45. **Johnson AM, Petherick A, Davidson S, et al.:** Transmission of HIV to heterosexual partners of infected men and women. Abstract 4058: IV International Conference on AIDS, Stockholm, June, 1988.

46. **Peterman TA, Stoneburner RL, Allen JR, Jaffe HW, Curran JW:** Risk of human immunodeficiency virus transmission from heterosexual adults with transfusion-associated infections. JAMA 259:55–58, 1988.

47. **Staszewski S, Schieck E, Rehmet S, et al.:** HIV transmission from male after only two sexual contacts. Lancet 2:628, 1987.

48. **Franzen C, Jertborn M, Biberfeld G, et al.:** Four generations of heterosexual transmission of LAV/HTLV III in a small Swedish town. II International Conference on AIDS, Paris, 1986.

49. **Padian N, Wiley J, Glass S, Marquis L, Winkelstein W:** Anomalies of infectivity in the heterosexual transmission of HIV. Abstract 4062: IV International Conference on AIDS, Stockholm, June, 1988.

50. **Lawrence DN, Jason JM, Holman RC, et al.:** Heterosexual transmission of HIV to female partners of HIV-infected U.S. haemophiliac men. Abstract 4009: IV International Conference on AIDS, Stockholm, June, 1988.

51. **Kamradt TGA, Niese D, Schneweis KE, Breckman HH, Kamps BS:** Heterosexual

transmission of HIV in haemophiliacs. Abstract 4008: IV International Conference on AIDS, Stockholm, June, 1988.

52. **Goedert JJ, Eyster ME, Ragni MV, Biggar RJ, Gail MH:** Rate of heterosexual HIV transmission and association with HIV-antigen. Abstract 4019: IV International Conference on AIDS, Stockholm, June, 1988.

53. **Fischl M, Fayne T, Flanagan S, et al.:** Seroprevalence and risks of HIV infection in spouses of persons infected with HIV. Abstract 4060: IV International Conference on AIDS, Stockholm, June, 1988.

54. **Padian N, Marquis L, Francis DP, et al.:** Male to female transmission of human immunodeficiency virus. JAMA 258:788–790, 1987.

55. **Padian N, Glass S, Marquis L, Wiley J, Winkelstein W:** Heterosexual transmission of HIV in California: Results from a heterosexual partner's study. Abstract 4020: IV International Conference on AIDS, Stockholm, June, 1988.

56. **De Vincenzi I:** Heterosexual transmission of HIV: A European community multicentre study. Abstract 4024: IV International Conference on AIDS, Stockholm, June, 1988.

57. **Staszewski S, Rehmet S, Hofmeister WD, et al.:** Analysis of transmission risks in heterosexual transmitted HIV infection. Abstract 4068: IV International Conference on AIDS, Stockholm, June, 1988.

58. **Sion FS, Morais De Sa CA, Rachid De Lacerda MC, et al.:** The importance of anal intercourse in transmission of HIV to women. Abstract 4007: IV International Conference on AIDS, Stockholm, June, 1988.

59. **Steigbigel NH, Maude DW, Feiner CJ, et al.:** Heterosexual transmission of HIV infection. Abstract 4057: IV International Conference on AIDS, Stockholm, June, 1988.

60. **Laga M, Taelman H, Bonneux L, Cornet P, Vercauteren G, Piot P:** Risk factors for HIV infection in heterosexual partners of HIV infected Africans and Europeans. Abstract 4004: IV International Conference on AIDS, Stockholm, June, 1988.

61. **Nzilambi N, Ryder R, Colebunders R, et al.:** Married couples in Zaire with discordant HIV serology. Abstract 4059: IV International Conference on AIDS, Stockholm, June, 1988.

62. **Carael M, Van de Perre PH, Lepage PH, et al.:** Human immunodeficiency virus among heterosexual couples in central Africa. AIDS 2:201–205, 1988.

63. **Handsfield HH.:** Gonorrhoea and uncomplicated gonococcal infection. In Holmes KK, Maidh PA, Sparling PF, Wiesner PJ (eds): Sexually Transmitted Diseases, New York: McGraw-Hill 1984, pp 205–220.

64. **Goedert JJ, Eyster ME, Biggar RJ, Blattner WA:** Heterosexual transmission of human immunodeficiency virus: Association with severe depletion of T Helper lymphocytes in men with haemophilia. AIDS Res Hum Retroviruses 3:355–360, 1987.

65. **Kreiss J, Carael M, Meheus A:** Role of sexually transmitted diseases in transmitting human immunodeficiency virus. Genitourinary Med 64:1–2, 1988.

66. **Cameron DW, D'Costa LJ, Ndinya-Achola JO, Piot P, Plummer FA:** Incidence and

risk factors for female to male transmission of HIV. Abstract 4061: IV International Conference on AIDS, Stockholm, June, 1988.

67. **Plummer FA, Cameron W, Simonson N, et al.:** Cofactors in male-female transmission of HIV. Abstract 4554: IV International Conference on AIDS, Stockholm, June, 1988.

68. **Holmberg SD, Stewart JA, Gerber R, et al.:** Prior herpes simplex virus type 2 infection as a risk factor for HIV infection. JAMA 259:1048–1050, 1988.

69. **Van de Perre P, De Clercq A, Cogniaux Hectere J, Nzaramba D, Butzler JP, Sprecher-Goldberger S:** Detection of HIV p17-antigen in lymphocytes but not epithelial cells from cervicovaginal secretions of women seropositive for HIV: Implications for heterosexual transmission of the virus. Genitourinary Med 64:30–33, 1988.

70. **Levy JA:** The transmission of AIDS: The case of the infected cell. JAMA 259:3037–3038, 1988.

71. **Centers for Disease Control:** Condoms for prevention of sexually transmitted diseases. MMWR 37:134–137, 1988.

72. **Johnson AM, Wadsworth J, Elliot P, et al.:** A pilot study of sexual lifestyles in a random sample of the population of Great Britain. AIDS 3:135–141, 1989.

73. **Kvalem IL, Sundet JM, Kjisnes R, et al.:** Is sexual behavior changing as a result of the HIV-epidemic? Abstract 8065: IV International Conference on AIDS, Stockholm, June, 1988.

74. **Anderson RM, May RM, McLean AR:** Possible demographic consequences of AIDS in devoloping countries. Nature 332:228–234, 1988.

75. **Anderson RM, May RM:** Epidemiological parameters of HIV transmission. Nature 333:514–519, 1988.

76. **Allen JA, Curran JW:** Prevention of AIDS and HIV infection: needs and priorities for epidemiological research. Am J Public Health 78:381–386, 1988.

77. **Rutherford GW, Woo JM:** Contact tracing and the control of human immunodeficiency virus infection. JAMA 259:3609–3610, 1988.

78. **Wykoff RF, Heath CW, Hollis SL, et al.:** Contact tracing to identify human immunodeficiency virus in a rural community. JAMA 259:3563–3566, 1988.

79. **Adler MW, Johnson AM:** Contact tracing for HIV infection. Br Med J 296:1420–1421, 1988.

DISCUSSION

DR. SHELTON: I noted that you did not mention anything about the effect of circumcision, or rather the lack thereof. Is that because you do not believe the lack of circumcision is a cofactor? If you do believe it is, maybe you could hazard some thoughts on what it means.

DR. JOHNSON: It is not that I do not believe it. There were so many aspects to cover, and I know there are other speakers who will cover many of the cofactors in greater detail.

Certainly there seems to be some evidence that circumcision is in some way protective. I think most of this evidence has come from central Africa. And, clearly, there are good biological reasons why. The foreskin, in particular, may be affected by genital ulceration.

I have not studied this evidence in great detail. I think the same problem applies in sorting out the relative risks of different cofactors. That is, in determining to what extent one individual risk factor is contributing, when one is looking at a series of factors that may influence transmission.

DR. ALEXANDER: In Africa, are the people who are circumcised of a different religious order? Would there be other factors associated with circumcision that might be a reason why the disease is less prevalent among these individuals?

DR. JOHNSON: I have never worked in Africa, so I do not want to comment on that. I think there is someone here who has done a lot of work in that field. Dr. Cameron, I think, would probably know more about that. I do know that there clearly are very great differences in cultural practices with regard to both female and male circumcision.

DR. HODGEN: You intimated with your last slide that there might be a genetic predisposition to infection. Although the data are less than satisfactory in quantity and quality, at this time would you ask us to accept that genetic heritage is a significant factor, or are we far from really knowing that?

DR. JOHNSON: I would say we are far from really knowing that, and I think we need to know far more about the behavioral determinants of all STD transmission. Some work looking at one or two genetic determinants was submitted to the *Lancet*. The paper was subsequently withdrawn. I know many other groups have been looking at HLA groupings and so on, but I am not aware of any clear evidence that genetic factors are a major component.

DR. KAMUNGOMA: I would like to know the exact role of genital ulceration in HIV transmission. In Kinshasa, Zaire, in one of our studies, we found a significant difference between HIV seronegative and HIV seropositive in relation to the presence of genital ulcers. But, in a cohort study we carried out 6 months ago, we did not find a significant difference between HIV seropositive and seronegative prostitutes.

DR. JOHNSON: I assume that this refers to whether the genital ulceration is the result of HIV infection or predates it. Certainly, in our study, we looked at data on herpes, which is the predominant genital ulceration in our country, and I find a significant relationship between history of herpes and HIV positivity. But, when one looks more closely at the data, I think the herpes manifestation, the ulceration, may be a result of HIV infection and not the other way around. Thus, one needs to be cautious, as you say, in examining which came first, the ulceration or the HIV disease.

3

Heterosexual Transmission: Infectivity and Risks

Nancy Padian

Despite more than 8 years of surveillance and study of the human immunodeficiency virus (HIV), many questions about the risk of the heterosexual transmission of HIV remain. The most striking question is why the descriptive epidemiology of acquired immune deficiency syndrome (AIDS) differs among continents. In various developing countries, including parts of Africa, Haiti, and Central and South America, AIDS follows the typical pattern of a bidirectional, heterosexually transmitted disease. In contrast, in developed countries, including the United States, Australia, and western Europe, the epidemic remains largely confined to homosexual men and needle-sharing intravenous drug users (IVDUs) [1]. The fundamental uncertainty underlying this observation is whether such differences will converge over time so that heterosexual transmission will contribute more to the epidemiology of countries such as the United States. The answer to this question rests on at least three issues: the infectivity of HIV; the relative efficiency of heterosexual transmission of HIV (transmission by gender: male to female and female to male); and the importance of various risk factors associated with transmission, including sexually transmitted diseases (STDs). In this chapter, I address each of these areas with the goal of clarifying parameters that help predict the magnitude of heterosexual transmission of HIV in the United States.

INFECTIVITY OF HIV AND NUMBER OF SEXUAL PARTNERS

Infection does not ensue following every exposure to an infectious pathogen; infectivity may be defined as the probability of infection

Heterosexual Transmission of AIDS, pages 25–34

given such exposure. However, to understand epidemic spread, and before considering infectivity, one must first assess the probability that a randomly chosen sexual partner will be infected. In areas characterized by a high prevalence of HIV infection, such as the U.S. homosexual community of San Francisco, where infection rates may be as high as 50% [2], number of partners and rate of partner change are highly associated with infection because the likelihood of choosing an infected partner is great [3]. Number of partners should be less significant in communities characterized by lower infection rates. Thus, among heterosexuals in San Francisco, number of partners per se is not associated with infection because the seroprevalence rates in this community are low [4,5]. Although the risk of number of partners is therefore not a constant, many researchers and mathematical modelers believe that rate of acquisition of new partners is the driving force behind epidemic growth [6,7]. One theory that accounts for the HIV epidemic among heterosexuals in Central Africa, but not in the United States, is that the number of new partners among African heterosexuals is greater than among U.S. heterosexuals [8].

A direct relationship exists between number of partners and infectivity rates. A low infectivity rate suggests that repeat exposure with an identified infected partner is more important than number of partners. Conversely, a high infectivity rate indicates that number of partners is quite significant because transmission is likely to occur with each new partner. Thus, number of partners as a risk factor varies in strength according to both the seroprevalence in the community from which the partner is selected and the infectivity rate of the pathogen. However, number of partners is never inconsequential; increasing number of partners increases the likelihood of selecting an infected partner and thus the likelihood that, given an infected partner, transmission will occur.

Transmission rates may be assessed either by per-partner infectivity or per-contact infectivity. Per-partner infectivity rate is defined as the probability that a random infected partner will transmit disease to a random uninfected partner. Choosing an infected partner does not guarantee that transmission will occur subsequent to exposure. Grant and coauthors [9] estimated per-partner infectivity rate in a sample of homosexual men. The parameters they used to generate the model were number of partners during a defined time period, prevalence of HIV at the beginning of the time period, and rate of seroconversions (new infections) during the time period. Their model yielded an infectivity rate of .102, with a 95% confidence interval of .043 to .160. In a heterosexual population, parameters would be defined differently and a different infectivity rate would result.

Per-contact infectivity rate is defined as the probability that transmission will occur given one true exposure to an infected partner. Early attempts to model per-contact infectivity assumed a constant infectivity rate that was homogeneous for all infected individuals and their sexual partners. Using this model, Padian and coauthors [10] modeled data from the female partners of infected men and determined that the per-contact infectivity rate for penovaginal intercourse was about .001. After observing varied transmission rates, with some individuals becoming infected after a few contacts and others remaining uninfected despite multiple exposures, Wiley and coauthors [6] reexamined the same data using a variable infectivity rate and determined that .001 was a low estimate; depending on factors related to variation in infectiousness or in susceptibility, infectivity could be higher.

These probabilities are sometimes misinterpreted to be cumulative risk. For example, the figure .001 has been interpreted to mean that 1000 exposures are required for transmission to occur. However, the probability is the same with each exposure. Multiple exposures simply mean that the likelihood that one exposure could result in transmission is increased. Thus one would expect documentation of some instances of transmission based on one contact, although this would be a rare event. Johnson and coauthors [11] did observe two reports of seroconversion after one exposure. Conversely, one would expect that multiple exposures could occur with no transmission. At this point, there is no way of knowing which exposure would result in transmission. Individual variations in either infectivity or susceptibility affect transmission probabilities.

TRANSMISSION RATES BY GENDER AND RISK GROUP

As of December, 1988, the U.S. Centers for Disease Control (CDC) reported 1,757 AIDS cases among the female partners of infected men or men at risk [12]. This figure represented 76% of all cases attributed to heterosexual contact and 2% of all cases. Data from male-to-female partner studies have been fairly consistent and cluster into two groups. Infection rates among the female partners of infected bisexual men, hemophiliac men, or men infected from contaminated blood transfusions vary from about 15% to 20%, depending on the study size and sample [13–15]. Rates among the female partners of male IVDUs or of men of central African origin are consistently higher, on the order of 40% to 100% [16,17].

Several hypotheses may explain the discrepancy in rates between these two types of studies. Female partners of IVDUs or of central African men may be more sexually active and thus may be at increased risk of infection. Alternatively, the presence of cofactors (discussed below), such as concurrent infections (particularly STDs), nutritional status, and general health, may be different among the different risk groups of men or their partners and could affect both infectivity and susceptibility. Other explanations include the possibility that men from one risk group are generally more efficient transmitters or that partners of IVDUs also have used drugs intravenously and thus have been exposed to HIV through shared drug-using instruments, although they may deny such use on interview. Regardless of the explanation, these differences highlight the importance of heterosexual transmission in areas characterized by a high prevalence of infection among IVDUs. Until these differences are better understood, findings should not be generalized across all partner studies or to all populations.

The efficiency of female-to-male transmission compared to male-to-female transmission remains in dispute. In contrast to 1,757 male-to-female transmissions as of December, 1988, the CDC reported only 539 AIDS cases among the male partners of infected women or of women at risk [12]. This figure represented 24% of all cases attributed to heterosexual contact and 0.6% of all cases. Results from female-to-male partner studies are far less consistent than results from male-to-female studies. Infection rates vary from observations of no infection among the male partners of infected women [18] to transmission that appears to be equally efficient bidirectionally [16, 17]. Because relatively few women are infected at this point in the epidemic (women represent about 8.5% of all reported AIDS cases) [12], male partners of infected women are difficult to find. Thus studies of female-to-male transmission are based on very small numbers, making large-scale generalizations inappropriate. Again, infection rates appear to be higher among the male partners of female IVDUs or of infected women of central African origin. Hypotheses constructed to explain this phenomenon are similar to those put forth to explain this discrepancy in male-to-female transmission.

Because fewer cases have been attributed to female-to-male transmission, risk factors for female-to-male transmission have not been delineated as carefully as they have been for male-to-female transmission. If certain risk factors are necessary for female-to-male transmission to occur, and if these factors are more prevalent in central Africa, this may partially explain that distinctly heterosexual transmission pattern.

TABLE 1. Demographic Risk Factors for Heterosexual Transmission

Gender[a]
Risk group of the index case[a]
Race[a]
Age
Socioeconomic class

[a]Statistically significant in at least one partner study.

FACTORS ASSOCIATED WITH TRANSMISSION

Tables 1–3 summarize risk factors for heterosexual transmission that have been examined primarily in heterosexual partner studies. In these studies, one can monitor transmission between an identified infected person and the uninfected partner while controlling for other sources of exposure; one can thus examine direct viral transmission between individuals. These risk factors can directly affect infectiousness, or susceptibility, or both, and thus transmission rates.

Risk factors for heterosexual transmission are shown in Table 1. Gender (efficiency of female-to-male compared to male-to-female transmission) and risk group of the index case (with rates of transmission from IVDUs being higher than rates from bisexual men or men infected from contaminated blood products) were found to be significant in at least one study. Padian and coauthors [18] found black and Latina female partners of infected men to have higher rates of infection than their white counterparts. This association could not be completely explained by controlling for other established risk factors.

Behavioral risks depicted in Table 2 are associated with sexual activity. Protective trends have been noted with condom use, although condoms do not confer risk-free status [19]. Stronger effects may be masked because reliable data about correct condom use are difficult to obtain, and seroconversions are rarely observed in a cohort of heterosexual couples with one infected partner. Although transmission has been documented through penovaginal intercourse in all partner studies, the practice of anal intercourse has also been shown to increase the chance of transmission [5,17].

Table 3 lists biological variables associated with infectiousness and susceptibilty. The first four variables—disease stage in the index case, CD4 lymphocyte count, positive HIV culture, and presence of P_{24} antigen—are surrogate measures for time of infection in the index case. The theory is that the longer an individual is infected, the more

TABLE 2. Behavioral Risk Factor for Heterosexual Transmission

Condom use[a]
Other types of contraception
Other partners in known risk group
Number of sexual partners
Type of sexual activities
Oral intercourse[a]
Anal intercourse
Vaginal intercourse
Intercourse during menstrual cycle
No. of acts of intercourse

[a]Statistically significant in at least one partner study.

TABLE 3. Biological Risk Factors for Heterosexual Transmission

Diagnosis (AIDS/symptomatic/(+)asymptomatic)[a]
CD_4 lymphocyte cell count[a]
HIV culture (peripheral blood mononuclear cells)[a]
P_{24} antigen assay[a]
Circumcision[a]
Bleeding during sex[a]
Sexually transmitted diseases and gynecological abnormalities[a]
Abnormal pap smear
Hysterectomy
Pregnancies

[a]Statistically significant in at least one partners study.

viremic and thus infectious he or she becomes. Although many studies [20,21] have confirmed this finding, results are not consistent across all studies, and additional studies using larger samples are needed.

Lack of circumcision as a risk factor was not observed first in a partners study. Rather, Cameron and coauthors [22] and Plummer and coauthors [23] first reported this observation in a study of Nairobian prostitutes and their clients. However, this finding was confirmed in a partners study [24].

Several of the biological factors reported in Table 3 might be related to infectiousness as well as to susceptibility. For example, bleeding during sex from trauma has been reported as a risk for heterosexual transmission [18]. Because blood contains virus, the open lesions from trauma during sexual intercourse could provide direct viral entry. This factor could actually facilitate transmission if either the infected or the uninfected partner experiences trauma.

Similarly, a concurrent infection from an STD could alter the protective mucosa, making transmission easier, or it could result in a proliferation of circulating lymphocytes that either could harbor and transport virus or act as target cells. Presence of genital ulcers has been postulated to account for much of the heterosexual transmission observed in central Africa [1,22]. Fischl and coauthors [24] also found that coinfection from herpes and gonorrhea facilitated transmission among couples examined in the United States. However, other studies [18,20,21] have not reported an association between STDs and HIV transmission. As with any risk factor, the prevalence must be great enough to permit an association to be observed. The lack of consistent findings across studies could be explained if STDs increase the chance that HIV transmission will occur without being necessary for this to happen.

Whether STDs are directly associated with transmission or are only markers for sexual activity is still unclear. This important question has yet to be resolved. If STDs are important cofactors and if their high prevalence in central Africa accounts for heterosexual transmission there, their control would be an effective part of an HIV prevention program.

CONCLUSIONS

More than 8 years into the AIDS epidemic, we are still posing many of the questions that we asked when statistics were first being compiled. Many of these questions speculate about the magnitude of heterosexual transmission worldwide. The central African model seems inappropriate to use to predict the epidemiology of HIV disease in the developed world. Few infectious diseases demonstrate the same transmission patterns across all geographic areas. As was discussed above, the prevalence of various risk factors may account for some differences in epidemiology.

Social and cultural factors are also important. Inadequate health care or unhygienic living conditions may affect susceptibility to disease. Although heterosexual transmission may not be widespread in the United States, we are observing "pocket" epidemics among the urban poor in areas characterized by prevalent intravenous drug use and STDs. These areas mimic many of the living conditions experienced by peoples in central Africa [1]. In any case, regardless of the probability of infection, risk must be tempered by the severity of the outcome. Although the chance of infection from HIV for middle and upper class individuals in the United States may be low, one must err on the side of caution. As long as transmission of HIV results in a lethal infection for which there is no cure, even a minimal risk is not worth taking. In addition, many of the precautions recommended to protect against AIDS transmission are viable ways to prevent transmission of other STDs.

REFERENCES

1. **Padian N:** Heterosexual transmission of acquired immunodeficiency syndrome: International perspectives and national projections. Rev Infect Dis 9:947–960, 1987.

2. **Winkelstein W, Samuel M, Padian N, et al.:** The San Francisco Men's Health Study, III: Reduction in human immunodeficiency virus transmission among homosexual/bisexual men in San Francisco, 1982–1986. Am J Public Health 77:685–689, 1987.

3. **Winkelstein W, Lyman D, Padian N, et al.:** Sexual practices and risk of infection by the human immunodeficiency virus: The San Francisco Men's Health Study. JAMA 257:321–325, 1987.

4. **Cohen J, Hauer L, Poole L, et al.:** Sexual and other practices and risk of HIV infection in a cohort of 450 sexually active women in San Francisco. Abstract WP. 57: III International Conference on AIDS, Washington, DC, 1987.

5. **Padian N, Marquis L, Francis D, et al.:** Male-to-female transmission of human immunodeficiency virus. JAMA 258:788–790, 1988.

6. **Wiley J, Herschkorn S, Padian N:** Heterogeniety in the probability of HIV transmission per sexual contact: The case of male-to-female transmission in penile-vaginal intercourse. Statist Med (in press).

7. **Anderson R, May R:** Epidemiological parameters of HIV transmission. Nature 333: 514–519, 1988.

8. **Hrdy D:** Cultural practices contributing to the transmission of human immunodeficiency virus in Africa. Rev Infect Dis 9:1109–1119, 1987.

9. **Grant R, Wiley J, Winkelstein W:** The infectivity of the human immunodeficiency virus: Estimates from a prospective study of a cohort of homosexual men. J Infect Dis 156:189–193, 1987.

10. **Padian N, Wiley J, Winkelstein W:** Male-to-female transmission of human immunodeficiency virus (HIV): Current results, infectivity estimates, and San Francisco population seroprevalence estimates. Abstract THP. 48: III International Conference on AIDS, Washington, DC, 1987.

11. **Johnson A, Petherick A, Davidson S, et al.:** Transmission of HIV to heterosexual partners of infected men and women. Abstract 4058: IV International Conference on AIDS, Stockholm, June, 1988.

12. **Centers for Disease Control:** AIDS weekly surveillance report, December 12, 1988.

13. **Peterman T, Stoneburner R, Allen J, et al.:** Risk of human immunodeficiency virus transmission from heterosexual adults with transfusion-associated infections. JAMA 259: 55–58, 1988.

14. **Jason J, McDougal J, Dixon G, et al.:** HTLV-III/LAV infection in hemophiliacs. Abstract: 26th Interscience Conference on Antimicrobial Agents and Chemotherapy, New Orleans, 1986.

15. **Padian, N, Winkelstein, W:** Heterosexual transmission of the AIDS virus in northern California. Abstract: 26th Interscience Conference on Antimicrobial Agents and Chemotherapy, New Orleans, 1986.

16. **Hira S, Wadhawan D, Nkowane B, et al.:** Heterosexual transmission of HIV in Zambia. Abstract 4006: IV International Conference on AIDS, Stockholm, June, 1988.

17. **Steigbigel N, Maude D, Feiner C, et al.:** Heterosexual transmission of HIV infection. Abstract 4057: IV International Conference on AIDS, Stockholm, June, 1988.

18. **Padain N, Greenblat R, Glass S, Dull I:** Clinical and immunological correlates of the heterosexual transmission of HIV. Abstract: 28th Interscience Conference on Antimicrobial Agents and Chemotherapy, Los Angeles, 1988.

19. **Fischl M, Dickinson G, Scott G, et al.:** Evaluation of heterosexual partners, children, and household contacts of adults with AIDS. JAMA 257:640–644, 1987.

20. **Goedert J, Eyster M, Ragni M, et al.:** Rate of heterosexual HIV transmission and associated risk with HIV-antigen. Abstract 4019: IV International Conference on AIDS, Stockholm, June, 1988.

21. **Laga M, Taelman H, Bonneaux L, et al.:** Risk factors for HIV infection in heterosexual partners of HIV infected Africans and Europeans. Abstract 4004: IV International Conference on AIDS, Stockholm, June, 1988.

22. **Cameron D, D'Costa L, Ndinya-Achola J, et al.:** Incidence and risk factors for female to male transmission of HIV. Abstract 4061: IV International Conference on AIDS, Stockholm, June, 1988.

23. **Plummer F, Cameron W, Simonsen N, et al.:** Co-factors in male-female transmission of HIV. Abstract 4554: IV International Conference on AIDS, Stockholm, June, 1988.

24. **Fischl M, Fayne T, Flanagan S, et al.:** Seroprevalence and risks of HIV infections in spouses of persons infected with HIV. Abstract 4060: IV International Conference on AIDS, Stockholm, June, 1988.

DISCUSSION

MR. SPIELER: First, in your ongoing study, do you have any data on the relationship between contraceptive methods and the risk of HIV transmission other than with the use of barrier methods? Second, you made a clear distinction that bleeding during sex, which apparently results from trauma, increases the risk of transmission. What about the risk of transmission from sex during menstrual bleeding?

DR. PADIAN: With regard to your first question, we are looking at other forms of contraception. Dr. Cameron will be discussing the role of oral contraception in transmission on the second day of the

Workshop. Interestingly enough, in my sample, there are not enough people practicing other forms of contraception to answer this question. Nevertheless, it is something we are continuing to examine, but not with much statistical power.

Concerning your second question, as with all others who are conducting partner studies of which I know, we see no increased risk with bleeding from menstruation. The risk is definitely the result of sex during bleeding associated with trauma. The way we ask the question is whether they have noticed that there has been bleeding from either their genitals or their partner's genitials during intercourse. This, of course, does not rule out the presence of microscopic lesions of which the couples are not aware that might occur from intercourse. So it is, at best, a crude look at the risk factor. But, it is a very strong predictor.

4

HIV Transmission From Hemophilic Men to Their Heterosexual Partners

Dale N. Lawrence, Janine M. Jason, Robert C. Holman, and John J. Murphy

The first reports of acquired immune deficiency syndrome (AIDS) or lymphadenopathy in heterosexual partners or children of human immunodeficiency virus (HIV)-infected hemophilic men [1–3] have been followed by progressively more systematic serologic and virologic surveys [4–26]. In the United States, the proportion of women at risk who have been tested for HIV antibody remains low [13]. Available information indicates that, at least through 1986, knowledge about HIV in hemophilic patients (and partners) was limited [27,28]. Prevention recommendations from governmental authorities [29–32] have increasingly been published in lay language [33–37]. Since late 1986, substantial government assistance, channeled through the Centers for Disease Control (CDC) and Health Resources and Services Administration (HRSA) to hemophilia treatment centers, has been available to improve awareness of recommendations and to encourage changes in sexual practices in compliance with the recommendations.

We reviewed the findings of HIV serosurveys and sexual practice correlations reported from U.S. and international studies. In addition, we documented that women with AIDS whose infection was attributed to heterosexual contact with an HIV-infected hemophilic man represent nearly 2% of all women infected heterosexually [38].

Heterosexual Transmission of AIDS, pages 35–53
Published 1990 Alan R. Liss, Inc.

TABLE 1. Detailed Reports of HIV Seroprevalence in Heterosexual Partners of HIV-infected Hemophilic Men (by last date of partner enrollment)

Survey dates (month/year)	Year published	Country (state)	Lead author	Number tested	Number (%) positive	95% Confidence interval[a]
11/82–3/84	1985	US (CA)	Kreiss	21	2 (9.5)	1.7–31.8
1984	1985	UK	Jones	36	3 (8.3)	2.2–23.6
1984	1986	UK	McVerry	14	0 (0.0)	0.7–26.8
1985	1986	Sweden	Biberfeld	40	4 (10.0)	3.3–24.6
2/86	1986	France	Allain	148	10 (6.8)	3.5–12.4
10/84–9/86	1987	US (PA)	Goedert	24	4 (16.7)	5.5–38.2
8/85–11/86	1986	US	Operskalski	56	12 (21.4)	12.0–34.8
9/84–12/86[b]	1988	US (MA)	Brettler	47	0 (0.0)	0.2–09.4
1986	1988	US (PA)	Ragni	21	4 (19.0)	6.3–42.6
7/85–2/87	1987	US (CA)	Padian	19	4 (21.0)	7.0–46.1
1/85–3/87	1987	US	CDC (Jason)	772	77 (10.0)	8.0–12.4
7/86–4/87	1988	US (NJ)	Kim	14	1 (7.1)	0.4–35.8
7/83–4/87	1989	US	Lawrence	56	5 (8.9)	3.3–20.4
7/84–11/87[b]	1988	US (NC)	Smiley	32	3 (9.4)	2.5–26.2
10/85–10/87	1989	France	Laurian	31	3 (9.7)	2.5–26.9
6/85–1/88[b]	1988	FRG	Kamradt	164	16 (9.8)	5.5–15.6

[a]Confidence interval around the point estimate of seroprevalence in percent [39].
[b]Information obtained through personal communication with author.

SEROPREVALENCE SURVEYS

Between January, 1985, and February, 1989, 16 detailed reports (Table 1) and five briefer reports (Table 2) provided HIV seroprevalence information for female sex partners of HIV-infected hemophilic men. Five non-U.S. studies described results from surveys conducted by regional hemophilia treatment centers [5,8,21,23,24]; three described results approximating a national survey of such partners [6,7,19]. Seven U.S. studies enrolled patients from predominantly one treatment center/region. Two other studies enrolled partners and couples through multicenter collaborations [11,26]; one survey collected reports of testing by physicians and treatment centers throughout the United States [13]. HIV-antibody testing of sex partners has been very limited when viewed from this national perspective.

Populations Studied

This review covers studies that enrolled 10 or more couples. In all studies, enrollment was based on the couples' willingness to partic-

TABLE 2. Brief Reports of HIV Seroprevalence in Heterosexual Partners of HIV-infected Hemophilic Men

Year abstract published	Country (state)	Lead author	Number tested	Number (%) positive	95% Confidence interval
1987	US (LA)	Andes	24	4 (14.8)	4.9–34.6
1988	Argentina	Muchinik	28	5 (17.9)	6.7–37.6
1988	Italy	Nosari	13	3 (23.1)	6.2–54.0
1988	Sweden	Schulman	18	1 (5.6)	0.3–29.4
1988	Brazil	Gonzaga	56	15 (26.8)[a]	16.2–40.5[a]

[a]Included enrollment of women with AIDS.

ipate. No studies provided precise information on the proportion of eligible HIV-infected sexually active men with a steady partner who had been willing to be enrolled.

Six studies mentioned the minimum duration of contact: 5 months, 6 months, 1 year, 2 years, 2 years, 3 years. Most women were enrolled from 1983 to 1987. Although several studies included one couple or more consisting of a hemophilic index man with AIDS [4,14,16,20], the index man of most couples was asymptomatically HIV-infected. Only one study [26] enrolled a majority of couples with an index man with AIDS. Three studies reported that progressive generalized lymphadenopathy (PGL) was observed in one or more of their infected seropositive spouses. Where stated, most couples consisted of an index partner with hemophilia A.

Questionnaire Data

Six surveys included a questionnaire to gather information on sexual practices and other behaviors or characteristics of the women for correlation with their serologic status [4,14,16,18,20,26]. Data on sexual practices included frequency of sexual relations, types of sexual contact (vaginal, oral, or anal), number of sex partners, and estimates of the frequency of condom use and other contraceptive methods. In two studies, the frequency of contacts and duration of probable exposures were used to estimate the total number of sexual encounters for each woman [20,26]. In a few studies, the hemophilic male partner completed a questionnaire. In the four studies [4,16,20,26] that compared information obtained from each member of the pair, results agreed.

Serologic Testing Methods

Most serologic testing used enzyme-linked immunosorbent assay (ELISA) methods, followed by confirmatory immunoblot testing. Two studies used Western blot testing exclusively [18,26]. A seronegative woman with a positive virus culture was included as seropositive by one group [18].

Exclusion of Persons With Other Risk Factors

Acknowledging other possible sources of HIV infection in the partners, one study [18] described two pairs of partners among whom intravenous (IV) drug abuse had also taken place; omitting these couples dropped this study's observed seropositivity rate by 40%. If infection through IV drug abuse is more efficient and its prevalence is increasing in the United States, we must exclude such couples. This risk must be reviewed with all partners enrolled in serosurveys.

Six studies [4,14,16–18,26] specified that needle-stick incidents (associated with assisting the hemophilic partner with factor infusions) either had not occurred or were not reported significantly more frequently by seropositive women.

Reported Seroprevalence: Statistical Analysis and Confidence Intervals (CIs)

Seroprevalence data from these studies are summarized in Tables 1 and 2. The associated error of estimation is reflected in the 95% CI for a single proportion, calculated by the method discussed by Fleiss [39] for extremes of a probability distribution. Most CIs are very wide, influenced by the small number of participants and the generally low prevalence.

Observed seroprevalences in the 11 U.S. studies were 0–21%. The largest study, a national survey of U.S. physicians and hemophilia treatment centers in mid-1987, showed a cumulative seroprevalence of 10.0% (95% CI 8.0% to 12.4%) among the 772 women for whom serologic information was available [13]. Exclusive of this study, the median seroprevalence for the other 10 U.S. studies was 9.5%. Six of eight European studies showed seroprevalences of 5.6–10.0%. A small study in the United Kingdom found a seroprevalence of 0%, one in Italy a seroprevalence of 23.1%. The 95% CIs included 10.0% in all the studies. A seroprevalence study from Brazil acknowledged the enrollment of women with AIDS.

One study provided point (in time) seroprevalence estimates [7]; most other studies enrolled women during periods extending up to 5 years. The cumulative seroprevalences reported for these full study periods do not take into account possibly important changes in the risk of seroconversion during shorter periods. Thus, a woman initially enrolled in a study during 1987 or 1988 and found to be seropositive might have been infected several years previously. Therefore, there may be a (horizontal) time scale-associated error for most published estimates as well as a sample size-determined error associated with the (vertical scale) seroprevalence estimates.

A potentially serious source of bias in heterosexual transmission studies is that women most likely to be exposed and infected may have been preferentially accessible, preferentially solicited for enrollment, or more willing to enroll because of factors correlated with their partners' likelihood of transmitting HIV. For example, if men with earlier (e.g., late 1970s) exposure to HIV-contaminated factor concentrates were more likely to have AIDS by 1985, their steady heterosexual partners would have had greater cumulative opportunities for exposure. In addition, the female partner of a man in deteriorating health may take him for frequent medical care. Any woman with malaise or lymphadenopathy would likely be enrolled and tested by most centers already engaged in such studies. Her inclusion in any study's cumulative findings would result in a seroprevalence estimate that does not truly represent all women at risk. Alternatively, symptomatic HIV-infected women might avoid enrollment. The potential for such bias is only infrequently discussed [22], but including or excluding even one or two such women would, in most studies, substantially alter the observed seroprevalence.

SEX PRACTICES AND OTHER CORRELATES OF INFECTION RISK

Two studies, one enrolling 42 and the other 56 women, each noted that one woman did not engage in vaginal intercourse. Information regarding intercourse during menses was rarely solicited; one study found no significant correlation between this practice and the women's serologic status [14]. In studies asking about oral-genital sex, approximately 45% to 60% of women reportedly engaged in this practice. Differentiating between active (fellatio) and passive (cunnilingus) roles was not possible from most questionnaires. Anal sex was reported infrequently [4,14,18,26] and was not significantly associated with seropositivity. Six studies reported on frequency of sexual relations [4,14,16,18,20,26]; five indicated no significant dif ference between the mean number of sexual encounters per month in seronegative and seropositive women. The numbers of women (and male partners) who reported a history of sexually transmitted disease (STD) (specified or unspecified) were so few in the five studies reviewing this issue [14,16,18,20,26] that no conclusion could be drawn regarding STDs as possible cofactors in HIV transmission in this risk group.

Condom Use

The proportion of women reporting at least some condom use by their male partners was 0–60%. Even studies observing percentages in the upper part of this range noted that the proportion with "consistent" use of condoms was usually much lower. Two studies stated that pregnancies had occurred [16,20], indicating that condoms were either not used or not used effectively. The CDC/National Hemophilia Foundation national survey of serologic status of sex partners of hemophilic men recorded 22 births in HIV-infected women [13].

One study noted that condom use was lowest among the most sexually active women; the authors estimated that 75% of sexual encounters by participating women had not involved condom use [26]. Only 18% of the women reported that their partners' almost always used condoms; these women were 30 to 49 years old.

Since exposure to semen during fellatio without condoms might allow HIV infection despite condom use during vaginal sex, the HIV-antibody status of women in one study was examined according to whether the women used "maximal preventive techniques," defined as the partner's use of condoms "nearly always" and avoidance of oral/genital sex [26]. None of five seropositive women used maximal preventive techniques; only four (13%) of 32 seronegative women did (Fisher exact test [two-tailed]; P = NS) [39].

Except for one study [25], seronegativity was not significantly correlated with consistent condom use [16,20,26]. The lack of evidence from these studies to support the protective value of condom use may be due to one or more of the following factors: 1) consistent condom use during the early period of infection was rare in most hemophilic men; 2) proper condom use was not documented in these studies of hemophilic couples; 3) the small studies rejected the null hypothesis of no benefit to condom use; 4) the studies were not prospective, and unreported changes in use patterns might have occurred; and 5) condom use was not highly effective.

Periods of Greatest Risk to the Heterosexual Partner

Periods of viremia and HIV antigenemia could be temporally associated with an increased risk of HIV transmission to unprotected partners. These periods might occur early, late, or intermittently [20] during the male partner's infection. The period of severe immunodeficiency has been proposed as the period of greatest risk [14]. Using the clinical status of the index partner at the time of enrollment, one study found that 5% of partners of asymptomatic men, but 11% of partners of HIV symptomatic [AIDS, AIDS-related complex (ARC), PGL] hemophilic men, were infected; this difference was not statistically significant [26]. The clinical stage and the degree of immunologic impairment are both correlated with interval since infection and, thus, the length of time the female partner was at risk for exposure; most studies were not able to stratify their analyses by duration of the male partner's infection. The hypothesis that antigenemia in the index partner might correlate with seropositivity in the other partner was not supported in one study [16].

Changes in Sexual Practices During 1984 to 1987

The enrollment periods for most published studies were largely completed before systematic HIV antibody testing of hemophilia patients or of their sex partners became widespread. None of these early studies contained a formal component to assess behavioral changes. Follow-up of initial patients enrolled in the CDC's study to determine subsequent serologic status of the women has been difficult. Reasons cited for failure to continue in the study include divorce or estrangement of the couples, embitterment with the medical community, and grief [26]. In one study, the information on sexual practices for the participants in 1986 and 1987 was compared to that for earlier participants (1983 to 1985); the median number of sexual contacts per month was slightly but not significantly lower [26].

Likelihood of Transmission per Sexual Encounter

If the typical hemophilic man had been infected by 1982–1983, condom use was not reducing the risk to his sex partner(s) during the first 3 or more years because condoms were rarely used. Nevertheless, despite hundreds of episodes of unprotected vaginal contact per couple, as well as frequent oral-genital sex, most studies have found HIV antibody in only approximately 10% of women.

Examining female partners of men in other risk groups, Padian estimated that the likelihood of transmission per exposure (vaginal intercourse) was 1 per 1,000 (95% CI 0–0.0024) [15]. Kim et al. [20] recently noted that, based on questionnaire data, 13 seronegative women had a calculated total of more than 2,500 sexual encounters without infection; on the other hand, he noted that one seropositive woman had reported a midrange sexual frequency, representing about 200 or fewer contacts [20]. Overall, this represented about 0.3 transmissions per 1,000 encounters.

The risk from vaginal intercourse is probably still subject to underestimation and overestimation biases. Certain biologic characteristics of certain index hemophilic men, or their respective partner(s), may favor transmission. Certainly, the role of genital ulcerative disease as a cofactor in heterosexual HIV transmission in Africa does not appear to be important for most U.S. hemophilic men and their partners.

Since many encounters reported on questionnaires could have occurred after HIV transmission but before serologic testing, the real risk of HIV transmission per exposure may be greater than 1 per 1,000. A study of heterosexual partners of men or women infected through blood transfusion showed that as few as one to eight vaginal sexual contacts were sufficient to transmit infection [40]. Prospective studies have recorded continuing instances of seroconversion [18].

It has been difficult to analyze the attributable risk of particular sexual practices: receptive anal intercourse, vaginal intercourse, active oral-genital sex (fellatio), and passive oral-genital sex (cunnilingus). Receptive anal intercourse has been infrequently reported, and oral-genital contact is highly correlated with vaginal intercourse. Largely based on studies of HIV transmission in homosexual men, many researchers believe that the rank order of risk, highest to lowest, is in the sequence listed above. Most calculations to date are based on vaginal intercourse risk without adjustment for frequency of condom use.

AIDS CASES IN FEMALE PARTNERS

The CDC maintains national surveillance of AIDS cases reported from state and territorial health departments. Twenty-seven women with AIDS who cited heterosexual contact with a hemophilic man as their sole risk factor were reported to CDC as of December 7, 1988 (Fig. 1). These women represented nearly 1.6% of all women with AIDS whose infection was acquired through heterosexual contact

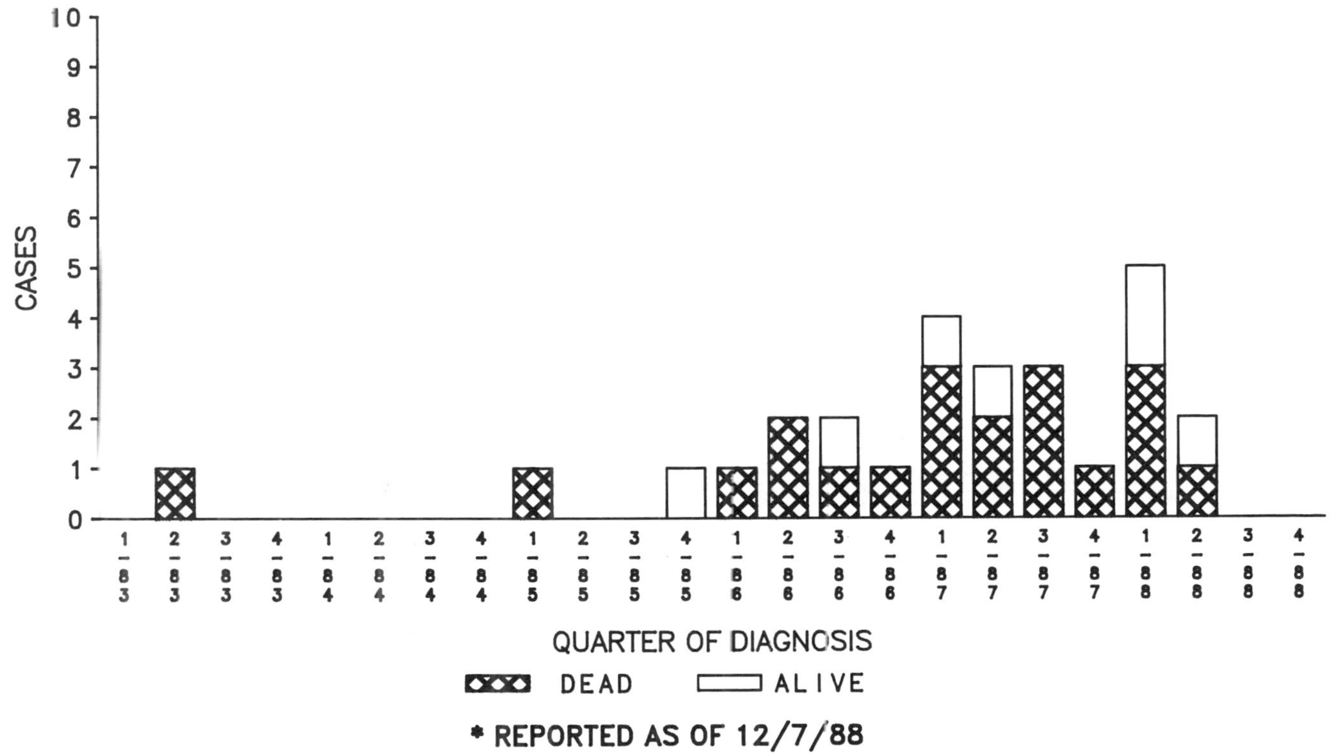

Fig. 1. U.S. cases of AIDS in female heterosexual partners of hemophilic men by quarter of diagnosis.

TABLE 3. Age Distributions of a Sample of Steady Heterosexual Partners of HIV-Infected U.S. Hemophilic Men and of Women With AIDS Contracted Through Heterosexual Exposure to HIV-Infected Hemophilic Men[a]

Age group (years)	Number of asymptomatic women (%)	Number of women with AIDS (%)
20–29	58 (38.2)	10 (37.0)
30–39	51 (33.6)	10 (37.0)
40–49	22 (14.5)	2 (7.4)
50–59	14 (9.2)	3 (11.1)
60–69	6 (3.9)	1 (3.7)
70+	1 (0.6)	1 (3.7)
All	152 (100.0)	27 (100.0)

[a]χ^2 goodness-of-fit test, P = NS [41].

[38]. The earliest case was diagnosed in June, 1983; seven (25.9%) were diagnosed in the first two quarters of 1988. Twenty-two (81.4%) have had *Pneumocystis carinii* pneumonia. The remaining five have had other opportunistic infections. None have had Kaposi's sarcoma. Based on ancillary information, approximately 70% of the hemophilic partners of the initial 11 women diagnosed were still asymptomatic at the time the women were diagnosed. Most women were married to their hemophilic partners at the time of infection and diagnosis. Limited information on sexual practices is available on only nine of the women. Among six who provided information about anal sex, two reported occasional receptive anal intercourse, during which condoms were not used.

The dates of infection were usually not known for either the women with AIDS or their hemophilic partners, although infection for two women must have occurred at least 5 years earlier. The duration of the sexual relationships ranged from months to decades.

The risk to female heterosexual partners began with the infection of their hemophilic male partners from contaminated factor concentrates. The dates of infection of the male partners are rarely known because periodic serologic testing of hemophilia patients did not become widespread until recent years.

Table 3 shows the age distribution of U.S. women with AIDS reported to the CDC through December 7, 1988. Also shown is the age distribution of adult female heterosexual partners of HIV-infected hemophilic men in the treatment center populations of Michigan, Colorado, and southern California (pooled data; Crudder S, Stabler

S, Gross J; personal communication). No remarkable age distribution differences are apparent. Since the frequency of sexual contact generally decreases with advancing years, while condom use peaks in the forties and declines in the postmenopausal years [26], a difference in the efficiency of transmission might not be apparent.

DISCUSSION

During the initial years of the AIDS epidemic, heterosexuals were not generally believed to be at substantial risk. Even today, the World Health Organization describes this route of transmission as more characteristic of the predominant transmission pattern in many lesser developed countries. Thus, recognition by hemophilic men of their potential as a source of infection to their heterosexual partners required a level of understanding and acknowledgment greater than that of the general public.

Another psychological barrier had to be overcome. In hemophilia patients and most other at-risk groups, AIDS was recognized as a fatal clinical entity before the discovery of the agent and development of serologic tests. In contrast, with few exceptions [1–3], the earliest information about risk of infection of heterosexual partners of hemophilic men came from seroprevalence studies among the asymptomatic women.

Unaware of the long latency period, respected authorities were still stating during the mid-1980s that the significance of a positive serology was uncertain in view of the small proportion of all "exposed persons" who had developed disease. In the virtual absence of AIDS cases, uninfected women may not have grasped the significance of the emerging seroprevalence studies.

Afraid of possible negative consequences of a positive serology and without any available therapeutic action to be taken if positive, most hemophilic men had not yet been tested. Although advised that they could be a source of infection to sexual partners, the couples lacked the added motivational impact of the hemophilic man's serologic results to adopt the recommended abstinence or "safer sex."

Therefore, as late as 1985–1986, a full 3 years after the estimated median date of infection of U.S. hemophilia patients, most women having sexual contact with an HIV-infected hemophilic man had not consistently adopted sexual practices associated with reduced risk of HIV transmission. Publications recommending drastic changes in sexual practices [29–31,33] were principally directed to health care professionals. In late 1986, major federal funding increases became available from the CDC and the Bureau of Maternal and Child

Health, HRSA, and thereby to regional hemophilia treatment programs and the National Hemophilia Foundation. The funds permitted rapid expansion of efforts to reach and motivate couples to discontinue high-risk sexual practices. By 1987–1988, information for health care professionals had been supplemented by many newly developed "consumer-oriented" publications [34–37].

Clearly, expanded enrollment of current and previous partners in counseling and testing programs would be advisable. Periodic evaluation of previously tested and counseled partners would allow assessment of the efficacy of the counseling. The techniques of the health educator have been adopted in efforts to reach out to the sex partners. Information gained from these studies of female sexual partners of typically monogamous hemophilic men are also valuable to public health officials attempting to anticipate the risks associated with male-to-female heterosexual spread within the "general" U.S. adult population.

SUMMARY

We reviewed 21 published reports of HIV serosurveys conducted during the past 5 years among the heterosexual partners of HIV-infected hemophilic men. Eleven described seroprevalences in partners of U.S. men; the remainder described findings in other countries. Sixteen studies (ten U.S.; six non-U.S.) provided detailed information on participant selection, serologic test methods, and sex practices. The largest U.S. study was a 1987 national telephone survey of U.S. physicians and hemophilia treatment centers. In this study, only 34% of the known female partners had been tested for HIV antibody; the prevalence was 10.0%. The median seroprevalence for the other 15 detailed studies, each involving 13 or more women, was 9.5%. The observed seroprevalences for these 15 studies were 0% to 21.4%. HIV seropositivity in the female partners did not significantly correlate with the reported frequency of sexual relations, condom use, history of STDs, or anal intercourse. The conclusions that can be drawn from these studies are limited by several methodologic problems, including the small numbers of participants, which compromised the studies' power to implicate potentially important risk factors.

REFERENCES

1. **Pitchenik AE, Shafron RD, Glasser RM, Spira TJ:** The acquired immunodeficiency syndrome in the wife of a hemophiliac. Ann Intern Med 100:62–65, 1984.

2. **Ratnoff OD, Lederman MM, Jenkins JJ:** Lymphadenopathy in a hemophiliac patient and his sexual partner [letter]. Ann Intern Med 100:915, 1984.

3. **Ragni MV, Urbach AH, Kiernan S, et al.:** Acquired immunodeficiency syndrome in the child of a haemophiliac. Lancet 1:133–135, 1985.

4. **Kreiss JR, Kitchen LW, Prince HE, Kasper CK, Essex M:** Antibody to human T-lymphotropic virus type III in wives of hemophiliacs: Evidence of heterosexual transmission. Ann Intern Med 102:623–626, 1985.

5. **Jones P, Hamilton PJ, Bird G, et al.:** AIDS and haemophilia: Morbidity and mortality in a well-defined population. Br Med J 291:695–699, 1985.

6. **Biberfeld G, Bottiger B, Berntorp E, et al.:** Tranmission of HIV infection to heterosexual partners but not to household contacts of seropositive haemophiliacs. Scand J Infect Dis 18:497–500, 1986.

7. **Allain J-P:** Prevalence of HTLV-III/LAV antibodies in patients with hemophilia and in their sexual partners in France [letter]. N Engl J Med 315:517–518, 1986.

8. **McVerry BA, Machin SJ, Galloway MJ, et al.:** HTLV-III antibody and T-cell subset ratios in haemophiliacs and their spouses. Br J Haematol 63:347–352, 1986.

9. **Jason JM, McDougal JS, Dixon G, et al.:** HTLV-III/LAV antibody and immune status of household contacts and sexual partners of persons with hemophilia. JAMA 255:212–215, 1986.

10. **McFadden T, Jason JM, Feorino P:** HTLV-III/LAV seronegative, virus negative sexual partners and household contacts of hemophiliacs [letter]. JAMA 255:1702, 1986.

11. **Operskalski E, and the Transfusion Safety Study Group:** Transmission of human immunodeficiency virus infection to household contacts of persons with congenital hematologic disorders. Abstract: 28th Annual Meeting, American Society of Hematology, December 6–9, 1986, San Francisco, p 131A.

12. **Andes WA, Rangan SR, deShazo RD, Daul CB:** The risks of heterosexual transmission of HIV in hemophiliac couples [abstract]. Clin Res 35:596A, 1987.

13. **Centers for Disease Control:** HIV infection and pregnancies in sexual partners of HIV-seropositive hemophilic men—United States. MMWR 36:593–595, 1987.

14. **Goedert JJ, Eyster ME, Biggar RJ, Blattner WA.** Heterosexual tranmission of human immunodeficiency virus: Association with severe depletion of T helper lymphocytes in men with hemophilia. AIDS Res Hum Retroviruses 3:355–361, 1987.

15. **Padian N, Marquis L, Francis DP, et al.:** Male-to-female transmission of human immunodeficiency virus. JAMA 258:788–790, 1987.

16. **Ragni MV, Gupta P, Rinaldo CR, Kingsley LA, Spero JA, Lewis JH:** Human immunodeficiency virus (HIV) transmission in female sexual partners of HIV antibody positive hemophiliacs. Public Health Rep 103:54–58, 1988.

17. **Brettler DB, Forsberg AD, Levine PH, Andrews CA, Baker S, Sullivan JL:** HIV isolation studies and antibody testing in household contacts and sexual partners of persons with hemophilia. Arch Intern Med 148:1299–1301, 1988.

18. Smiley ML, White GC, Becherer P, et al.: Transmission of human immunodeficiency virus to sexual partners of hemophiliacs. Am J Hematol 28:27–32, 1988.

19. Kamradt TGA, Niese D, Schneweis KE, Brackmann HH, Kamps BS: Heterosexual transmission of HIV in hemophiliacs. Abstract 4008: IV International Conference on AIDS, Stockholm, June, 1988.

20. Kim JC, Raska K III, Clemow L, et al.: Human immunodeficiency virus infection in sexually active wives of infected hemophilic men. Am J Med 85:472–476, 1988.

21. Schulman S, Johnsson H, Albert J, Loogna K, Kramer Y. A 3-year follow-up of sexual partners of HIV-positive haemophiliacs. Abstract 96: Annual Meeting, World Federation of Hemophilia, Madrid, May, 1988.

22. Gonzaga AL, Bonecker C, Vargens Jr. AIDS in sexual partners of hemophilic patients. Abstract 256: Annual Meeting, World Federation of Hemophilia, Madrid, May, 1988.

23. Muchinik G, Campestri R, Perez Bianco R, et al.: Heterosexual Transmission of HIV Infection. Abstract 158: Annual Meeting, World Federation of Hemophilia, Madrid, May, 1988.

24. Nosari AM, Barbarano L, Caimi TM, et al.: Antibodies to human immunodeficiency virus (HIV) in haemophilia, von willebrand's disease and their heterosexual partners: Updating. Abstract 228: Annual Meeting, World Federation of Hemophilia, Madrid, May, 1988.

25. Laurian Y, Peynet J, Verroust F. HIV infection in sexual partners of HIV-seropositive patients with hemophilia [letter]. N Engl J Med 320:183, 1989.

26. Lawrence DN, Jason JM, Holman RC, Heine P, Evatt BL, and the Hemophilia Study Group: Sex practice correlates of human immunodeficiency virus transmission and acquired immunodeficiency syndrome incidence in heterosexual partners and offspring of U.S. hemophilic men. Am J Hematol 30:68–76, 1989.

27. Hargraves MA, Jason JM, Chorba TL, et al.: Hemophiliac patients knowledge and educational needs concerning acquired immunodeficiency syndrome. Am J Hematol 26: 115–134, 1987.

28. Wasserman K, Wilson PA: Psychosocial impact of AIDS. Abstract 19A: 39th Annual Meeting, National Hemophilia Foundation, Omaha, October 9–10, 1987.

29. Centers for Disease Control: Prevention of acquired immune deficiency syndrome (AIDS). MMWR 32:101–104, 1983.

30. Centers for Disease Control: Recommendations for assisting in the prevention of perinatal transmission of human T-lymphotropic virus type III/lymphadenopathy-associated virus and acquired immunodeficiency syndrome. MMWR 34:721–726,731–732, 1985.

31. Centers for Disease Control: Additional recommendations to reduce sexual and drug abuse-related transmission of human T-lymphotropic virus type III/lymphadenopathy-associated virus. MMWR 35:152–155, 1986.

32. Centers for Disease Control: Condoms for prevention of sexually transmitted diseases. MMWR 37:133–137, 1988.

33. **National Hemophilia Foundation:** AIDS Update: Hemophilia and Acquired Immune Deficiency Syndrome (AIDS): Intimacy and Sexual Behavior. New York: National Hemophilia Foundation, 1985.

34. **National Hemophilia Foundation:** Hemophilia Information Exchange: Intimacy, Sexuality and Hemophilia. New York: National Hemophilia Foundation, 1987.

35. **Waterbury M, Gray GL, Scott J, Kessler CM, Sachse K:** Safer Sex: Guidelines for the Prevention of Transmission of the AIDS Virus. Washington, DC: Children's Hospital National Medical Center, 1987. Nimorwicz P: What Women Should Know about HIV Infection AIDS and Hemophilia. New York: National Hemophilia Foundation, 1988.

36. **Nimorwicz P:** What Women Should Know About HIV Infection, AIDS and Hemophilia. New York: National Hemophilia Foundation, 1988.

37. **Levine SB:** Let's Talk About Sex. New York: National Hemophilia Foundation, 1988.

38. **Centers for Disease Control:** AIDS Weekly Surveillance Report—United States, December 5, 1988.

39. **Fleiss JL:** Statistical Methods for Rates and Proportions. New York: John Wiley & Sons, 1981, pp 13–15.

40. **Peterman TA, Stoneburner RL, Allen JR, Jaffe HW, Curran JW:** Risk of human immunodeficiency virus transmission from heterosexual adults with transfusion-associated infections. JAMA 259:55–58, 1988.

41. **Snedecor GW, Cochran WG:** Statistical methods. Ames, Iowa: The Iowa State University Press, 1980, pp 75–78.

DISCUSSION

DR. ALEXANDER: In general, what is the life span of a hemophiliac? Is it the same as the general population?

DR. LAWRENCE: No, it is not yet as long as the general population. Prior to the advent of factor VIII concentrate therapy, which was the vehicle of infection for most of the U.S. hemophilia patients, the average age, or the median age, of hemophilia patients in this country was about 10 years. And, with the advent of this therapy that forestalled life-threatening accidents and spontaneous bleeds, these patients gained 10 years. This was a dramatic improvement.

And, as with the assault of AIDS upon other risk groups in this country, it came at a time when their lives had been totally turned around in a very positive sense of what their own identity was going to be, and their future, their job potential, their marriage potential, their lifestyle, and so on. The infection came as a devastating new awareness to them as well.

DR. MAYER: An issue that I think other speakers will be dealing with is the idea that one may become more infectious with the progression of HIV infection. That is, people with AIDS, people who are symptomatic, may be more likely to transmit the virus to their spouses, although your data suggests that this may not be the case with hemophiliacs. Did you take a critical look at numbers of sexual exposures to try to get at the issue of infectiousness in the course of the relationships between the hemophiliacs and their spouses?

DR. LAWRENCE: Only about three studies have been conducted that, fortuitously, had available serological testing from the late 1970s onward. These studies allowed some estimation of the mid-point of probable infection in the hemophiliac male partner.

Dr. Ragni was among the first to publish this work. Dr. Eyster had some data, and Dr. Kim of New Jersey did also. From these studies, we have some idea when seroconversion occurred. Also, a study that I carried out was helpful in this regard. The difficulty is that the women who are infected, and have developed AIDS, may well have been infected in the early part of that time frame, so that infection in 1978, 1979, or 1980 would be far more likely to result in a diagnosis today than an infection that occurred only from 1982 to 1984 or more recently. Therefore, because of the incubation period, the latency period from exposure to the diagnosis of AIDS, the women who have been infected more recently are not going to be represented proportionately in our model. And I think that, until we know partner pair by partner pair, we are going to be in difficult straits estimating whether the number of sexual contacts cumulatively was a 100 or 500 or 1,000 in determining when infection took place. So I am not comfortable with most of my estimates, and maybe with most others too.

Regarding the early versus late period of highest risk, there are a few opinions. You have the group who believe that the early period of a man's infection seems to be the most viremic. You have the group believing that the pre-terminal illness is the most infectious period. And, you have those who take the middle ground, saying there is a probability function operating throughout the whole period, maybe with a correlation between HIV virus circulation and antigenemia. I cannot take a strong position. I think we have to keep both ends, and maybe the middle as well, in our thinking.

DR. WITKIN: Is there any relationship between HIV transmission and fertility? Has that been examined?

DR. LAWRENCE: In terms of pregnancies that have occurred, Dr. Janine Jason has correlated work from around the country that, tragically, shows the hemophiliac patient population—in disregard to the "official medical publications" or in ignorance of them—has operated from a very deep instinctual desire to rush ahead of the HIV virus transmission and have a family and share all the other features of parenting. I think those unfortunate couples have quite often engaged in a conscious effort to have a child. And, we have seen a higher fertility rate, according to Dr. Jason's findings, among the hemophilia adult population than almost any other segment of the U.S. population. In terms of HIV reducing or increasing fertility, certainly I have no idea if it reduces fertility. I have no information that there is any increase in spontaneous abortion in these couples. And, for your interest, as of December 7, 1988, we now have six cases of AIDS in the offspring of women who were infected in this way, either by the current partner and father of the child or by a previous partner. So I cannot address the true issue you have raised, but there may be some useful correlates in my reflections.

DR. HODGEN: Am I correct in assuming from your remarks that the infectivity of these men was present very early after their acquisition of the virus because they had no symptoms and they thought they were well?

DR. LAWRENCE: Well, yes. In fact, right up through about 1986 or even afterwards, most couples, perhaps only dimly aware that there was something called seroprevalence, but unaware that there were any AIDS cases, continued almost totally unprotected sexual intercourse. And among those couples whose cohabitation included the early years—I will call them the late 1970s and very early 1980s—when the vast number of hemophiliac men seroconverted, we know at least two of the women who had seroconverted, among, say, 15 I investigated and for whom had detailed information, had contact with a man only 5 years or more ago. Therefore, it had to have been fairly early in his viremic or infected period relative to today.

DR. HODGEN: Would anything in the data since that time allow you to expect that these men could be infecting women even before they are seropositive?

DR. LAWRENCE: I see no reason that that would not be true. It certainly seems to me that viremia during the so-called window period before seroconversion would be at least as hazardous, if not more so, than immediately thereafter.

DR. CONE: You mentioned a phrase on which I wonder if you could expand. The phrase about female partners who "share in their fate." This made me think about the large proportion of gay and bisexual men who fail to use condoms even when they know the insertive partner is seropositive. I am wondering if that phrase applies equally to these groups of people?

DR. LAWRENCE: Well, when I wrote that phrase last night, I wondered if it would be too flamboyant. But I think that there is something to this. I think that a woman who gives herself to a relationship with a man who traditionally only a decade or 15 years ago would have been almost unable to hold a job (30% unemployment rate); to a man who often has to survive with therapy every 3–4 days; to a man who may be stricken by a life-threatening bleed or hospitalizations at any moment, for years and years; to a man whose general life span has been foreshortened, is probably not a typical spouse—or is certainly a remarkable candidate for the role.

I think that the interaction of that psychology and this disease needs to be explored very, very carefully, at least in this group, and to some extent maybe in other groups as well.

Having come from an infectious disease background, including tropical medicine, and having worked in some aspects of leprosy, I was certainly aware of, and impressed with, the stories of spouses joining the infected man at a leper colony. So this is no new phenomenon, certainly, but I think that its impact today on what this Workshop is trying to accomplish, and worldwide, is a very important one, at least for some segments. And if it pertains to other risk groups, I hope we can address that without destroying the bonds of intimacy that are operating and have supported at least two lives, if not those of their children and the rest of society.

DR. PETERMAN: I liked your slide showing the ages of the sexual partners of these men. And I am particularly interested in older women who may be postmenopausal. The possibility of more traumatic sexual intercourse with women who have perhaps atrophic vaginitis may increase the transmission rate. You did not find any evidence for that in your study, but I wonder if confounding factors might be found in this data, such as are older men with hemophilia less likely to have been infected early compared to younger men?

DR. LAWRENCE: It is very hard to answer that question. First of all, as you probably remember from conversations we have had in the past, I was intrigued that the first men with AIDS and hemophilia whom I visited were generally elderly, and most of them were married. Then, the first spouse pair I visited were both elderly. The woman died of AIDS shortly after the visit. And I began to wonder whether there was an efficiency of transmission from atrophic vaginitis or other things that, unfortunately, are not on our questionnaires, and often are not in the medical histories. So, I developed the hypothesis that maybe the elderly women were rapidly moving on to AIDS in disproportionate numbers. That would make sense in perhaps both groups. But I see the age profile of women living with infected men is not yet significantly different from the profile of ages of women with AIDS. What I do not know is whether the infection rate is proportionate, by age group, to that for women in the next stage, AIDS. Since I cannot believe that sexual practices per week or per month are as common in elderly women as they are in younger people, it is entirely possible that there is a reciprocal relationship between the numbers of sexual contacts in elderly women and the efficiency of transmission. I know that the women beyond the age of 50 in my study were not using condoms at all; they had no need to for family planning reasons. On the other hand, I assume the reason is family planning. There is a totally separate explanation. If you had a sudden sweep of infection through all ages of the men, and, therefore, an exposure opportunity in all ages of the paired women, if the probability of transmission was exactly 10% over the first couple of months (the midrange of most estimates), we would see that pattern more or less. I do not know which of these explanations is correct.

5

Facilitators of HIV Transmission During Sexual Contact

Thomas A. Peterman

The risk of acquiring human immunodeficiency virus (HIV) infection during sexual contact depends on the risk of having an infected partner and the risk of transmission of infection. Factors that influence transmission should be studied for two reasons. First, studies may suggest new ways to prevent transmission. For example, if genital ulcer disease facilitates HIV transmission, reducing the prevalence of genital ulcers would reduce the risk of HIV transmission. Second, facilitators of transmission may influence the future of the epidemic. For example, if infectiousness increases in late stages of infection, future transmission patterns may be different.

Potential facilitators can be studied in many ways, including the use of animal models or the study of human pathophysiology. This paper concentrates on epidemiologic studies of the role of sexually transmitted diseases (STDs) as facilitators of HIV transmission. The ideal epidemiologic study would compare the risk of transmission for persons who are alike except for the presence or absence of a single possible facilitator. Although this research design is ethically and logistically impossible, the alernatives should be assessed to see how closely they approach the ideal.

FACILITATORS THAT INCREASE SUSCEPTIBILITY

Susceptibility relates to whether sufficient virus can enter cells to establish an infection. Many factors could influence susceptibility, and susceptibility could vary by type of sexual activity because of

Heterosexual Transmission of AIDS, pages 55–68

differences in the effectiveness of the epithelial barriers of the rectum, vagina, and mouth. Similarly, an infection or trauma that damages the epithelial barrier could facilitate entry of the virus. Theoretically, conditions that increase the availability of target cells at the exposure site could increase susceptibility, as could genetic differences in target cells or natural barriers to infection.

Type of Sexual Contact

The high rates of transmission among homosexual men suggest that HIV may be transmitted more efficiently by anal intercourse than by other types of sexual contact. However, many confounders are possible, including the frequency of intercourse, number of sexual partners, and prevalence of infection in those partners. The susceptibility of the rectal versus the vaginal mucosa is probably best studied by looking at the partners of HIV-infected persons. Padian and coauthors [1] found that women who practiced anal intercourse with their infected partners were 2.3 times more likely to be seropositive than women who had only vaginal intercourse. Many other investigators have found relative risks between 2 and 3 in similar partner studies [2–4]. Although this difference in risk is not large, it may be larger for persons having sexual intercourse many times during a short period of time.

Information about the risk of transmission by oral sex is currently insufficient. Kingsley and coauthors [5] found no infected men who reported only oral-genital contact, but the sample size was small and their HIV-exposure status was not known. More recent studies [6–8] of homosexual men suggest that transmission by oral sex is becoming increasingly important as these men change their sexual practices. Additional studies of the efficiency of transmission during oral-genital contact are needed to help in advising gay men, and to determine the likelihood of transmission in other groups (e.g., crack [cocaine] users) who commonly practice oral sex.

STDs

Several early studies suggested that people with genital ulcers may be more susceptible to HIV infection. Quinn et al. [9] reported a cross-sectional study of the prevalence of HIV infection in a Baltimore STD clinic. This study included a brief anonymous questionnaire and serologic tests for HIV and syphilis. HIV seropositivity was more common in men with vs. without history of syphilis [58/281 (20.6%) vs. 112/2,437 (4.6%)], men with positive vs. negative syphilis serology

[58/203 (28.6%) vs. 113/2,513 (4.5%)], and men with vs. without a history of genital herpes [7/52 (13.5%) vs. 163/2,666 (6.1%)]. After adjusting for race and reported homosexual activity, the odds ratios (ORs) for all relationships fell, although they remained statistically significant for a history of syphilis (OR = 2.0) and for a positive serologic test (OR = 3.3). Women with a history of syphilis or serological evidence of past syphilis were not significantly more likely to have HIV antibody. These findings suggest that genital ulcers increase susceptibility, but the study was not designed to assess that hypothesis. Since little information was available about the partners of participants, and none about which infection came first, it is unknown whether this correlation is due to an association with HIV infection in the partners or to differences in susceptibility during sexual contacts.

HIV infection was associated with syphilis and herpes simplex virus type 2 (HSV-2) in two cross-sectional studies of homosexual men reported by Stamm and coauthors [10]. The first looked at serum from 200 men in an acute proctitis study from 1983 to 1986. After adjustment for number of sexual partners, infection with HIV was associated with a history of syphilis (OR = 3.4), positive syphilis serology (OR = 8.4), and antibody to HSV-2 (OR = 3.3). The other study looked at 110 homosexual men who were seen for HIV screening. After controlling for number of sexual partners, men who were seropositive were more likely to have HSV antibody (OR = 8.5) or positive syphilis serology (OR = 9.9). Although these studies showed an association between HSV-2 and HIV, which infection came first is not clear. Furthermore, without knowing the HIV exposure histories of the two groups, it is not clear if HSV is a facilitator for transmission or a marker for exposure to HIV.

Prior HSV-2 infection was suggested as a risk factor for HIV infection in a study by Holmberg and coauthors [11]. This study of hepatitis B involved testing serum samples collected from a cohort of men. HIV seroconverters were matched with controls who did not seroconvert. HIV seroconverters were more likely to have HSV-2 at the time the third specimen was drawn (32/47, 68%) compared to men who remained HIV seronegative (26/57, 46%). Among those who were HSV-2 negative on the first specimen, seroconversion to HSV-2 occurred for 11 (42%) of 26 HIV seroconverters compared to five (14%) of 35 men who remained HIV-seronegative. The association with HSV-2 remained after controlling for age, number of sexual partners, and percentage of sexual acts involving receptive anal intercourse. This study had the advantage of being able to determine that HSV-2 seroconversion (the time at which genital ulcers are most common) occurred at about the same time as the HIV seroconversion, but the actual frequency of genital ulcers is not known. A history of genital herpes was reported by five (16%) of 32 men with both HSV-2 and HIV compared to three (12%) of 26 men with HSV-2 alone.

One group of investigators in Nairobi, Kenya, has contributed several valuable studies. One of the first papers, by Kreiss and coauthors [12], included a cross section of prostitutes who registered at a research clinic or at an AIDS research clinic between February and April, 1985. Prostitutes classified as low-status were more likely to be seropositive (42/64, 66%) than those classified as high-status (8/26, 31%). After stratification, no association was found between HIV serology and duration of prostitution or number of sexual encounters per year. However, there was an increased relative risk associated with sexual exposure to men from other African countries, and seropositive women were more likely to have current infection with gonorrhea [relative risk (RR) 3.8], genital ulcers (RR 3.3), or positive syphilis serology (RR 2.5). The association with STD could mean either that the partner who transmitted the STD was more likely to have HIV infection or that the coinfected person was more susceptible or more infectious.

A cross-sectional study, reported by Simonsen and coauthors [13], looked at 340 men who went to a Nairobi STD clinic and reported the source for their STD as a prostitute from the high-risk area described in their earlier studies. Thirty-eight (11%) of the 340 men had HIV antibody. HIV-seropositivity rates were higher in men who did vs. did not travel out of Kenya [6/19, (32%) vs. 32/321 (10%)], men who were uncircumcised vs. circumcised [17/87 (20%) vs. 21/253 (8%)], men with vs. without previous prostitute contact [34/259 (13%) vs. 4/81 (5%)], men with vs. without a history of genital ulcers [24/82 (29%) vs. 14/258 (5%)], and men with vs. without a current diagnosis of genital ulcer [24/162 (15%) vs. 14/178 (8%)]. There was no significant association with lifetime number of partners, past or present urethritis, or another STD. This study could not determine the HIV-exposure histories of the men visiting the clinic. The authors controlled for this by adjusting for the reported number of exposures to the prostitutes (one vs. more than one), but whether this adjustment controlled for HIV exposure is unclear. A second problem is the uncertainty about which came first, HIV infection or genital ulcers. Finally, the relationship to circumcision may be confounded by other factors; most uncircumcised Kenyan men come from the area bordering Uganda and Tanzania, countries where HIV infection is more common.

A prospective study in the area of Nairobi of prostitutes with a high incidence of STDs was reported by Plummer and coauthors

[14]. Histories and laboratory studies of women who developed HIV antibody during the study were compared to those of women who remained seronegative. Among the 595 prostitutes considered for the study, 196 (33%) were initially HIV antibody negative. Of these 196 women, 83 seroconverted and 41 remained seronegative for at least 12 months. Genital ulcer disease occurred in 60% of seroconverters and 45% of seronegative women, but HIV seroconverters had more frequent episodes (mean 0.11 vs. 0.04 episodes per month). Women who seroconverted also were more likely to have positive cultures for *Chlamydia trachomatis* (32/81, 40%) compared to women who did not seroconvert (6/39, 15%). Gonococcal infection, syphilis serology, and cervicitis did not show significant relationships to HIV. This study also found that women who seroconverted were more likely to have a history of oral contraceptive use (32/83, 39%) compared to seronegative women (7/41, 17%), and they were less likely to report any condom use (14/76, 18%) compared to women who remained seronegative (28/41, 68%). This study, being prospective, was able to show that ulcers often preceded HIV infection. However, HIV exposure history still was not available.

Trauma

Trauma during sexual intercourse obviously could lead to breaks in the mucosal barriers, but what is considered traumatic sex? Many studies have asked about bleeding during sex, but this is a rather crude assessment of trauma. If any sexual contact that disrupts the mucosal barrier is considered traumatic, trauma could be frequent and difficult to detect. Several variables could influence the likelihood of tears. A study [15] of the wives of HIV-infected transfusion recipients found that older women were more likely to seroconvert than younger women. Perhaps this finding relates to atrophic vaginitis and more trauma during sex. Dry sex is considered desirable in certain areas of Africa. Repeated sexual encounters in a short period of time, such as those taking place in some gay bath houses, may also result in more mucosal tears. These observations suggest hypotheses that will be very difficult to study. They also demonstrate some complex interactions that may influence the likelihood of sexual transmission.

Genetic Differences

Genetic differences could play a role in susceptibility, although there is little evidence to suggest that they do. One study [16] suggested that susceptibility may be related to a gene for group-specific component, but others [15] found no association with this factor. The possibility of genetic differences is intriguing, especially from an immunologic standpoint.

FACILITATORS THAT INCREASE INFECTIOUSNESS

Conditions that increase infectiousness basically are those that increase viral shedding. Shedding could be facilitated by genital ulcers or a genital discharge of infected cells. Bleeding during menses or following trauma might also increase the amount of virus present in genital secretions. Other conditions that influence viremia generally also might increase shedding during sexual contact. For example, infectiousness might be higher early in infection, before a person develops antibody. Similarly, transmissibility could increase late in infection, when a person begins to develop antigen excess. Concomitant infections or other stimulants of the immune system might also stimulate HIV replication, increase viremia, and increase infectiousness.

STDs

In most reported studies of STDs as facilitators of HIV transmission, effects on susceptibility are difficult to distinguish from effects on infectiousness. However, one study, by Cameron and coauthors [17], primarily addressed infectiousness. This study enrolled men who attended a Nairobi STD clinic and who reported that the source of their infection might be a prostitute from an area where most prostitutes were known to be infected with HIV. Of the 422 men who enrolled, 51 (12%) were initially HIV seropositive. Seroconversion was seen in 24 (8%) of 293 men who were followed. HIV seroconversion was more common in men who reported prostitute contact at least monthly vs. less than monthly [12/82 (15%) vs. 12/211 (6%)], presented with genital ulcer disease vs. other STDs [21/150 (14%) vs. 3/143 (2%)], and were uncircumcised vs. circumcised [18/70 (26%) vs. 6/213 (3%)].

To measure the risk of seroconversion after a single contact in which an STD was acquired, evaluation was limited to men who reported a single sexual contact with a prostitute and who did not acquire a new genital ulcer disease in the follow-up period. Six of the 101 men meeting these criteria were initially seropositive. Seventy-three others returned for follow-up, six (8%) of whom seroconverted. Seroconversion was more common in men with genital ulcers vs. urethritis [6/37 (16%) vs. 0.36 (0%)] and in men who were uncircumcised vs.

circumcised [5/27 (19%) vs. 1/46 (2%)]. Thus, if the partners of these men were equally likely to be infected with HIV, men who acquired a genital ulcer were more likely to acquire HIV infection because their partners had a genital ulcer when they had sexual contact.

Bleeding

Theoretically, menstrual bleeding could increase the amount of HIV in cervical secretions and thus increase infectiousness. Studies to date [4,18] usually have found no such relationship, but they have lacked sufficient power to draw conclusions.

Viremia

A third way that infectiousness might increase is through a general increase in the amount of replicating virus in the infected person. Early in infection, before antibody is produced, there is relative antigen excess. Theoretically, HIV viremia may be higher during periods of antigenic stimulation by other infections [19]. HIV antigen excess also occurs late in infection as the immune system begins to deteriorate. Two epidemiologic studies [18,20] have suggested that HIV transmission may be more common in the late stages of disease. Goedert and coauthors [18] found that men with hemophilia who transmitted infection to their wives were more likely to be in the late stage of their infection, as measured by a low T4 count or the presence of HIV antigen. Some studies [20] have found similar results; others [21,22] have not. It is too early to say how much the stage of illness influences infectiousness, if at all, but transmission clearly can occur at any stage.

CONCLUSIONS

Few things can be said with certainty about facilitators for HIV transmission, but this should not stop us from acting on what we do know. Anal intercourse probably transmits infection more efficiently than vaginal intercourse, but the difference is not large enough to explain the current distribution of disease nor to influence markedly the risk of heterosexual transmission. On the other hand, the risk of transmission by oral sex might be considerably lower. If so, changing from anal to oral intercourse could have a major impact on homosexual transmission.

Genital ulcer disease is another probable facilitator, but multiple sources of bias and confounding make it difficult to determine the magnitude of the effect. Obviously, individuals should be advised not to have sexual intercourse when they have genital ulcers. More importantly, intervention studies are needed to see how programs that target genital ulcers affect HIV transmission. This type of study probably can be carried out only in African countries that have a high incidence of treatable genital ulcers and HIV infection.

In the United States, we need to learn who is acquiring HIV infection and the possible contribution of STD facilitators. Easily treatable genital ulcer diseases (syphilis and chancroid) are relatively rare in the United States. However, there may be persons with a high incidence of both genital ulcers and HIV infection for whom intensive efforts to treat syphilis would decrease HIV transmission.

Finally, sexual transmission of HIV can occur only when an infected and an uninfected partner have sexual contact. Individuals probably would be less likely to start a sexual relationship with someone whom they knew was infected with HIV. However, determining the infectious status of a partner is extremely difficult. We need to develop better ways to help people know when a potential partner is infected.

REFERENCES

1. **Padian N, Marquis L, Frances DP, et al.:** Male-to-female transmission of human immunodeficiency virus. JAMA 258:788–790, 1987.

2. **Sion FS, Morais de Sa CA, Rachid de Lacerda MC, et al.:** The importance of anal intercourse in transmission of HIV to women. Abstract 4007: IV International Conference on AIDS, Stockholm, June, 1988.

3. **De Vincenze I:** Heterosexual transmission of HIV: A European community multicentre study. Abstract 4024: IV International Conference on AIDS, Stockholm, June, 1988.

4. **Steigbigel NH, Maude DW, Feiner CJ, et al.:** Heterosexual transmission of HIV infection. Abstract 4057: IV International Conference on AIDS, Stockholm, June, 1988.

5. **Kingsley LA, Detels R, Kaslow R, et al.:** Risk factors for seroconversion to human immunodeficiency virus among male homosexuals. Lancet 1:345–349, 1987.

6. **Mayer KH, Degruttola V:** Human immunodeficiency virus and oral intercourse. Ann Intern Med 107:428–429, 1987.

7. **Greenblatt RM, Osmond D, Moss A, Samuel M, Shabosky S, Winkelstein W:** Behaviors associated with incident HIV infection among homosexual men in San Francisco. Abstract 4086: IV International Conference on AIDS, Stockholm, June, 1988.

8. **Rozenbaum W, Gharakhanian S, Cardon B, Duval E, Navarette MS, Coulaud JP:** HIV transmission by oral sex. Abstract 4562: IV International Conference on AIDS, Stockholm, June, 1988.

9. **Quinn TC, Glasser D, Cannon RO, et al.:** Human immunodeficiency virus infection among patients attending clinics for sexually transmitted diseases. N Engl J Med 318: 197–203, 1988.

10. Stamm WE, Handfield HH, Rompalo AM, Ashley RL, Roberts PL, Corey L: The association between genital ulcer disease and acquisition of HIV infection in homosexual men. JAMA 260:1429–1433, 1988.

11. Holmberg SD, Stewart JA, Gerber AR, et al.: Prior herpes simplex virus type 2 infection as a risk factor for HIV infection. JAMA 259:1048–1050, 1988.

12. Kreiss JK, Koech D, Plummer FA, et al.: AIDS virus infection in Nairobi prostitutes: Spread of the epidemic to East Africa. N Engl J Med 314:414–418, 1986.

13. Simonsen JN, Cameron DW, Gakinya MN, et al.: Human immunodeficiency virus infection among men with sexually transmitted diseases: Experience from a center in Africa. N Engl J Med 319:274–278, 1988.

14. Plummer FA, Simonsen JN, Cameron DW, et al.: Cofactors in male-female sexual transmission of HIV. Submitted for publication.

15. Peterman TA, Stoneburner RL, Allen JR, Jaffe HW, Curran JW: Risk of human immunodeficiency virus transmission from heterosexual adults with transfusion-associated infections. JAMA 259:55–58, 1988.

16. Eales L-J, Nye KE, Parkin JM, et al.: Association of different allelic forms of group specific component with susceptibility to and clinical manifestation of human immunodeficiency virus infection. Lancet 1:999–1002, 1987.

17. Cameron DW, Simonsen JN, D'Costa LJ, et al.: Genital ulcer disease and lack of male circumcision are cofactors in female to male sexual transmission of human immunodeficiency virus. Submitted for publication.

18. Goedert JJ, Eyster ME, Ragni MV, Biggar RJ, Gail MH: Rate of heterosexual HIV transmission and associated risk with HIV-antigen. Abstract 4019: IV International Conference on AIDS, Stockholm, June, 1988.

19. Quinn TC, Piot P, McCormick JB, et al.: Serologic and immunologic studies in patients with AIDS in North America and Africa. JAMA 257:2617–2621, 1987.

20. Laga M, Taelman H, Bonneux L, Cornet P, Vercauteren G, Piot P: Risk factors for HIV infection in heterosexual partners of HIV infected Africans and Europeans. Abstract 4004: IV International Conference on AIDS, Stockholm, June, 1988.

21. Padian N, Wiley J, Glass S, Marquis L, Winkelstein W: Anomalies of infectivity in the heterosexual transmission of HIV. Abstract 4062: IV International Conference on AIDS, Stockholm, June, 1988.

22. Horsburgh CR Jr, Seage G, Mayer K, Schable C: Transmitters of HIV are not identified by persistent serum antigen or antibody patterns. Abstract 4565: IV International Conference on AIDS, Stockholm, June, 1988.

DISCUSSION

DR. FORREST: You said that only 12% to 16% of people who tested positive for herpes simplex had reported that they had, in fact, had the infection. I wonder if you could say more about whether you think this is due to their lack of willingness or to their lack of recognition? This is especially important when you talk about helping people identify whether their partners might be infected. Certainly one cofactor is the presence of another STD, and if you are saying that many people may not even recognize that they have herpes simplex, this presents problems in trying to identify it in a partner.

DR. PETERMAN: That is a good point. Herpes II infection is often asymptomatic, although if you investigate people who have herpes you can see lesions. If you work closely with them, you can get them to recognize that they have flare-ups of genital lesions. However, there is some subclinical ulceration, the role of which I think is not clear. But it is a good point that if we are trying to make an association with an STD that we cannot recognize, it is going to make it more difficult.

DR. ARYA: Apart from male circumcision, female circumcision is practiced in vast areas of Africa. The role that this plays as a risk factor for the transmission of AIDS in that part of the world, I suppose, still has not been investigated.

Now, I will point out that in certain rural areas in Arabia, skin cutting is practiced for all sorts of ailments. This is executed by traditional healers using techniques that cause extensive exudation and secondary infection. This has been responsible for the increased prevalence of hepatitis B and cancer in wide areas. At the moment, these areas have been classified as pattern III for HIV transmission, but, once AIDS reaches there, I am sure these practices will have an important role to play.

DR. PETERMAN: I think that is a good point. We need to know more about that.

DR. BURNHILL: I am wondering whether genital ulcerations are not getting a bad rap in a peculiar way. I am convinced that there is a relationship between genital ulcers and the risk of getting HIV. There is also a relationship with human papilloma virus (HPV). I wonder if it is not because 1) people with painful ulcerations tend to be able to give those histories and obviously are exposed to more disease, or 2) more disturbing, whether there is some immunodeficiency that makes it more likely to get papilloma virus or herpes virus and AIDS, which is difficult to measure.

I work mainly with lower genital tract disease, and I can tell you that, by far, most partners of people with HPV or herpes do not have visible lesions. We have not looked sufficiently at susceptibility to disease as a clue to transmission.

DR. PETERMAN: I agree that this is a tremendously complex area, and I do not think we should oversimplify it by saying "yes" or "no" to the question about genital ulcers as risk factors. There are a lot of concerns that need to be raised.

One thing about genital ulcer disease that separates it from a generalized immunodeficiency in susceptible people is that there is an intervention for genital ulcers and there is not for general immunodeficiencies in a population. I think that by conducting studies in some African countries with an intervention to decrease genital ulcer disease we can, perhaps, answer the question about the role it plays and see if the control of genital ulcers reduces HIV transmission.

DR. PHANUPHAK: Are there any studies either in Africa, the United States, or elsewhere indicating if postcoital vaginal douching, or thorough vaginal washing, is a risk factor or protective factor for HIV transmission?

DR. PETERMAN: I am personally not aware of any such studies, although, in some of the early studies of gay men, douching was found to be associated with HIV transmission. But these men had sexual contact after that, and it was thought that perhaps the douching would disrupt the genital mucosa or the rectal mucosa and facilitate transmission in that way. I am not familiar with any studies, though, that look at postcoital douching in women.

DR. GUINAN: I would like you to comment on the contribution of circumcision to heterosexual transmission compared with all the other risk factors. I would guess that it is relatively small. But the way it is presented, and because the data are statistically significant, it would appear to be much more important than perhaps it might be. And I question any suggestion of an intervention that might not be appropriate; that is, to start circumcising all males. In the history of STD, for the hundreds of years we have known about it, circumcision has always been identified as protective. But, every one of those studies, when analyzed, was faulty. They lacked sexual activity data or were not controlled for sexual partners, or socioeconomic groups, or other factors. Therefore, none of them really holds true. There was really no good evidence. Now, the data presented here are much better in that they control not only for sexual partners but for the biggest risk factor, exposure to someone who is infected.

If you look at that cohort study of people who, as I understood it, were exposed to HIV-positive people, the seroconversion rates in the circumcised vs. uncircumcised are flawed because the numbers of uncircumcised are much greater than circumcised. I would say that in Africa the burden of circumcision is probably relatively small because of all the other risk factors. The role of circumcision as a risk factor needs to be put into better perspective.

Also, what are the factors leading to circumcision in Africa? Are they socioeconomic? Do you have to pay for circumcision? Who gets circumcised, and why and when in their life do they get circumcised? Many people have been circumcised late in life because they believe that it will protect them from disease. I think that these things are very important to delineate.

DR. PETERMAN: You bring up a lot of good points. The first thing I would like to clarify is that none of these studies really knows if the people studied were exposed to HIV or not. The studies in Kenya asked the men if they had sex with a group of prostitutes, and this group of prostitutes has a seropositivity rate of about 80–85%. So, we do not know for sure whether these men had sex with an infected person, although when the rate is that high it is fairly likely.

The question about circumcision was, I think, fairly well discussed by Simonsen in his paper. He pointed out that the men in Kenya who are circumcised tend to come from areas bordering Uganda and Tanzania, where rates of HIV infection may be higher. Therefore, there are a lot of possible confounders, and I would hesitate to speculate on the role of circumcision, much less on its contribution to HIV transmission. I think there are a lot of possible confounders in terms of who gets circumcised, and who circumcised and uncircumcised men have sex with.

DR. SHELTON: I would like to address that same point. I think you are being a bit hard on the Nairobi study; I view it a bit differently. The men in the second Nairobi study had sex with a cohort of prostitutes among whom something like 80–90% were HIV-positive. I do not know if there were data on the actual number of exposures, but I think that the prevalence rate is a fairly good index that there was some degree of exposure. It strikes me that this is a case when, if you are concerned about potential bias explaining an observation, it becomes incumbent upon you to try and figure out if there were some confounding variables that would explain why there was such a fairly large difference. What to me is somewhat remarkable is the very status and relationship that was observed. I cannot see that degree of strength washing out easily in terms of systemic bias. So I view that study a bit differently, I suppose, in my interpretation.

DR. PETERMAN: I have never been to Nairobi, and I think if you ask circumcised and uncircumcised men who they have had sex with, you might have trouble getting a good answer because of cultural problems. I think there is room for a lot of possible confounders.

I want to bring up the point that we have to consider how much evidence it takes to make some sort of public health recommendation. And for something like genital ulcer disease as a risk factor for transmission, as an academician, I could argue against all those studies, but, as a public health person, I say we need to get rid of genital ulcer disease anyway, and the evidence is sufficient to make that recommendation right now.

For circumcision, the issue, I think, is a little bit different, and I personally might ask for a bit more data before I would recommend circumcision for all men in Africa.

DR. PUDNEY: Do you have any indication that infection with cytomegalovirus (CMV) might increase the transmission of HIV?

DR. PETERMAN: I think that Scott Holmberg looked at CMV in his study, and no association was found. I think the problem was that the infection rate was so high that it was difficult to look at in that group.

DR. HOLMBERG: Correct. Our study did not find such an association, but there is a study of male homosexual partners in Boston and the preliminary data suggest that CMV increases infectiousness.

DR. HARRIS: I would like to ask Dr. Peterman and possibly Dr. Heymann one question. Our informal policy on genital ulcer disease at the Agency for International Development (AID) is that we want to see it erased. We think that better management of STDs, in general, is a good idea, but we have limited resources and we are not going to focus on that until somebody conducts a study showing that the reduction of genital ulcer disease through a treatment program also reduces the transmission of HIV. I would like you to comment on whether you think our position is reasonable. I would be interested in hearing from Dr. Heymann if the WHO program has any studies planned to address this issue; AID does not right now.

DR. PETERMAN: Well, I cannot make the decision for you, but I will say that it is complicated by a number of things. One is the alternatives that you have for reducing HIV transmission, and the other is the length of time it will take to demonstrate effectiveness in one of these studies.

I think you are probably more aware than I am of the difficulty of doing an intervention study in an African country when one is looking for efficacy. I think that intervention studies should be set up in such a way that they can generate this information. But, at the same time, I am hesitant to say that we should wait until they are completed in all areas and under all circumstances before making decisions. It is a complex problem.

DR. HEYMANN: I think genital ulcerative disease is something that needs to be treated. Prevention of genital ulcer disease certainly should be a priority because it is also a possible way of preventing HIV infection.

Regarding your second point about whether any studies were planned, such studies are very difficult. It is difficult to establish the attributable risk in a disease in which many different factors are involved. We are planning to assemble a group of experts to try to determine the best methodologies for such studies and how to eliminate variables. We are also working with Family Health International to try to develop some of these protocols.

6

Changing Behavior: Barrier Methods in High-Risk Populations

Malcolm Potts and Paul J. Feldblum

Acquired immune deficiency syndrome (AIDS), viewed from a pathophysiologic perspective, is a relatively simple disease, but, viewed in the human context, AIDS is a complex problem. Since this new infection is sexually transmitted, AIDS appears first in individuals who have the largest number of sexual partners. The paramount problems in this dreaded disease are not virology—the molecular details are understood; nor prevention—the limited choices are starkly simple; nor surveillance—the data are more than sufficient to scare us. Rather, the key issues are institutional, bureaucratic, and political. The patterns of sexual activity that epidemiologists call "variance from the mean" are viewed by some decision-makers as "perversion."

We face two problems in trying to change the behavior of and provide barrier methods for high-risk populations: 1) understanding the advantages and disadvantages of barrier methods and identifying problems associated with their distribution and acceptance and 2) securing the freedom of action necessary to implement programs of education and service.

SEXUAL BEHAVIOR

It is self-evident that individuals who have many sexual partners are both more likely to acquire human immunodeficiency virus (HIV) infection and to transmit it to others. Epidemiological models show that a given number of sexual acts distributed among a small number

Heterosexual Transmission of AIDS, pages 69–79

of persons, each with many sexual partners, presents more risk to the individuals involved and to the remaining community than the same number of coital acts distributed among a large number of persons, each with a small number of sexual partners during a lifetime. Thus, the most sexually active persons affect the epidemic in disproportion to their number in the population.

Several computer models of HIV spread [1,2] agree on the following four predictions.

1. HIV infection through contaminated blood, although tragic, is not a major factor in the epidemic.
2. Casual sexual partnerships may give rise to a self-sustaining epidemic, but spread will be slow.
3. Groups with high-risk behaviors will greatly accelerate the spread of HIV infection throughout the remainder of society.
4. A reduction of high-risk behaviors not only protects the lives of the individuals involved in those behaviors but has the potential to slow significantly the spread of the epidemic throughout society.

Like other polygamous or promiscuous primates, such as gorillas or chimpanzees, *Homo sapiens* are sexually dimorphic (males are 15% to 20% heavier than females), and the testis/body ratio in males is high, as in other primates that mate frequently, compared with genuinely monogamous apes, such as gibbons [3]. In many societies past and present, most men have more sexual partners during a lifetime than most women. The extra partners for a substantial number of men come from a small number of women who provide sexual services for money. One consequence of this pattern is that men tend to get sexually transmitted diseases (STDs), and by inference AIDS, from casual sexual encounters, whereas most women's infections tend to come from steady partners.

The sexual practices of homosexual men and homosexual women differ greatly. At least until recently, gay men have tended to seek frequent erotic outlets with a large number of partners. Lesbian women tend to establish more stable long-term relationships in which erotic contract is less significant [4].

The distribution of the number of lifetime sexual partners is asymmetrical, with a small number of persons having many partners and a majority of individuals having a few partners (Fig. 1). Recent data [5] from the United Kingdom suggest that, although one-third of women under age 30 years have had one lifetime sexual partner, the

TABLE 1. Factors Influencing Condom Failure Rates[a]

	Cigarette smoking by women			
	Never a smoker	Ex-smoker	Current smoker	χ^2
Number of failures	282	92	222	
Crude pregnancy rate per 100 woman-years	2.7	3.6	3.8	15.7 (0.001)
Adjusted rate	2.7	3.5	3.8	16.5 (0.001)

[a]Reproduced from Vessy et al. [10] with permission of the publisher.

majority of women (85%) have not had more than one new partner in the past year. The same study also suggests that women who begin intercourse under the age of 16 years have more frequent intercourse and more sexual partners as teenagers and through their twenties than do women who begin intercourse after age 16 years.

USE OF BARRIER METHODS

How likely are groups that are at high risk of acquiring and transmitting HIV to use barrier methods? A review of the use of barrier methods as contraceptives may help to answer this question.

Worldwide, an estimated 40 million couples rely on condoms for family planning, only 13 million of whom are in the Third World. Seven times as many men use condoms in Japan as in the whole of Africa, where fewer than one man in 200 uses condoms [6]. However, social marketing programs for condoms are highly successful in Bangladesh, India, and Colombia; they are likely to be the most cost-effective way to reach low-risk populations in Third World countries.

Before the widespread use of pills and intrauterine devices (IUDs), barrier methods of contraception were the major method of family planning in western countries. In 1959, a Population Investigation Committee survey of a sample of U.K. couples found that 48% had ever used condoms and 36% were current users. In the same survey, one in eight users relied on the diaphragm. In the United States, at the same time, 31% of couples interviewed in the Family Growth in Metropolitan America Study [7] were using condoms. The use of condoms diffused from the upper to lower socioeconomic strata in the first half of the twentieth century in western countries. At the time of maximum post-war condom use in Europe and North America, the method was popular among blue-collar workers and professionals, and often appealed to couples with clearly defined sexual

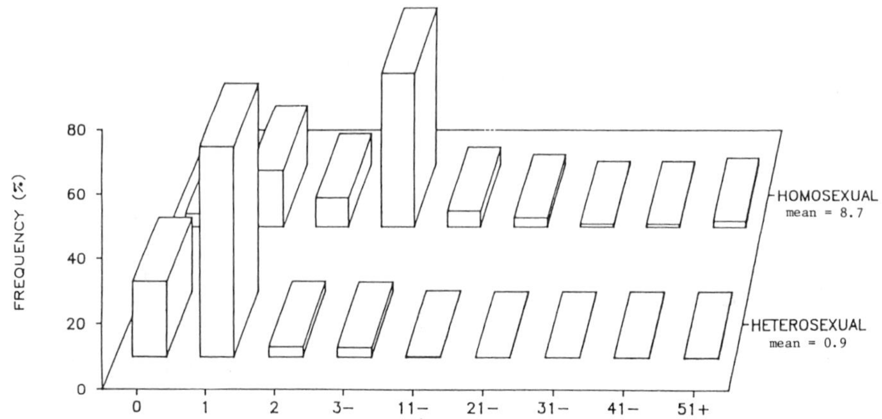

Fig. 1. Mean number of sexual partners per year, April 1986.

roles within marriage [8]. Diaphragms were primarily a middle class method. Among U.S. women using contraception in 1982, 8.3% used a diaphragm, and, interestingly, use was greater among unmarried women (13.4%) than among currently married women (6.7%) [9].

The contraceptive effectiveness of barrier-method use increases with duration of use and probably also correlates with certain aspects of personality (Table 1). For example, users who smoke have a higher failure rate for condoms than non-smoking users [10]. It seems logical that these same characteristics correlate with barrier-method use in the case of HIV or other sexually transmitted disease (STD) transmission.

The harsh reality is that individuals with the largest number of sexual partners—prostitutes and gay men—often live on the fringes of society. Prostitutes, in particular, are caught up in a cycle of poverty. At greatest risk are the poorest, most exploited prostitutes, those who have the most partners in a unit interval of time. Prostitutes often have little education, unstable family lives, and few alternative employment opportunities; they live in substandard, overcrowded housing, often smoke, and sometimes use hard drugs. Indeed, the current U.S. crack epidemic is producing a new type of prostitute who exchanges sex for drugs. Many U.S. women become prostitutes to pay for intravenous drugs, and drug abuse through injection is probably the main way they acquire HIV infection (Shedlin M, personal communication). In short, the target for barrier-

TABLE 2. Epidemiological Characteristics and Changes in Sexual Behavior of Greek Registered Prostitutes (1984–1987)[a]

Characteristics	1985	1987
Median age (years)	38.4	37.8
Duration of prostitution (median years)	13.0	8.0
Mean number of sexual contacts per month	1,140.0	960.0
Use of condoms (%)	66.0	97.9
Acceptance of clients from central Africa (%)	6.5	0
Incidence of syphilis (%)	17.1	3.2
Incidence of gonococcal infection (%)	14.0	0

[a]Reproduced from Papevangelou et al. [16] with permission of the publisher.

method use is precisely those persons who are least likely to use barrier methods of contraception.

PROGRAMS

Important changes can occur in response to realistic interventions. Gay men in the United States and Europe began to educate themselves about AIDS as they became aware of the disease. A slowing of HIV acquisition [11] and a fall in STDs suggest that these gay men are having fewer partners and are using condoms more carefully [12]. In Britain, the mean annual number of partners of homosexual men fell from 10.5 in April, 1986, to 4.8 in January, 1987 [13,14]. At one STD clinic in London, the gonorrhea prevalence rate fell from 15.3% in 1982 to 5.1% in 1986 [15]. The use of persons with AIDS as peer educators seems to have been an important factor in behavior changes among gay men.

Western prostitutes already use condoms quite well. In New York, condom use is widespread for oral and vaginal intercourse, but prostitutes still have unprotected intercourse with their "pimps," who often use drugs. However, interventions to educate and to distribute condoms to prostitutes have changed some behaviors in a relatively short time (Table 2) [16]. North and Chantler (see, respectively, Chapters 23 and 25, this volume) discuss the potential role of spermicides in women at high risk for HIV infection.

Barrier methods must be promoted in all appropriate ways. Persons at highest risk for HIV infection may not read newspapers nor listen to the radio, and prostitutes often work during prime-time television hours. Although conventional promotion (i.e., at clinics or workplace or through social or commercial marketing) is essential to validate the method and is a cost-effective way to reach the most people, more direct, face-to-face strategies must be pursued among high-risk groups. Every effort must be made to empower prostitutes to take greater control of their lives [17]. Decriminalization of prostitution must be considered.

HIV can spread at a devastating rate among prostitutes. In Nairobi, prevalence jumped from 7% in 1980 to over 80% in 1987. In Tamil Nadu, India, 10 of 102 prostitutes tested were HIV-positive [18]; in Thailand, 23 of 892; and, in the Philippines, only five of 3,500, but in the absence of contradictory evidence, it is prudent to assume that prevalence may increase as it has in Africa.

Relatively few interventions have been made to slow HIV transmission in Third World prostitutes. Health education has been conducted with one group of prostitutes in Nairobi who have been followed for years [19]. The adjusted relative risk of acquiring HIV among prostitutes who claimed to use condoms was 0.11 (Cameron DW, in preparation). Family Health International (FHI) has begun interventions among prostitutes in Ghana; Cameroon; Mali; Burkina Faso; and Juarez, Mexico. One approach to high-risk behavior interventions among prostitutes is to train selected ones to teach their peers about AIDS and about ways to prevent the spread of HIV infection. The preferred approach is to persuade women to give up prostitution, and sometimes this happens. But most prostitutes are poor and support children; they cannot leave the business and must be taught to protect themselves. Some change in prostitute and client behavior can be achieved relatively quickly. Prior to peer counseling and free condom distribution in Yaounde, Cameroon, 53% of 125 prostitutes used condoms with their clients "from time to time" or more frequently. During the intervention, almost all the women accepted condoms, and, when questioned 3 months later, 96% of those available for follow-up reported that they were using condoms "from time to time" or more frequently.

Building on experience already gained, FHI's AIDSTECH program is developing 26 intervention projects with high-risk behavior groups in countries such as Burundi, Kenya, Nigeria, Senegal, Tanzania, Zaire, Zimbabwe, Dominican Republic, eastern Caribbean, Ecuador, El Salvador, Peru, Philippines, and Thailand (as well as those countries mentioned earlier). In most of these countries, high-risk behavior group interventions will begin as small projects, will be reviewed and modified as experience is gained, and will be expanded into large-scale programs and replicated as quickly as resources permit. Planning for program expansion and replication must be an integral part of intervention activities.

Improving the diagnosis and treatment of STDs, especially of genital ulcers, may also prove to be an effective and important intervention that will reduce HIV transmission. Oral antibiotic treatment for chancroid is relatively straightforward [20].

The objective assessment of interventions with prostitutes will be difficult [21]. Indicators of program success vary from intervention to intervention but commonly include measurement of at least one of the following indicators: improvement in knowledge of AIDS and how it is transmitted, decreased prevalence of STDs among target groups, decreased incidence of HIV infection among target groups, compliance with condom use, and number of referrals or visits to the STD treatment site. Validating the effectiveness of intervention programs with high-risk groups will be important. Prostitutes, in particular, are exploited persons who often respond enthusiastically to genuine offers of help. We suspect that they may overreport condom use to please the project staff.

ISSUES

In the last analysis, the problem may not be as much in education and condom distribution as in obtaining the freedom to act and in generating the political will to initiate programs and replicate successful ones. Barrier methods have their limitations, and effort and patience will be needed to achieve wide use by high-risk populations. A key problem is that unpopular minorities often are at greatest risk of HIV infection, whereas those who control society's resources, whether in a democracy or a more centralized state, intuitively respond to the expressed or implied needs of the majority. This issue is relevant to foundations and to nongovernmental, governmental, and intergovernmental agencies that plan interventions. Therefore, we have a conflict. From one point of view, interventions with high-risk populations are a public health opportunity. HIV is a fragile virus and even a modestly successful program of protection with barrier methods can have a powerful impact. Communities of prostitutes and gay men are primarily urban, concentrated in limited areas, few in number, and easily identified. Offering help to those most likely to acquire and transmit the disease is scientifically conservative.

From another viewpoint, such interventions are a policy maker's nightmare. The accusation that a foundation or tax money is promoting prostitution or a gay lifestyle is discomforting to even the most concerned member of a national AIDS committee or the most experienced administrator of international aid. Some decision makers either want to deny certain lifestyles or are reluctant to recognize that these lifestyles spread the disease. The attention given to cleaning up the blood supply reflects a counterpoint: contaminated blood endangers society in general, so all of society responds enthusiastically. Indeed, people who get AIDS through blood transfusion are perceived as innocent.

In many ways, experience with AIDS is a speeded-up rerun of the global family planning experience. For 10–15 years, some nations denied they had a population problem. As a consequence, population growth is out of control today in countries as different as China and Kenya. Similarly, Uganda, Zaire, the United States, and many other countries denied for 12–36 months that they had an AIDS problem. Consequently, the problem today is more difficult and more expensive.

CONCLUSIONS

The World Health Organization (WHO) leadership in this area is appropriately called the Global Programme on AIDS. Important support is available from the European economic community and a number of bilateral programs, including the Agency for International Development (A.I.D.) and the AIDSTECH/AIDSCOM programs supported by A.I.D.

Enough is known about intervention with prostitutes and gay men to begin to replicate interventions in every exposed group. Although attention must be paid to parts of India, Southeast Asia, and Latin America, emphasis in the next 12 months should be on Africa. We must set up a global strategy even though we need more information about the most acceptable and cost-effective way of making such interventions available.

In reality, most interventions are in the pilot project stage. Any intervention, particularly in the Third World, takes time to start. Therefore, we must begin the necessary initiatives in the next 12 months, and expect to modify them as we gain experience from the earlier pilot projects. The behavior of our institutions must change if we are to succeed in changing the behavior of high-risk groups. The international community has made available more than $60 million for AIDS programs in the Third World (Bialy G, personal communication). A modest part of these resources probably can cover high-risk groups in much of the world. The success or failure of the use of available resources can be determined by how many cases of HIV transmission are prevented.

The vast majority of people, even prostitutes, worldwide are not infected with AIDS. Barrier methods are the closest thing we have to a "vaccine." The public health policies used to distribute vaccines must be applied to the distribution of barrier methods to populations at high risk. To eliminate smallpox, the world needed a well managed global program that tracked down the disease in the most remote parts of the poorest countries. To slow the spread of AIDS, we must have a similar global strategy that is comprehensive in its plan and well managed in its execution and that covers all groups with high-risk behaviors.

ACKNOWLEDGMENTS

Partial support of this work was provided by Family Health International (FHI), with funds from the U.S. Agency for International Development. The views expressed in this paper are the authors' own and do not necessarily reflect those of A.I.D.

REFERENCES

1. **Auvert B, Moore M, Bertrand WE, et al.:** Dynamics of HIV infection and AIDS in a central African city. Int J Epidemiol (in press).

2. **Anderson RM, May RM:** Epidemiological parameters of HIV transmission. Nature 333:514–519, 1988.

3. **Tuttle RH:** Apes of the World. New Jersey: Noyes Publications, 1986.

4. **Tripp CA:** The Homosexual Matrix. New York: Signet, 1975.

5. **UK Family Planning Research Network:** Patterns of sexual behavior among sexually experienced women attending family planning clinics in England, Scotland and Wales. Br J Fam Plan 14:74–82, 1988.

6. **Sherris JD, Lewison D, Fox G:** Update on condoms—Products, protection, promotion. Popul Rep Series H, 6, 1982.

7. **Peel J, Potts M:** Textbook of Contraceptive Practice. Cambridge: Cambridge University Press, 1969.

8. **Deys CM, Potts M:** Condoms and things. In Schering Workshop on Contraception: The Masculine Gender. Adv Biosci 10:287–293, 1972.

9. **Bachrach CA:** Contraceptive practice among American women, 1973–1982. Fam Plan Perspect 16:253–259, 1984.

10. **Vessy MP, Villard-Mackintosh L, McPherson K, Yeates D:** Factors influencing use-effectiveness of the condom. Br J Fam Plan 14:40–43, 1988.

11. **Winkelstein W, Wiley JA, Padian NS, et al.:** The San Francisco men's health study: Continued decline in HIV seroconversion rates among homosexual/bisexual men. Am J Public Health 78:1472–1474, 1988.

12. **Schechter MT, Craib KJP, Willoughby B, et al.:** Patterns of sexual behavior and condom use in a cohort of homosexual men. Am J Public Health 78:1535–1538, 1988.

13. **Anderson RM:** The epidemiology of HIV infection: Variable incubation plus infectious periods and heterogeneity in sexual activity. In press.

14. **AIDS Advertising Campaign:** Report on Four Surveys During the First Year of Advertising 1986–87. London: British Market Research Bureau, 1987.

15. **Carne CA, Weller IVD, Johnson AM, et al.:** Prevalence of antibodies to human immunodeficiency virus, gonorrhea rates and changed sexual behavior in homosexual men in London. Lancet 1:656, 1987.

16. **Papevangelou G, Roumeliotou A, Kallinikos G, Papoutsakis G, Trichopoulou E, Stefanou TH:** Education in preventing HIV infection in Greek registered prostitutes. J AIDS 1:386–389, 1988.

17. **Scibelli P:** Empowering prostitutes: A proposal for internation legal reform. Harvard Women's Law J 10:119–157, 1987.

18. **Simoes EAF, Babu PG, John TJ, et al.:** Evidence for HTLV-III infection in prostitutes in Tamil Nadu (India). Indian J Med Res 85:335–338, 1987.

19. **Ngugi EN, Plummer FA, Simonsen JN, et al.:** Prevention of transmission of human immunodeficiency virus in Africa: effectiveness of condom promotion and health education among prostitutes. Lancet 2:887–890, 1988.

20. **Ndinya-Achola JO, Nasanze H, Fransen L, et al.:** Three day oral course of augmentin to treat chancroid. Genitour Med 62:202–204, 1986.

21. **Abramson PR:** Sexual assessment and the epidemiology of AIDS. J Sex Res 25:323–346, 1988.

DISCUSSION

DR. PADIAN: I was wondering if you could comment on using prostitutes as educators? I have read several articles lately that talk about the importance of instituting prevention programs among prostitutes. Because prostitutes themselves are effective educators, they could be used to disseminate information on methods to prevent transmission.

DR. POTTS: I think that is very true. After all, condoms have been around since the sixteenth century, and they were initially used for protection against STDs. They then got into family planning and contraceptive use.

We have to empower prostitutes, first of all, to work as units. We want situations where every prostitute in a brothel says, "You cannot have sex unless you use a condom." Then I think we can get rapid change. And men who use condoms in those situations may also learn that it is not a totally bad or difficult thing to use a condom.

I would like to think we can have educational programs for the clients of prostitutes, but they are so diffuse; they are between 10% and 50% of all men, and are difficult to reach. So, with limited resources, I suggest targeting the women, educating them, and giving them the necessary supplies; we should not make them scapegoats, but, in my opinion, this is the most effective thing that the virus is telling us we can do in 1989.

DR. WILLIAMSON: I want to make a comment comparing working with prostitutes in the United States and in the developing world. I think it is easier to work with prostitutes in the developing world because they do not have the tangle of pathologies that you sometimes find in the United States. They are not drug users. They are not partners of drug users. They are not as stigmatized as in the United States. They are not minorities. Very often they are widows. They are women with children, and, I think, they are more receptive to health education than U.S. prostitutes. Nevertheless, there have been successes with prostitutes in the United States. But I think the work we have done shows that prostitutes in developing countries are very receptive to these education programs, and we have not encountered the obstacles that people said we would encounter.

DR. POTTS: I agree entirely. My wife and I were in a brothel 2 weeks ago in Mexico; the women were so receptive. They said, "Thank you for coming." They came from extended families, and they had not been raped when they were 9 years old, or sexually abused in some terrible way. They were really very responsive. Although this is a difficult area, I have every confidence that now is the time to move out in a global program, and that this is, I believe, the best use of our resources. I think that this meeting is going to refine how we do those things. I am merely saying that the program implementors should start working with prostitutes; they should be wise and realize that we are going to make a lot of mistakes and that we are probably going to get some political flak, but, in my experience, not as much as people believe.

7

Biology of Retroviruses

Kenneth D. Somers

Retroviruses were discovered in the early 1900s, when it was demonstrated that chicken leukemia and sarcomas could be transmitted to chickens by cell-free filtrates. Since then, retroviruses have been isolated from a variety of species (Table 1). Interest in retroviruses was spurred rapidly by two independent lines in inquiry: 1) the discovery of human T-cell lymphotrophic viruses, HTLV-I and HTLV-II, as the etiologic agents of adult T-cell leukemia and hairy cell leukemia, respectively [1,2]; and 2) the demonstration that the activated cellular oncogenes detected in a variety of human and animal tumors are the cellular homologs of retroviral oncogene(s) [3]. The sudden emergence of acquired immune deficiency syndrome (AIDS) has stimulated interest in retroviruses generally and in human immunodeficiency viruses (HIV) specifically [4–6].

CLASSIFICATION

Retroviruses belong to the family Retroviridae. Three subfamilies are recognized: Oncovirinae (the RNA tumor virus group), Lentivirinae (visna/maedi viruses), and Spumavirinae.

1 Oncovirinae include the oncogenic retroviruses or RNA tumor viruses. Members infect human, mammalian, avian, and reptilian species and induce sarcomas, leukemias, lymphomas, and carcinomas in susceptible hosts. HTLV-I and HTLV-II are human oncogenic members of this subfamily.

2 Lentivirinae include retroviruses that induce slowly developing disease characterized by a long incubation period and protracted clinical course. Visna virus, the prototype lentivirus, causes an encephalitis or pneumonia of sheep. Other members of the lentivirus family include equine infectious

Heterosexual Transmission of AIDS, pages 81–91

TABLE 1. Retrovirus Distribution

Class	Species
Teleostei	Fish
Reptilia	Snakes
Aves	Chickens, pheasants, turkeys, ducks
Mammalia	Mice, rats, hamsters, guinea pigs
	Cats, mink
	Pigs, deer, sheep, goats, cattle, horses
	Monkeys
	Humans

anemia virus, caprine arthritis-encephalitis virus, feline immunodeficiency virus, simian immunodeficiency viruses, and HIV. Unlike the oncogenic retroviruses, lentiviruses cause nontransforming and cytopathic infections.

3 Spumavirinae include members present in a number of mammalian species (felines, bovines, nonhuman primates, and humans) and cause persistent infections without clinical disease in their natural hosts. Spumaviruses induce cytopathic effects in cell culture characterized by foamy degeneration and vacuolization of infected cells.

PROPERTIES

Generic properties of retroviruses are summarized in Table 2. Retroviruses are spherical, enveloped virions, 80–120 nm in diameter, containing an icosahedral nucleocapsid. The genome consists of two identical molecules of single-stranded, positive-sense RNA of 5–10 kb in size. Retroviruses contain a virion-associated reverse transcriptase (RNA-dependent DNA polymerase), which catalyzes the synthesis of a double-stranded DNA copy of the viral RNA genome. Virions are assembled and mature by budding from the plasma membrane.

LIFE CYCLE

The retroviral life cycle is illustrated in Figure 1. Retroviruses initiate infection by attachment to receptors on susceptible target cells. In the case of HIV, virus attachment to target cells is mediated by the high-affinity binding of the HIV envelope glycoprotein gp120 with the target cell CD4 molecule. Thus phenotypic expression of the CD4 antigen determines the cell and tissue tropism of HIV. Following

TABLE 2. Properties of Retroviruses

Spherical, enveloped virions, 80–120 nm in diameter
Genome consists of two molecules of single-stranded, positive-sense RNA, 5–10 kb in size
Contain virion-associated reverse transcriptase
Virions assemble and mature by budding from plasma membrane

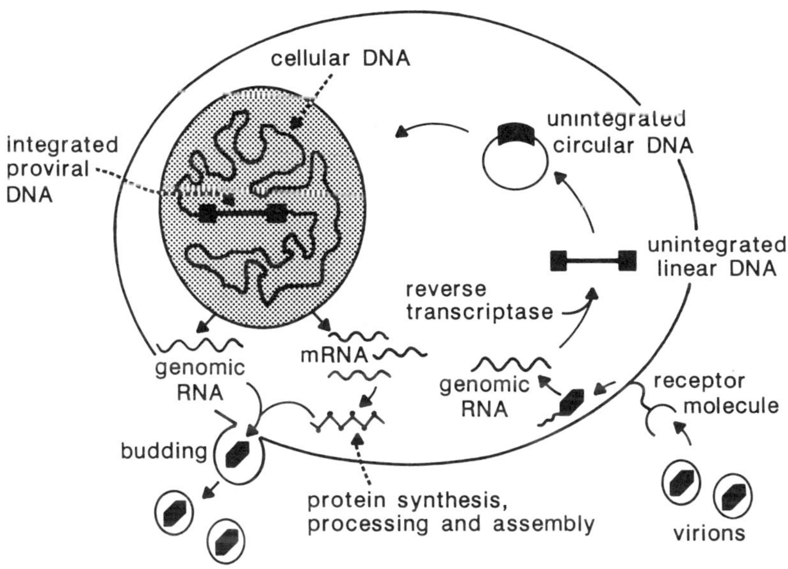

Fig. 1. Retrovirus life cycle.

attachment, the virus is believed to gain entry to cells by fusion of the viral envelope with the cell membrane. Direct fusion of the virus and the cell membrane is thought to be mediated by the transmembrane portion (gp41) of the virus envelope protein. Subsequent to entry, the internalized virus core is uncoated, and genomic RNA is transcribed to double-stranded DNA by the enzyme reverse transcriptase. Newly synthesized viral DNA can exist in a linear or circularized form and may remain in an unintegrated form or be integrated into the host chromosomal DNA. Integration is required for transforming retroviruses (e.g., HTLV-I and HTLV-II). However,

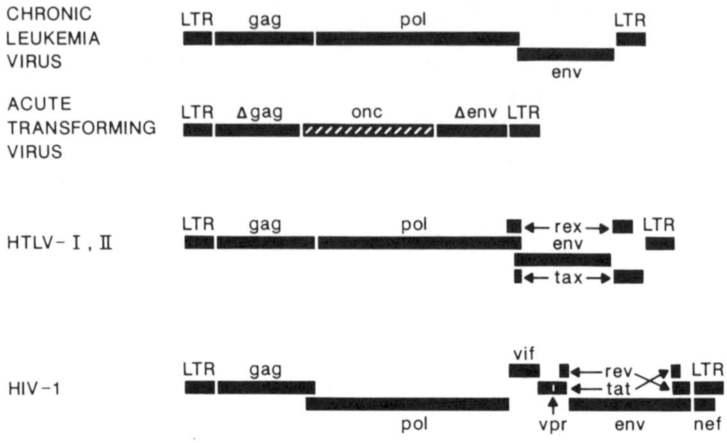

Fig. 2. Genomic organization of retroviruses.

the accumulation of large amounts of unintegrated viral DNA is an unusual feature of cytopathic HIV infections [7]. Efficient expression of multiple copies of unintegrated viral DNA may be an important factor in cell killing by HIV [8]. Integrated proviral DNA behaves like a cellular gene and is transcribed by cellular RNA polymerase II to yield full-length genomic RNA and viral mRNA. Subgenomic mRNAs are translated into virus-specific proteins that have either structural, enzymatic, or regulatory functions. Newly synthesized viral genomic RNA, envelope, and core proteins assemble at the cell surface, and new virions are released by budding from the cell membrane.

GENOMIC ORGANIZATION

Genomic structure of the proviral DNA form of representative retroviruses is illustrated in Figure 2. Integrated proviral DNA is flanked by long terminal repeats (LTRs), which do not code for any proteins but contain sequences for regulating RNA transcription from the genome. Specifically, LTRs contain enhancer and promoter elements and the 5′ cap site for initiation of RNA synthesis. In addition, LTRs contain sequences for termination of transcription and polyadenylation, features relevant to the 3′ LTR. Three genes are common to all replication-competent retroviruses: *gag* codes for virion core proteins; *pol* codes for virion-associated catalytic proteins (reverse transcriptase, integrase, and protease); and *env* codes for viral envelope proteins. Nondefective chronic leukemia viruses, typified by murine and avian leukemia viruses, contain the three essential genes required for replication. Chronic leukemia viruses replicate efficiently in cultured cells but do not induce cellular transformation. In vivo, these viruses induce a variety of leukemias after a long latent period of several months. The mechanism of oncogenicity by these viruses derives from the integration of viral DNA adjacent to a cellular protooncogene. This event, called insertional activation or promoter insertion [9], places the cellular protooncogene under the influence of the strong transcriptional control elements of the provirus and serves to up-regulate expression of the protooncogene. Uncontrolled or inappropriate expression of the cellular protooncogene is thought to be critical to leukemogenesis by these viruses.

Acute transforming retroviruses are defective for replication, induce leukemias or sarcomas in weeks or a few months, and transform cells in culture. The exception to this general rule is Rous sarcoma virus, which is a nondefective, acutely transforming virus. All defective, acutely transforming retroviruses have suffered a loss of one or more genes necessary for replication. These viruses are now known to have acquired an oncogene(s) responsible for transformation in vitro and tumor formation in vivo. Retroviral oncogenes derive from cellular protooncogenes and are thought to have been captured as a consequence of recombination of a nontransforming retrovirus with a cellular protooncogene [10]. The transduced oncogene is actively transcribed using the proviral LTR and frequently exhibits structural modifications or mutations that contribute to altered function.

The human retroviruses HTLV-I and -II form a third category. These viruses are replication-competent and can both immortalize and transform T lymphocytes in vitro. HTLV-I and -II do not contain an oncogene but contain two regulatory genes, *tax* and *rex* [11,12]. The *tax* gene is a strong trans-activator of viral gene expression. The *rex* gene protein (Rex) acts to regulate the production of viral structural proteins and represses regulatory genes. The *tax* gene product (Tax) activates expression of cellular regulatory sequences as well as viral LTR sequences. Demonstration that Tax can up-regulate expression of genes encoding interleukin-2 (IL-2) and the IL-2 receptor in T lymphocytes [13] suggests that the Tax protein may play a role in leukemogenesis by inducing abnormal or autonomous cell proliferation, which may be a step necessary in tumor progression.

The fourth group of retroviruses, HIV, is the most complex retrovirus recognized (Fig. 3). In addition to the three structural genes (*gag*, *pol*, and *env*), the HIV genome has at least six novel genes, three of which (*tat*, *rev*, and *nef*) have known regulatory functions [11,12].

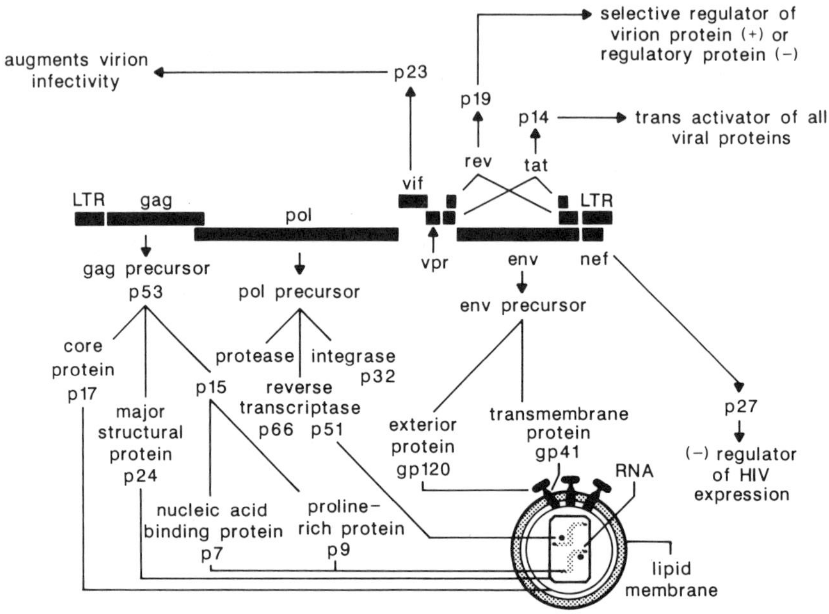

Fig. 3. Gene map and protein products of HIV-1.

The function of the remaining genes is either unknown (*vpr, vpx*), or augments virus infectivity and virus transmission in vitro (*vif*). HIV mutants defective in *vif* gene function were 100–1,000-fold less infective than wild-type virus [14,15].

The *tat* gene is a positive trans-activator of all viral proteins and is essential for virus growth [16]. The Tat protein acts to provide the virus with a positive feedback loop and greatly increases the pace of virus growth. The *rev* gene acts to repress regulatory genes but upregulates genes for viral structural proteins, thus favoring viral growth. Point mutants in the *rev* gene fail to synthesize virus structural proteins and are defective in virion production [17]. The *nef* gene encodes a negative regulatory factor that down-regulates virus replication. *nef* Gene mutants overproduce viral RNA and mature virus [18], suggesting that the normal function of the *nef* gene product (Nef) is to apply the brake on HIV gene expression. Repression of HIV growth by Nef may contribute to the development of virus latency. Investigation of HIV genome structure has revealed a group of regulatory genes that suggest a complex network of controls that function in the life cycle and pathogenesis of HIV.

GENETIC VARIATION OF HIV

Substantial genetic variation is observed among different isolates of HIV-1 and HIV-2, particularly in the envelope gene [19,20]. Similar genomic diversity is common to lentiviruses of primates and sheep [21,22]. The degree of sequence variation is most profound in the *env* gene coding for the exterior glycoprotein gp120, where 20% amino acid sequence differences have been observed in different isolates [23]. Recent studies indicate that individual isolates of HIV-1 are composed of populations of genetically and biologically distinct variants [24,25]. As many as 17 genotypically distinct viruses were identified by restriction endonuclease mapping in sequential isolations from two infected individuals [24]. A similar analysis of HIV-1 isolates obtained from the same individual 16 months apart showed a progressive change in the viral genome with time. The evidence indicates that genotypic variation of HIV can occur in vivo and that this change is rapid and extensive. The significance of HIV variation in viral pathogenesis is uncertain, but the capacity for rapid genetic change is likely to contribute to antigenic variation of HIV and the ability of the virus to evade the immune response. In addition, genomic variation of HIV may lead to altered cell tropism and altered virulence. The heterogeneity of gp120 has frustrated efforts to exploit this external virion protein in vaccine development. However, despite the extensive variability of the HIV envelope, conserved domains are interspersed between regions of hypervariability. These conserved regions are likely to be important for virus structure and attachment to susceptible cells and may serve as targets for prevention and therapy of HIV infection. Continued investigation of the complex HIV life cycle may identify additional targets that are vulnerable to therapeutic strategies.

REFERENCES

1. **Poiesz BJ, Ruscetti FJ, Gazdar AF, Bunn PA, Minna JD, Gallo RC.** Detection and isolation of type C retrovirus particles from fresh and cultured lymphocytes of a patient with cutaneous T-cell lymphoma. Proc Natl Acad Sci USA 77:7415–7419, 1980.

2. **Kalyanamaran VS, Sarngadharan MG, Robert Guroff M, et al.:** A new subtype of human T-cell leukemia virus (HTLV-II) associated with a T cell variant of hairy cell leukemia. Science 218:571–573, 1982.

3. **Bishop, JM:** Cellular genes and retroviruses. Annu Rev Biochem 52:301–354, 1983.

4. **Dalgleish A, Malkovsky M:** Advances in human retroviruses. Adv Cancer Res 51: 307–360, 1988.

5. **Shaw GM, Wong Staal F, Gallo RC.** Etiology of AIDS: Virology, molecular biology,

and evolution of human immunodeficiency viruses. In DeVita VT Jr, Hellman S, Rosenberg SA (eds): AIDS: Etiology, Diagnosis, Treatment, and Prevention. Philadelphia: J.P. Lippincott Co., 1988.

6. **Fauci AS:** The human immunodeficiency virus: Infectivity and mechanisms of pathogenesis. Science 239:617–622, 1988.

7. **Shaw GM, Hahn BH, Arya SK, Groopman JE, Gallo RC, Wong-Staal F:** Molecular characterization of human T-cell leukemia (lymphotropic) virus type III in the acquired immune deficiency syndrome. Science 226:1165–1171, 1984.

8. **Somasundaran M, Robinson HL:** Unexpectedly high levels of HIV-1 RNA and protein synthesis in a cytocidal infection. Science 242:1554–1557, 1988.

9. **Hayward WS, Neel BG, Astrin SM:** Activation of a cellular *onc* gene by promoter insertion in ALV-induced lymphoid leukosis. Nature 290:475–480, 1981.

10. **Bishop JM:** Viral oncogenes. Cell 42:23–38, 1985.

11. **Gallo R, Wong-Staal F, Montagnier L, Haseltine WA, Yoshida M:** HIV/HTLV gene nomenclature. Nature 333:504, 1988.

12. **Varmus H:** Regulation of HIV and HTLV gene expression. Genes Dev 2:1055–1062, 1988.

13. **Siekevitz M, Feinberg MB, Holbrook N, Wong-Staal F, Greene WC:** Activation of interleukin 2 and interleukin 2 receptor (Tac) promoter expression by the trans-activator *(tat)* gene product of human T-cell leukemia virus, type I. Proc Natl Acad Sci USA 84: 5389–5393, 1987.

14. **Fisher AG, Ensoli B, Ivanoff L, et al.:** The *sor* gene of HIV-1 is required for efficient virus transmission in vitro. Science 237:888–892, 1987.

15. **Strebel K, Daughterty D, Clouse K, Cohen D, Folks T, Martin MA:** The HIV "A" *(sor)* gene product is essential for virus infectivity. Nature 328:728–730, 1987.

16. **Dayton AI, Sodroski JG, Rosen CA, Goh WC, Haseltine WA:** The *trans*-activator of the human T cell lymphotropic virus type III is required for replication. Cell 44:941–947, 1986.

17. **Sadaie MR, Benter T, Wong-Staal F:** Site-directed mutagenesis of two trans-regulatory genes (*tat*-III, *trs*) of HIV-1. Science 239:910–913, 1988.

18. **Luciw PA, Cheng-Mayer C, Levy JA:** Mutational analysis of the human immunodeficiency virus: The *orf*-B region down-regulates virus replication. Proc Natl Acad Sci USA 84:1434–1438, 1987.

19. **Coffin JM:** Genetic variation in AIDS viruses. Cell 46:1–4, 1986.

20. **Zagury JF, Franchini G, Reitz M, et al.:** Genetic variability between isolates of human immunodeficiency virus (HIV) type 2 is comparable to the variability among HIV type 1. Proc Natl Acad Sci USA 85:5941–5945, 1988.

21. **Schneider J, Hunsman G:** Simian lentiviruses—The SIV group. AIDS 2:1–9, 1988.

22. **Narayan O, Zink MC, Huso D, et al.:** Lentiviruses of animals are biological models of the human immunodeficiency viruses. Microbial Pathogen 5:149–157, 1988.

23. **Starcich BR, Hahn BH, Shaw GM, et al.:** Identification and characterization of conserved and variable regions in the envelope gene of HTLV-III/LAV, the retrovirus of AIDS. Cell 45:637–648, 1986.

24. **Saag MS, Hahn BH, Gibbons J, et al.:** Extensive variation of human immunodeficiency virus type-1 in vivo. Nature 334:440–444, 1988.

25. **Fisher AG, Ensoli B, Looney D, et al.:** Biologically diverse molecular variants within a single HIV-1 isolate. Nature 334:444–447, 1988.

DISCUSSION

DR. ADA: In the last 8 months, I have heard a number of presentations by people talking about the basic biology of the retroviruses, but I do not think I have heard one quite as concise and clear as what Ken just gave us. Now is your opportunity to ask the questions you have always wanted to ask somebody about the properties of this virus; not a simple virus, as one of the earlier speakers said, but really one of the most complex viruses and one subject to regulating influences that we did not suspect a few years ago.

DR. ALEXANDER: You talked about one individual from whom 17 viral variants were isolated. Is that because mutation of the virus occurs within the body or because he was exposed to 17 different types?

DR. SOMERS: Probably both, but I think the prevailing idea is that the virus can mutate significantly.

DR. ANDERSON: You commented but did not spend much time on the endogenous retroviruses. There is considerable evidence from animal models that endogenous retroviruses are expressed at high frequency in the reproductive tissues in the placenta and the male reproductive tract. I have combed the literature for reports on endogenous retrovirus expression in the male reproductive tract in humans and have not found much. Can you comment on endogenous retroviruses in the human?

DR. SOMERS: I am not aware of much evidence for endogenous retroviruses in humans. Murray Gardner is going to speak this morning and probably will have something to say about endogenous retroviruses in animals.

I am aware of a few studies that provide some structural electron microscopic evidence for endogenous retroviruses. There are some human genes that seem to be related to endogenous retroviruses. Only some of the components, like the glycoproteins, are made.

These genes may play a role in human disease or in human development, but there is very little information.

DR. JOHN: Do these genetic variations give any biological property advantages to the virus other than perhaps escape from neutralization?

DR. SOMERS: That is an interesting question. Obviously, one implication of the profound variations seen in the envelope gene region is that there would be antigenic variation; that is, variation in the proteins that make up the gp120, allowing the virus to evade the immune response. Obviously, efforts to develop a vaccine have been thwarted in large part by this variation in the HIV gp120 region.

I should point out, however, that there are regions interspersed between these hypervariable regions that seem to be conserved among HIV in the gp120, and it is thought by some that these conserved regions may still function as targets for vaccination or therapy. Also, some of the regulatory genes that I talked about very briefly also may serve as targets that may be vulnerable to various intervention strategies.

DR. CONE: Concerning the receptor binding sites, do all of the different isolates still bind to CD4?

DR. SOMERS: I do not know the answer to that. To my knowledge, they do. I do not know if there are variants that are mutated and have lost the ability to attach via CD4.

DR. ADA: There are several reports. I do not know that any are published stating that, in fact, virus has been recovered from cells that do not have messenger RNA CD4.

DR. CONE: That would suggest that there are other binding sites, but it would not rule out that the virus still infected the cells via CD4 in other cells.

DR. ADA: Well, they may have, but they may also have been taken, say, by antibody complexes to cells that have HIV receptors or competent receptors. But I think this is an area that needs to be investigated more closely.

DR. SODROSKI: I would like to comment on the CD4 question. I think the immunogenic studies have indicated that the regions of HIV-I, HIV-2, and SIV that have been implicated in CD4 binding are relatively well conserved among different geographic isolates, as well as the different viruses, all of which use CD4 as a receptor. So there is fairly good conservation of those regions, which makes them reasonably good targets. Unfortunately, in addition to being conserved, the regions also seem to be buried within the gp120 molecule. They may not be easy to access for antibody attachment.

With respect to the question of whether there is another receptor for HIV, I think that there is no evidence at this point for another means of entry by this virus into cells. Granted, antibody enhancement of HIV uptake has been seen in macrophage-like cells, yet it is still not clear that the mode of entry into any cell type is CD4-independent. More work has to be done to strengthen any claim that there is another means of entry of this virus that is biologically relevant or efficient relative to the CD4-dependent entry.

DR. JOHN: The chromaffin cells of the gut of the large intestine and small intestine have receptors for the virus, but we do not believe it is CD4. We think it is something else.

DR. WITKIN: Is it known what cell types have integrated the HIV genome and how many copies are integrated into the host DNA?

DR. SOMERS: To my knowledge, the cell types that are susceptible will have HIV DNA integrated in them. I am not sure of the copy number. I suspect it is variable.

DR. MATA: Are there differences either in the amount of receptors per cell or in the quantity of the receptors to percentage antigen?

DR. SOMERS: There is evidence that the CD4 receptor density varies with the cell type. T4 lymphocytes may have more CD4 molecules than macrophages, which may in turn have considerably more CD4 receptors than gut cells.

8

Natural History of Animal Retroviruses: An Overview

Murray B. Gardner

The family of retroviruses consists of four subfamilies: oncoviruses, D-retroviruses, lentiviruses, and spuma- (foamy) viruses.

1 The oncoviruses induce chronic lymphoma and leukemia in chickens, mice, cats, cattle, gibbon apes, monkeys, and humans, and the mammary tumor viruses of mice (MTV) induce breast tumors [1]. These chronic leukemia viruses infrequently recombine with cellular protooncogenes to give rise to acute leukemia and sarcoma viruses in chickens, mice, cats, and monkeys, but these highly oncogenic recombinant viruses are not infectious in nature [2].
2 The D-retroviruses induce fetal immunosuppression in macaques [3].
3 The lentiviruses induce chronic inflammatory conditions of brain, lung, and joints in sheep and goats [4]; hemolytic anemia in horses [5]; lymphocytosis in cattle [6]; and immunodeficiency in cats [7], monkeys [8], and humans [9].
4 The spuma- (foamy) viruses present as latent infection in many species (chickens, sheep, cattle, cats, monkeys, chimpanzees, and humans). These viruses induce cytopathic effects in vitro but apparently are not associated with any disease [10].

The D-retroviruses, lentiviruses, and spumaviruses have not been shown to recombine with cellular genes. Although future investigations may link them to diseases in animals and humans, the spumaviruses are not considered further in this review.

Heterosexual Transmission of AIDS, pages 93–105

TABLE 1. Infectious Retroviruses[a]

Animal	Virus nomenclature	Type of disease
Oncoviruses		
Chickens	Avian leukosis virus (ALV)	Leukemia
Mice	Murine leukemia virus (MuLV)	Leukemia, neuroparalysis immunodeficiency
	Mammary tumor virus (MTV)	Breast cancer
Cats	Feline leukemia virus (FeLV)	Leukemia, aplastic anemia immunodeficiency
Gibbon apes	Gibbon ape leukemia virus (GaLV)	Leukemia
Cattle	Bovine leukemia virus (BoLV)	Leukemia
Monkeys	Simian T-lymphotropic virus (STLV)	Leukemia
Humans	Human T-lymphotropic virus (HTLV)	Leukemia
D-retroviruses		
Macaques	Simian AIDS retrovirus (SRV)	Immunodeficiency
Lentiviruses		
Sheep	Visna virus (VV)	Demyelination, pneumonitis
Goats	Caprine arthritis encephalitis virus (CAEV)	Pneumonitis, arthritis, mastitis, encephalitis
Horses	Equine infectious anemia virus (EIAV)	Hemolytic anemia
Cattle	Bovine immunodeficiency virus (BIV)	Lymphocytosis
Cats	Feline immunodeficiency virus (FIV)	Immunodeficiency
Monkeys	Simian immunodeficiency virus (SIV)	Immunodeficiency
Humans	Human immunodeficiency virus (HIV)	Immunodeficiency

[a]This list of infectious retroviruses is representative but not inclusive.

Table 1 lists the animals, virus nomenclature, and types of disease associated with infectious retroviruses. Under natural conditions, these agents are relatively nonpathogenic. Under special conditions, such as crowding in captivity in closed breeding colonies or forced inbreeding, these agents can become pathogenic and induce disease outbreaks.

This review emphasizes the route of transmission of the infectious oncoviruses and lentiviruses. Most of these retroviral infections, with the probable exception of simian immunodeficiency virus (SIV), are not directly relevant to the heterosexual transmission of human immunodeficiency virus (HIV) because the sexual transmission of retroviruses in animals is distinctly uncommon. However, this means of retrovirus transmission has historical precedence in mice [11,12], and this model is briefly described.

VIRUS TRANSMISSION

Infectious retroviruses of the oncovirus and lentivirus subfamilies are transmitted in nature by three major pathways: horizontal transmission between individuals of the same generation, vertical epigenetic transmission from mother to offspring, and vertical genetic transmission from both parents to offspring [1]. Table 2 presents a summary of these routes of transmission in animals and humans. The viruses are spread by blood and body secretions, both cell-free and cell-associated, primarily in lymphoid cells and monocytes/macrophages. When the virus is highly expressed in vivo, as is seen with the leukemia of chickens, mice, and cats, cell-free spread is most common. When the virus is largely latent, as with the leukemia viruses of cattle and humans and the lentiviruses of animals and humans, cell-associated spread is most common. Although the D-retroviruses of macaques are low titered and primarily cell-associated in lymphoid tissues and blood, they are spread primarily in a cell-free form because of their high concentration as free particles in saliva.

HORIZONTAL TRANSMISSION

Horizontal transmission is the most common route of spread of infectious oncoviruses and lentiviruses in nature. All retroviral diseases of outbred animals and human beings are associated with an exogenous virus spread, either cell-free or cell-associated or both. Although spread is primarily by horizontal transmission, vertical infection by maternal epigenetic transmission also occurs. The specific avenue of horizontal transmission differs among the animal retroviruses, but all require close physical contact, with exchange of body fluids such as blood, saliva, milk, or semen. The lentiviruses, HIV and possibly SIV, appear unique among all the retroviruses

TABLE 2. Transmission of Infectious Retroviruses[a]

		Horizontal			Vertical epigenetic		
Animal	Virus	Contact	Sexual	Experimental	Congenital	Milk	Vertical genetic
Chicken	ALV	+[a]	–	+	⊕	NA	+
Mouse	MuLV	+	+	+	+	⊕	⊕
	MuMTV	–	+	+	?	⊕	⊕
Cow	BoLV	⊕	?	+	⊕	+	–
	BIV	?	?	+	?	?	–
Cat	FeLV	⊕	?	+	+	+	–
	FIV	⊕	?	+	?	?	–
Sheep	VV	⊕	?	+	?	⊕	–
Goat	CAEV	+	?	+	?	⊕	–
Horse	EIA	⊕	?	+	?		–
Monkey	SRV	⊕	?	+	+	+	–
	STLV	?	?	?	?	?	–
	SIV	?	?	+	?	?	–
Ape	GaLV	?	?	+	?	?	–
Chimpanzee	HIV	–	?	+	+	–	–
Human	HTLV	?	+	+	?	⊕	–
	HIV	–	⊕	+	+	+	–

[a]+, Transmission documented by this route, with the major routes circled; –, no transmission detected by this route; ?, lack of data, but not necessarily lack of transmission by this route.

because of their primary sexual route of horizontal spread. Aerosol or insect transmission of animal retroviruses is far less common, and casual transmission does not occur. In general, retroviruses spread inefficiently in nature and are species-specific. Only occasionally in evolution has cross-species spread of some retroviruses apparently occurred. Examples include the apparent cross-species transmission millions of years ago of an endogenous retrovirus of baboons (BaEV) to cats (RD114) and of an endogenous murine leukemia virus (MuLV) of south eastern Asian mice to gibbon apes (GaLV) [13]. Evidence is not convincing for the infection of human beings with any animal retrovirus, despite ample and continuing searches. This is important since it should reassure lay persons who continue to be concerned about possible infection of humans with feline leukemia virus (FeLV), bovine leukemia virus (BoLV), and, more recently, SIV. However, the close genetic similarity of HIV-2 to some SIV strains suggests a possible monkey (i.e., sooty mangabey)- to-human transmission in more recent times.

Exposure to infected saliva via biting, scratching, or grooming is the major route of spread of avian leukosis virus (ALV) in chickens,

FeLV and FIV in cats, and SRV (D-retrovirus) in macaques. Infection from saliva is a much less frequent mode of MuLV spread in laboratory mice and probably does not occur in wild mice. Apparently, prolonged close contact with respiratory secretions is how visna virus spreads in sheep. Exposure to blood-sucking insects and contaminated needles used for herd vaccination are the major routes of spread of BoLV in cattle and equine infectious anemia virus (EIAV) in horses. Exposure to infected semen or, less commonly, vaginal secretions is a major route of spread of HTLV and HIV in humans. Sexual transmission is the suspected route of spread of simian T-lymphotropic virus (STLV) and SIV in the natural nonhuman primate hosts, but this remains to be established. The finding that seroconversion to SIV in colony-bred sooty mangabeys occurs only after they reach sexual maturity provides indirect evidence in support of sexual transmission of SIV in its natural host. The recent demonstration by Marx (see Chapter 11, this volume) that SIV can be transmitted experimentally across the intact vaginal or urethral mucosa of susceptible macaques by exposure to cell-free or cell-associated virus in tissue culture fluid provides additional support for the sexual transmission of SIV. However, only under special circumstances in mice has a sexual route of retrovirus (MuLV or MTV) transmission been directly demonstrated [11,12].

The infectiousness and pathogenicity of all retroviruses shown in Table 1 (except STLV) have been demonstrated in the laboratory by the experimental inoculation of virus in tissue extracts, blood, or tissue culture fluids into cells in vitro or animals in vivo. Infection and disease have been induced with many biologically and molecularly cloned oncoviruses (e.g., ALV, MuLV, MTV, FeLV, SRV), but none of the molecularly cloned SIV strains has been pathogenic. In humans, blood stream spread of human T-lymphotropic virus (HTLV) and HIV via intravenous drug abuse and blood transfusions has provided additional evidence of the infectivity of both viruses and the pathogenicity of HIV. HIV has also been spread, albeit infrequently, to health care workers by contaminated needles [14] and to at least one laboratory worker by exposure to contaminated culture fluid [15].

VERTICAL EPIGENETIC TRANSMISSION

Vertical transmission of infectious ALV to chicken embryos via the productively infected maternal oviduct is a common route of spread of this virus in nature. Congenital transmission, transplacentally and, more importantly, via milk or colostrum is the major route of spread of MuLV in feral mice, MTV in laboratory and feral mice, and caprine arthritis encephalitis virus (CAEV) in goats. Congenital transmission is also a minor but significant route of spread of BoLV, FeLV, SRV, and HIV in cattle, cats, macaques, and humans, respectively. Milk transmission appears to be the major route of HTLV spread. By contrast, lentiviruses probably seldom spread vertically in animals or human beings. However, transplacental spread of HIV-1 has been observed in one HIV-1-infected pregnant chimpanzee.

VERTICAL GENETIC TRANSMISSION

This route of spread of infectious retroviruses applies only to the oncoviruses and occurs only in inbred mice that have been selectively bred to yield a high incidence of lymphoma or breast cancer [16]. Examples include the AKR mouse strain, in which 100% of the animals develop thymic lymphomas by 1 year of age because they inherit several copies of an infectious MuLV provirus, and the GR mouse strain, in which 100% of the mice develop breast cancers because they inherit infectious MTV proviruses. The genetic transmission of infectious virogenes is an artifact of intense inbreeding and does not occur in any outbred species, including, of course, humans. However, numerous oncovirus-related genes are present in the genomic DNA of all vertebrates, including humans. Some of these virogenes give rise to complete virions, which are noninfectious and nonpathogenic for their species although they may grow experimentally in cells of other species (xenotropic). Examples include the xenotropic MuLVs of mice (AT124), cats (RD114), and baboons (BaEV). Most of the endogenous vertebrate virogenes are defective and do not produce virus particles. In chickens and wild mice, certain inherited functional proviral env genes (e.g., FV-4) prevent leukemia or neuroparalysis by a receptor-interference mechanism [17]. Inherited virogenes also may be an important source of genetic information for activation of nearby cellular genes or for recombination with the exogenous oncoviruses of their respective species. The recombinant viruses may show altered cellular tropism or enhanced virulence compared to the parental virus. Examples of recombinant retroviruses include the mink cell focus (MCF) MuLVs of AKR and related inbred mice and the subgroup B and C strains of FeLV in domestic cats; each of these recombinant viruses is associated with an altered cell tropism and enhanced pathogenicity compared to the parental virus strains. However, recombination of exogenous and endogenous virogenes has not been demonstrated in most outbred-species, including wild mice and humans. Therefore, this recombi-

TABLE 3. Effect of Infectious Retroviruses on the Immune System

Tolerance	Congenital infection with: A. Leukemia viruses of chickens and mice B. D-retroviruses of macaques[a] C. Lentiviruses of monkeys and humans[a]
Autogenous immunity	Postnatal infection with: A. Leukemia viruses of chickens, mice, cats, cows, monkeys, apes, humans B. D-retroviruses of macaques C. Lentiviruses of sheep, goats, horses, cows, cats, monkeys, humans
Immune suppression	Postnatal infection with: A. Leukemia viruses of mice, cats, humans B. D-retroviruses of macaques C. Lentiviruses of cats, monkeys, humans

[a]Inconclusive data at present.

nation event also appears to be an artifact of inbreeding or of the presence of high in vivo levels of replicating retroviruses. Endogenous lentiviral-related genes have not been demonstrated in the DNA of any species, and the origin of these viruses remains uncertain. Recombination between exogenous oncoviruses and lentiviruses (or spumaviruses) has also not been found in nature.

AUTOGENOUS IMMUNITY

The possible effects of infectious retroviruses on the immune system are summarized in Table 3. All retroviruses can stimulate a humoral and cellular immune response in their natural hosts when they are acquired after development of immune competence. Host cell genes that are part of the histocompatibility complex influence the strength of the immune response to specific viral antigens and account for considerable individual variation in non-inbred animals. Other host cell genes control virus entry at the cell surface (e.g., FV-4 in some feral mice) or virus replication inside the cell (e.g., FV-1 in inbred mice). The CD4 gene on T-helper lymphocytes of human and nonhuman primates encodes the receptor for HIV and SIV and makes these cells a primary target of infection, leading to profound immune suppression. The prenatal expression of endogenous oncovirogenes (as occurs in chicken, mice, and cat embryos) leads to a relative postnatal immunological tolerance to these virogene proteins because they are recognized as "self." This is especially true of the ALV, MuLV, and FeLV group-specific core antigens. Recognition of this relative immunological tolerance to core antigens and detection of this antigen in fetal tissues in the absence of infectious virus was the basis of the viral oncogene hypothesis by Huebner and Todaro [18]. This hypothesis led to the discovery of cellular oncogenes and opened up an immense field of scientific inquiry [2,19].

Immunologic tolerance also occurs when the virus is congenitally acquired before or at birth, as seen with ALV in chickens and MuLV in wild mice. Exposure to the virus after waning of maternal passive immunity and the development of immune competence induces an immune response and is particularly effective in limiting the extent of natural or experimental infection with ALV in chickens, MuLV and MTV in mice, FeLV in cats, and D-retrovirus in macaques. This age-related resistance to infection is not as apparent with the lentivirus infections of animal and humans. In the oncovirus and D-retrovirus animal virus systems (i.e., MuLV, MTV, FeLV, SRV), natural protective immunity (i.e., elimination of infectious virus) correlates with presence of high-titered humoral immunity (neutralizing antibody), and viral vaccines that induce neutralizing antibody effectively prevent persistent infection and disease [20,21]. Passive immunity with immune sera or immunoglobulin has also been effective in these models. The failure, to date, of naturally occurring or vaccine-induced humoral or cellular immunity to protect against lentiviruses, particularly SIV and HIV, presents the dilemma of explaining virus persistence despite a vigorous immune response. The challenge is to devise a strategy to prevent or contain this infection.

MECHANISM OF RETROVIRUS INDUCED ONCOGENESIS AND CYTOPATHOLOGY

The oncoviruses induce cancer by both indirect and direct mechanisms [22]. Indirect mechanisms include general immune suppression and chronic antigenic stimulation. Direct mechanisms include transduction of cellular protooncogenes, cis-activation of cellular protooncogenes by promoter or enhancer insertion, and trans-activation of cellular genes by viral trans-activating proteins. The viral long terminal repeats (LTRs), in particular the enhancer regions, are often primary determinants of the target cell for leukemic transformation [23].

The oncoviruses and lentiviruses induce cell death by both indirect and direct mechanisms [3]. Direct mechanisms include the cytoplasmic accumulation of viral DNA or viral proteins, leading to cell lysis by membrane damage or syncytia induction. Retrovirus infection often leads to superinfection interference, whereby chronically infected cells resist further infection and remain viable. Failure of this process may be responsible for the cytopathic effects observed in massively reinfected cells [24]. Indirect cytopathic mechanisms include release of suppressor factors and the induction of an autoimmune process directed at virally altered target cells in the immune system, central nervous system, and elsewhere. Further discussion of these mechanisms of pathogenesis is beyond the scope of this chapter. Much remains to be learned about these molecular mechanisms. Hopefully, this knowledge will lead to more effective therapy and prevention.

MURINE MODEL FOR HETEROSEXUAL TRANSMISSION OF MuLV

Choice of an animal model for the heterosexual transmission of retrovirus and related contraceptive research is limited by the infrequency of this route of retrovirus spread in species other than humans (Table 1). The possible heterosexual transmission of SIV appears promising and relevant to humans, but it has not been demonstrated in either natural or experimental monkey hosts. The only proved examples of sexual spread of retrovirus in animals are the type C leukemia viruses (MuLV) and the type B mammary tumor viruses (MTV) of mice *(Mus musculus)*.

The strain of MuLV used for sexual transmission studies was derived from wild mice *(M. musculus)* habitating a squab farm near Lake Casitas (LC) in southern California [25]. These feral mice are characterized by a high level of infectious MuLV and proneness to pre-B-cell lymphomas and a neurotropic hind limb paralysis. The MuLV is congenitally acquired at birth, primarily via milk, and leads to a lifelong systemic infection with viremia and immunological tolerance specifically to the virus [11]. Since general immune competence is intact, these animals do not develop an acquired immune deficiency syndrome (AIDS)-like disease. Bidirectional, heterosexual transmission of MuLV was first shown in matings between viremic LC wild mice and uninfected C57L inbred mice and was later confirmed in matings between IRW inbred male mice infected experimentally with LC MuLV and uninfected female IRW mice. C57L inbred mice are free of infectious MuLV but are very susceptible to the MuLVs of LC wild mice. Venereal infection of C57 female partners was proved by the isolation of virus from the sera, vaginal swabs, and tissue extracts of six to eight C57L females after mating with viremic LC males. About 50% of the firstborn hybrid litters were viremic, increasing to 90% in the second and third litters; virus was isolated from the progeny only after the C57 mother became venereally infected. The F1 progeny were congenitally infected with the LC MuLV via maternal milk, as had occurred in the LC mice in nature. The progeny were susceptible to the same pre-B-cell lymphomas and neurotropic lower limb paralysis as occurred naturally in aging MuLV-infected LC mice. Sexual transmission of LC MuLV also occurred, but less readily, when viremic LC females were bred to C57L males. After breeding with viremic LC females, two of seven C57L males became infected, as shown by isolation of virus from liver, spleen, or serum. As expected, breeding of C57L mice to uninfected LC wild mice was associated with absence of sexual transmission of LC-MuLV.

By contrast, a similar horizontal sexual transmission of MuLV did not occur in matings between viremic LC mice and uninfected wild mice from the LC or another trapping area or between viremic LC mice and susceptible NIH Swiss laboratory mice. These findings indicated that sexual transmission of infectious MuLV seldom, if ever, occurs naturally among LC wild mice, but, under experimental conditions, it can become an efficient means of horizontal virus spread from LC wild mice to certain strains of highly susceptible inbred mice.

This observation was confirmed by the demonstration that IRW inbred male mice experimentally infected with LC MuLV or the related Friend strain of MuLV (F-MuLV) could efficiently transmit virus sexually to about 50% of their uninfected IRW female partners [12]. The viremic males contained high concentrations of infectious virus in semen and saliva. Venereal infection resulted in the production of antiviral antibody in the female recipients without viremia or clinical disease. However, infectious MuLV was detectable in the spleens of these females as long as 8 months after infection. Transmission of virus from infected IRW females to IRW males was not detectable, but less efficient horizontal transmission of virus between adult males apparently occurred by fighting and exchange of infected blood or saliva.

The rate of sexual transmission of LC-MuLV in these IRW matings (approximately 50%) makes this a potentially useful model for testing antiretroviral drugs. Using IRW inbred mice rather than wild mice for these studies offers the advantages of greater ease of handling and of breeding in captivity. This model is the subject of chapter 9 (this volume).

SUMMARY

This review describes the routes of transmission of infectious retroviruses in animals, types of associated host immune response, and associated diseases. As a model for sexual transmission and related contraceptive research relevant to AIDS, the SIV-infected macaque is promising. A murine model of retrovirus sexual transmission is also described. Whether mice can be used effectively to study contraceptive modalities remains to be seen.

REFERENCES

1. **Weiss R, Teich N, Varmus H, Coffin J:** Taxonomy in retroviruses. In: RNA Tumor Viruses. Cold Spring Harbor, NY, Cold Spring Harbor Laboratory, 1985, pp 25–207.

2. **Gardner MB:** Historical background. In Stephenson JR (ed): Molecular Biology of RNA Tumor Viruses. New York: Academic Press, 1980, pp 1–46.

3. **Gardner MB, Luciw P, Lerche N, Marx P:** Non-human primate retrovirus isolates and AIDS. In Perk K (ed): Immunodeficiency Disorders and Retroviruses. New York: Academic Press, 1988, Vol 32, pp 171–226.

4. **Haase AT:** Pathogenesis of lentivirus infections. Nature 322:130–136, 1986.

5. **Cheevers WP, McGuire TC:** Equine infectious anemia virus: Immunopathogenesis and persistence. Rev Infect Dis 7:83–88, 1985.

6. **Gonda MA, Brun MJ, Carter SG, et al.:** Characterization and molecular cloning of a bovine lentivirus related to human immunodeficiency virus. Nature 330:388–391, 1987.

7. **Pedersen NC, Ho E, Brown MJ, Yamamoto JK:** Isolation of a T-lymphotropic virus from domestic cats with an immunodeficiency-like syndrome. Science 235:790–793, 1987.

8. **Daniel MD, Letvin NL, King NW, et al.:** Isolation of T-cell tropic HTLV-III-like retrovirus from macaques. Science 228:1201–1204, 1985.

9. **Gallo RC, Montagnier L:** AIDS in 1988. Sci Am 259:40–48, 1988.

10. **Hooks JJ, Detrick-Hooks B:** Spumaviriae: foamy virus group infections: Comparative aspects and diagnosis. In Kurstak E, Kurstak C (eds): Comparative Diagnosis of Viral Diseases. New York: Academic Press, 1981, Vol 4, pp 519–618.

11. **Gardner MB, Chiri A, Dougherty MF, Casagrande J, Estes JD:** Congenital transmission of murine leukemia virus from wild mice prone to the development of lymphoma and paralysis. J Natl Cancer Inst 62:63–70, 1979.

12. Portis JL, McAtee FJ, Hayes SF: Horizontal transmission of murine retroviruses. J Virol 61:1037–1044, 1987.

13. Todaro GJ: Interspecies transmission of mammalian retroviruses. In Stephenson JR (ed): Molecular Biology of RNA Tumor Viruses. New York: Academic Press, 1980, pp 47–76.

14. Friedland GH, Klein RS: Transmission of the human immunodeficiency virus. N Engl J Med 317:1125–1135, 1987.

15. CDC: Update: Human immunodeficiency virus infections in health-care workers exposed to blood of infected patients. MMWR 36:285–289, 1985.

16. Pincus T: The endogenous murine Type C viruses. In Stephenson JR (ed): Molecular Biology of RNA Tumor Viruses. New York: Academic Press, 1980, pp 77–130.

17. Gardner MB, Rasheed S, Pal BK, Estes JD, O'Brien SJ: Akvr-1, a dominant MuLV restriction gene is polymorphic in leukemia-prone wild mice. Proc Natl Acad Sci USA 77:531–535, 1980.

18. Huebner RJ, Todaro GJ: Oncogenes of RNA tumor viruses as determinants of cancer. Proc Natl Acad Sci USA 64:1087–1094, 1969.

19. Bishop JN: Viral oncogenes. Cell 42:23–38, 1987.

20. Gardner MB, Pedersen N, Marx P, Luciw P, Gilden R: Vaccination against virally induced animal tumors. In Reif AE, Mitchell MS (eds): Immunity to Cancer. New York: Academic Press, 1985, pp 605–617.

21. Marx PA, Pedersen N, Lerche N, et al.: Prevention of simian acquired immune deficiency syndrome with a formalin-inactivated type D retrovirus vaccine. J Virol 60:431–435, 1986.

22. Weiss R, Teich N, Varmus H, Coffin J: RNA Tumor Viruses. Cold Spring Harbor, NY: Cold Spring Harbor Laboratory, 1985, pp 785–998.

23. Golemis E, Li Y, Fredrickson TN, Hartley JW, Hopkins N: Distinct segments within the enhancer region collaborate to specify the type of leukemia induced by nondefective Friend and Moloney viruses. J Virol 63:328–337, 1989.

24. Temin HM: Mechanisms of cell killing of cytopathic effects by retroviruses. Rev Infect Dis 10:399–405, 1986.

25. Gardner MB: Type C viruses of wild mice: Characterization and natural history of amphotropic, ecotropic and xenotrophic MuLV. Curr Top Immunol Microbiol 79:215–259, 1978.

DISCUSSION

DR. SODROSKI: Could you comment on whether the immune response in macaques makes a difference in the pathogenesis of SIV.

DR. GARDNER: Yes, it does. Indeed, the animals that make a vigorous immune response live longer. Animals that have poor immune responses usually die within 2–3 months. These animals have more syncytia and more virus, and the virus quickly overwhelms them. The animals that do make good neutralizing antibodies live on, but they do not survive more than a year or two. Then the virus wins. T-cell immunity is there. We can demonstrate T-cell proliferation to monocytes pulsed with the SIV antigen. It correlates with the early period when the immune system is fighting back, but does not get the job done. If we could find a way to keep the immune system functioning and prevent the double-edged sword from turning the other way and making autoantibodies, we would be a long way ahead. And that, of course, is what Salk is trying to do with their immunogenic approach, which, by the way, we tried on the monkey without success. Perhaps the virus is too strong a factor in the monkey system to be a fair counterpart to the human.

DR. SOMERS: Do animals that get sick fast have a poor humoral and cellular immune response?

DR. GARDNER: Yes. They are anergic. The T4 cells disappear, whereas otherwise they plateau and then eventually drop.

DR. HESS: In any of these successful animal models, is there the equivalent of Kaposi's sarcoma (KS)?

DR. GARDNER: Generally speaking, no. The type D virus often results in a disease called retroperitoneal fibrosis, and subcutaneous fibromatosis, which is a prolific growth of fibroblasts and the like; whether it is, indeed, a counterpart to KS has not been determined. The HIV-1 TAT transgenic mouse that has a fibrosarcoma-like lesion, might be the counterpart.

DR. WILLIAMSON: There were quite a few reasons for promoting breast milk. Do you think that breast feeding by HIV-positive mothers is a cause for alarm?

DR. GARDNER: I think breast milk is surely a potential route. I think that, with HTLV, it is a major route, perhaps equal to sex. But in the case of HIV, I think it is still anecdotal. Whether you should nurse if you are HIV-positive is the question. I think it might be injudicious to nurse if you have an alternate way of getting milk to your baby.

9

Sexual Transmission of a Murine Retrovirus: Host and Viral Determinants

John L. Portis, Frank J. McAtee, and Stanley F. Hayes

Although retroviruses can be transmitted vertically through stable provirus integration in the germ line, horizontal transmission appears to be the most important mode of spread of these viruses within a population of susceptible hosts. In the mouse, the transmission of several retroviruses from mother to offspring in the milk is well documented [1–3]. One such virus, found in feral mice, was first isolated by Gardner and coinvestigators [4] in the Lake Casitas region of southern California. This group of viruses (called collectively WM-E) causes a neurodegenerative disease after a long incubation period (up to 1 year) in the wild [4–6]. WM-E appears not to be carried in the germ line [7] but is maintained in the population through maternal transmission. This mechanism of transmission was proved in a classic epidemiologic study of foster-nursing [1]. That study also found that males could transmit the virus to females through sexual contact. Given the importance of sexual transmission in the spread of the human immunodeficiency virus (HIV) and the human T-lymphotropic virus type I (HTLV-I), this system appeared to offer promise as a model for studying sexual transmission of retroviruses.

DEFINITION OF THE MODEL

We have studied horizontal virus transmission in some detail using a molecular clone of the WM-E, called pBR-NE8, provided by

Heterosexual Transmission of AIDS, pages 107–114
Published 1990 Alan R. Liss, Inc.

Jolicoeur et al. [8]. Neonatal mice inoculated intraperitoneally develop a viremia after a few days that persists throughout life. These inoculated mice are immunologically tolerant of the viral antigens, probably due to the immaturity of their immune system at the time of inoculation [9]. Between 12 and 16 weeks of age, the mice develop clinical signs of neurologic disease [8]. If they survive for more than 5 months, 10–20% develop granulocytic or lymphocytic leukemia. However, mice inoculated with WM-E after 6 days of age mount a brisk immune response [10] and do not become viremic. These mice are infected, as demonstrated by low levels of infectious centers in their spleens [11], but the immune system prevents further spread of the virus and the animals remain asymptomatic.

To study horizontal transmission of this virus among adult mice, we designed an enzyme-linked immunosorbent assay (ELISA) to detect the WM-E-specific antibody response exhibited by adult inoculated mice. The rest of this section summarizes our published findings [11], which contain details of the experimental design. IRW (inbred Rocky Mountain white) neonatal mice (<48 hr old) were inoculated, and the viremic males were used as breeding partners at the age of 8–10 weeks. Mice of this age are sexually mature but have not yet developed neurologic disease. Viremic males were exposed to uninfected adult IRW females for a period of two estrous cycles (10 days) and then removed. The females were bled 2–3 weeks later, and their sera were assayed for WM-E-specific antibody. A high frequency of pregnancy (70–90%) was observed, and 50–70% of the female mice seroconverted. We obtained similar results with "superovulated" females that had been exposed to viremic males for only 18 hr. As expected, none of these adult-inoculated females exhibited a viremia, but low levels of WM-E-specific infectious centers ($<20/10^6$ cells) were detected in the spleens of these mice as long as 8 months after exposure to the infected males.

Males also transmitted the virus to other males when caged together for 10 days. However, female-to-female and female-to-male transmission was inefficient (<10% after a 10 day exposure) despite the fact that neonatally inoculated females exhibit serum virus titers comparable to neonatally inoculated males. Thus males appear to be the primary source of infectious virus in this system. Interestingly, viremic males that had been rendered chemically anosmic (without sense of smell) did not transmit the virus, indicating that infection required close contact (i.e., fighting or sexual behavior) and was not due to fomites from contaminated bedding, feed, or aerosols.

An analysis of external secretions indicated that saliva, semen, and uterine fluids all contained high levels of infectious virus [10^3–10^4 focus-forming units (FFU)/ml], but semen consistently contained the highest titers. We used immunohistochemistry on frozen sections to determine which cells were producing the virus. Due to the expression of endogenous envelope proteins within the male and female reproductive tracts [12], identification of WM-E necessitated the use of WM-E-specific monoclonal antibodies that are nonreactive with endogenous viral proteins [13]. These studies indicated that WM-E is expressed within epithelial cells of the salivary glands (acinar cells), uterus, and cervix (squamous and columnar epithelium). In the male reproductive tract, virus was expressed by Leydig cells in the interstitium of the testis and by columnar epithelial cells of the ductal system. Abundant viral protein was also found in the duct lumina. No evidence of virus expression was seen in the seminiferous tubules, which contain the germinal cells.

Transmission by saliva through the mucosal surfaces of the oral cavity appears unlikely for two reasons. First, several attempts to transmit infection by feeding saliva were unsuccessful. Second, although oral contact is observed among all mice irrespective of sex, only males efficiently transmit the virus. Saliva could be a source of infection through biting, since parenteral infection of adult mice is readily achieved. This is the most likely route of male-to-male transmission, since males caged together often fight. However, males often bite females during sexual contact as well.

The strongest evidence that male-to-female transmission does not occur by the parenteral route comes from studies of AKR mice. Females of this mouse strain are highly resistant to infection by viremic IRW males even after repeated exposure, yet AKR mice are as susceptible as IRW to parenteral inoculation [13], becoming persistently infected and producing a long-lasting specific anti-WM-E-antibody response. Adult AKR females express high levels of endogenous retroviral envelope protein within the female reproductive tract. This protein is expressed ubiquitously by epithelial cells from the vagina to the oviducts as well as by smooth muscle cells of the cervix and uterus. Since the endogenous virus of AKR mice has been shown to interfere with infection by WM-E in vitro, specific receptor blockade within the female reproductive tract is a likely mechanism of resistance.

MECHANISM OF SEXUAL TRANSMISSION

Electron microscopic studies of semen revealed high levels of cell-free virus often associated with (but not budding from) spermatozoa

[11]. The association between retroviruses and spermatozoa was first noted by Levy et al. [14] in a study of the endogenous viruses of NZB and AKR mice. To determine if spermatozoa were necessary, the effect of vasectomy on virus transmission was assessed. Surprisingly, vasectomized viremic male IRW mice were as efficient in transmitting WM-E to superovulated females as were the unmanipulated controls (Portis JL, unpublished observations). Thus this study indicates that specific association of the retrovirus with spermatozoa is unimportant in horizontal transmission of WM-E and suggests that females are likely infected by either cell-free virus or virus-infected somatic cells in the seminal fluid.

Using immunohistochemistry, we attempted to identify cells in the female reproductive tract that are initially infected. Frozen sections taken from superovulated IRW females 48 hr after exposure to viremic males were studied. No epithelial or stromal cells expressing WM-E glycoprotein were found, possibly due to sampling error. However, soon after ejaculation, there is a massive outpouring of mononuclear cells into the uterine lumen, and these cells may serve as the portal of entry for the virus. Such a mechanism would be consonant with the importance of mononuclear inflammatory cells in HIV infection [15,16].

VIRAL SEQUENCES THAT INFLUENCE EPITHELIAL CELL TROPISM WITHIN THE MALE REPRODUCTIVE TRACT

Although WM-E is transmitted with high efficiency from viremic males to females, other murine retroviruses are not. IRW males neonatally inoculated with Friend murine leukemia virus (F-MuLV) exhibit a high level of viremia as adults, but their capacity to transmit the virus to females is limited. Although transmission does occur, the frequency is low compared to WM-E ($<10\%$ on first exposure). When the sites of virus expression in viremic IRW mice were studied by immunohistochemistry, F-MuLV envelope glycoprotein, like WM-E, was detected in epithelial cells of the salivary gland and by Leydig cells of the testis. However, unlike WM-E, F-MuLV envelope glycoprotein was not expressed by epithelial cells of the uterus or the epididymis, and little F-MuLV glycoprotein was detected in the duct lumen [11]. These studies indicated that the efficiency of male-to-female virus transmission correlates with the expression of virus by epithelial cells within the ductal system of the male reproductive tract.

We recently constructed chimeric viruses between WM-E and F-MuLV to map the sequences that determine this difference in

TABLE 1. Virus Expression by Ductal Epithelium Determined by *pol-env* Region of WM-E Genome

Virus[a]		Testis[b]		Epididymis[b]	
LTR *gag-pol*	*pol-env*	Seminiferous tubules	Leydig cells	Ductal epithelium	Duct lumen
F-MuLV	F-MuLV	−	+	−	−
WM-E	WM-E	−	+	+	+
WM-E	F-MuLV	−	+	−	−
F-MuLV	WM-E	−	+	+	+

[a]F-MuLV is a molecularly cloned retrovirus FB29 [17]. WM-E is a molecular clone (15-1) isolated in our laboratory. Both are infectious and produce a viremia in mice after neonatal inoculation.

[b]Immunofluorescence on frozen sections was used to determine cellular localization of the respective viruses. Sections were stained with monoclonal antibodies specific for either WM-E [13] or F-MuLV [18] envelope glycoprotein and developed with fluorescein conjugates as described [11].

tropism. FB-29, a molecular clone of F-MuLV [17], is expressed exclusively in stromal, but not epithelial, elements of the epididymis; 15-1, a molecular clone of WM-E (Portis JL, unpublished observation), is expressed in epithelial cells of the epididymis. We exchanged a *pol-env* sequence encompassing 630 bases at the 3′ end of the *pol* gene and extending to a site 92 bases 5′ of the *env* termination codon. Neonatal IRW mice inoculated with both the parental and chimeric viruses developed a viremia (10^4–10^5 FFU/ml serum) within 1 week of infection. Immunohistochemical studies of viral glycoprotein distribution within the male reproductive tract are summarized in Table 1. The difference between F-MuLV and WM-E with respect to virus expression by the columnar epithelial cells lining the epididymis can be mapped to the *pol-env* region. This finding is not surprising since tropism in other nonretroviral systems appears to be controlled by the interaction between specific cell surface receptors and viral coat proteins. Although the murine retroviruses clearly gain entry into cells through membrane receptors [19–21] (which have not been chemically characterized), the existence of cell-type-specific receptors is disputed. Much of the specificity exhibited by murine retroviruses appears to be a function of cell-specific enhancer elements within the long terminal repeat (LTR) [22–24]. The current mapping studies clarify that the LTR of both WM-E and F-MuLV can function within the epithelial cells of the epididymis, but virus expression is seen only in the presence of *pol-env* sequences from WM-E. This suggests that specific receptors for the WM-E envelope glycoprotein may be expressed by epithelial cells of the reproductive tract.

CONCLUSIONS

The major drawback to this model is that mice infected as adults by WM-E do not develop disease. The host mounts a brisk immune response to the virus, and no further spread of virus occurs, although a low level productive infection can be detected in the spleen. Mice so infected are not viremic and do not transmit the virus further, either to their offspring or to other adults. Thus this type of infection is a "dead end."

However, several features make this model an attractive system for further study. Horizontal transmission of WM-E is highly efficient, and sexual contact appears to be an important component of this transmission. Mouse strains differ in their susceptibility to sexual transmission, suggesting the existence of host resistance genes. Retroviruses differ in the efficiency with which they are sexually transmitted, and this difference correlates with the cellular tropism of the respective viruses within the male reproductive tract. This difference in cellular tropism can be mapped to specific sequences within the retroviral genome. Thus sexual transmission has both host and viral genetic determinants, and both can be manipulated readily in the mouse.

REFERENCES

1. **Gardner MB, Chivi A, Dougherty MF, Casagrande J, Estes JD:** Congenital transmission of murine leukemia virus from wild mice prone to the development of lymphoma and paralysis. J Natl Cancer Inst 62:63–69, 1979.

2. **Jaenisch R:** Retroviruses and embryogenesis: Microinjection of Moloney leukemia virus into midgestation mouse embryos. Cell 19:181–188, 1980.

3. **Melief CJM, Louie S, Schwartz RS:** Esotropic leukemia viruses in cogenic C57BL mice: Natural dissemination by milk-borne infection. J Natl Cancer Inst 51:1243–1254, 1973.

4. **Gardner MB, Henderson BE, Officer JE, et al.:** A spontaneous lower motor neuron disease apparently caused by indigenous type-C RNA virus in wild mice. J Natl Cancer Inst 51:1243–1254, 1973.

5. **Andrews JM, Gardner MB:** Lower motor neuron degeneration associated with type C RNA virus infection in mice: Neuropathological features. J Neuropathol Exp Neurol 33: 285–307, 1974.

6. **Oldstone MBA, Lampert PW, Lee S, Dixon FJ:** Pathogenesis of the slow disease of the central nervous system associated with WM 1504 E virus. Am J Pathol 88:193–212, 1977.

7. **Barbacid M, Robbins KC, Aaronson SA:** Wild mouse RNA tumor viruses. A nongenetically transmitted virus group closely related to exogenous leukemia viruses of laboratory mouse strains. J Exp Med 149:254–266, 1979.

8. **Jolicoeur P, Nicolaiew N, Desgroseillers L, Rassart E:** Molecular cloning of infectious viral DNA from esotropic neurotropic wild mouse retrovirus. J Virol 45:1159–1163, 1983.

9. **Huebner RJ, Sarma PS, Kelloff GJ, et al.:** Immunological tolerance to RNA tumor virus genome expressions: significance of tolerance and prenatal expressions in embryogenesis and tumorigenesis. Ann NY Acad Sci 181:246–271, 1971.

10. **Hoffman PN, Robbins DS, Morse HC:** Role of immunity in age-related resistance to paralysis after murine leukemia virus infection. J Virol 52:734–738, 1984.

11. **Portis JL, McAtee FJ, Hayes SF:** Horizontal transmission of murine retroviruses. J Virol 61:1037–1044, 1987.

12. **Del Villano BC, Nave B, Croker BP, Lerner RA, Dixon FJ:** The oncornavirus glycoprotein gp 69/71: A constituent of the surface of normal and malignant thymocytes. J Exp Med 141:172, 1975.

13. **McAtee FJ, Portis JL:** Monoclonal antibodies specific for wild mouse neurotropic retrovirus: Detection of comparable levels of virus replication in mouse strains susceptible and resistant to paralytic disease. J Virol 56:1018–1022, 1985.

14. **Levy JA, Joyner J, Borenfreund E:** Mouse sperm can horizontally transmit type C viruses. J Gen Virol 51:439–443, 1980.

15. **Gartner S, Markovits P, Markovitz DM, Kaplan MH, Gallo RC, Popovic M:** The role of mononuclear phagocytes in HTLV-III/LAV infection. Science 233:215–219, 1986.

16. **Filice G, Cereda PM, Varnier OE:** Infection of rabbits with human immunodeficiency virus. Nature 335:366–369, 1988.

17. **Sitbon M, Sola B, Evans L, et al.:** Hemolytic anemia and erythroleukemia, two distinct pathogenic effects of Friend MuLV: Mapping of the effects to different regions of the viral genome. Cell 47:851–859, 1986.

18. **Chesebro B, Wehrly K, Cloyd M, et al.:** Characterization of mouse monoclonal antibodies specific for Friend murine leukemia virus-induced erythroleukemia cells: Friend-specific and FMR-specific antigens. Virology 112:131–144, 1981.

19. **Portis JL, McAtee FJ, Evans LH:** Infectious entry of murine retroviruses into mouse cells. Evidence of a postadsorption step inhibited by acidic pH. J Virol 55:806–812, 1985.

20. **Rein A, Schultz A:** Different recombinant murine leukemia viruses use different cell surface receptors. Virology 136:144–152, 1984.

21. **Delarco J, Todaro GJ:** Membrane receptors for murine leukemia viruses: Characterization using the purified viral envelope glycoprotein, gp71. Cell 8:365–371, 1976.

22. **Chatis PA, Holland CA, Silver JE, Frederickson TN, Hopkins N, Hartley JW:** A 3′ end fragment encompassing the transcriptional enhancers of nondefective Friend virus confers erythroleukemogenicity on Moloney leukemia virus. J Virol 52:248–254, 1984.

23. **Desgroseillers L, Jolicoeur P:** Mapping the viral sequences conferring leukemogenicity and disease specificity in Moloney and amphotropic murine leukemia viruses. J Virol 52:448–456, 1984.

24. **Short MK, Okenquist SA, Lenz J:** Correlation of leukemogenic potential of murine retroviruses with transcriptional tissue preference of the viral long terminal repeats. J Virol 61:1067–1072, 1987.

10

Sexual Transmission of an AIDS-Like Disease in the Cat

Richard A. Cone, Thomas R. Moench, and Kevin J. Whaley

We are developing new methods for prophylactic contraception that will use antibodies to immunize passively and protect the skin and mucus epithelia of sexual partners against the exchange of sperm and pathogens of sexually transmitted diseases (STDs). In this chapter we report preliminary data from an animal model we are developing to test these new methods for blocking the sexual transmission of acquired immune deficiency syndrome (AIDS). Our data demonstrate efficient vaginal transmission of feline immunodeficiency virus (FIV) infection in the cat. Also, in our first test of an available prophylactic contraceptive method in this animal model, a contraceptive jelly with nonoxynol-9 (N-9)—a widely used spermicidal detergent—significantly blocked vaginal transmission of FIV.

Since sexual transmission has not been documented in the natural transmission of FIV, our first goal was to determine whether vaginal inoculation with FIV pathogens would transmit disease. Our second goal, the main point of this report, was to determine whether an existing vaginal contraceptive method can block the vaginal transmission of FIV.

MATERIALS AND METHODS

Choice of Animal Model

We selected the cat model because FIV is a lentivirus closely related to the human immunodeficiency virus (HIV), and it induces a

Heterosexual Transmission of AIDS, pages 115–121

natural (endemic) disease in cats markedly similar to AIDS in humans [1–3]. FIV, like HIV, readily infects T cells. Hence, in this animal model, we can test two of the most likely pathogens now suspected for sexual transmission of AIDS, namely, free virus and infected T cells.

Pathogen Inoculation

A single vaginal inoculation with FIV pathogens was given to each of ten cats, five of which had been treated with contraceptive jelly prior to the inoculation. We used the highest, most infectious titer of pathogens we could readily prepare and the largest dose we thought would be retained in the vagina. The inoculum consisted of 2,000,000 feline T lymphoblasts infected with FIV (isolate V_{1p} Baltimore). This isolate is serologically identical to the prototype Petaluma isolate, demonstrates magnesium-dependent reverse transcriptase (RT) activity, and shows typical lentivirus morphology on electron microscopy [1,3]. The culture had a supernatant RT activity of 250,000 cpm/ml, and about 10% of the cells showed viral antigens by immunoperoxidase staining. The inoculum was delivered in 0.1 ml growth medium.

Choice of Prophylactic Contraceptive

We chose to test N-9 since this detergent is now used in many vaginal contraceptives and since it has been shown in vitro to be highly potent for inactivating HIV [4–6] as well as sperm and many other STD pathogens (see Chapter 23, this volume). We selected a contraceptive jelly containing 5% N-9 (Ramses contraceptive jelly) since this product could be readily adapted for use in the cat. This 5% jelly is sold to be used alone or with a diaphram. To be as comparable as possible to the human dose of this jelly when used without a diaphram, 5 ml, we used 0.2 ml, or 1/25 the human dose, based on the following approximate cat/human ratios: trunk length (1/2–1/3), mass (1/30), volume of ejaculate (1/100), and sperm/ejaculate (1/5). As in human use, nearly the entire dose was readily retained within the vagina.

Prior to delivering the inoculum, or jelly followed by the inoculum, we tranquilized each cat with ketamine. In half the animals, prior to delivering the inoculum, we delivered the contraceptive jelly using a method similar to that used by humans by delivering the jelly with a blunted pipet tip lubricated with a small amount of the jelly. The tip was inserted until it gently pressed against the cervix, and then

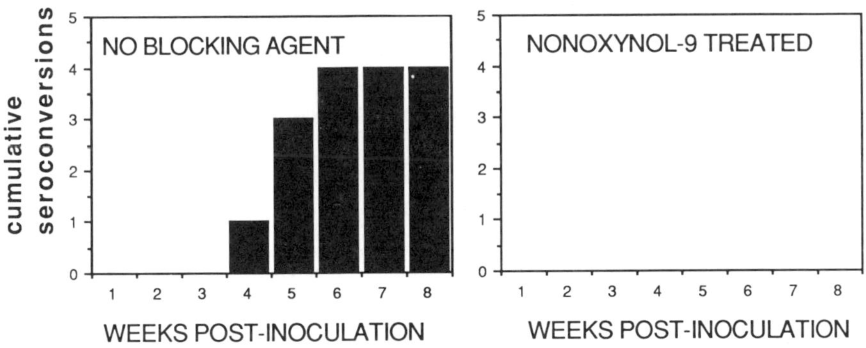

Fig. 1. Number of cats infected with FIV as a function of time after a single vaginal inoculation with FIV pathogens.

slightly withdrawn before the jelly was slowly expelled. The tip was then gently stirred to insure that the jelly would be well distributed. Finally, in all 10 animals, a small amount of jelly was rubbed onto the vulva to help prevent oral exposure to active inoculum when the animals cleaned themselves after the procedure.

The inocula were delivered using a similar blunted pipet tip, inserted until it pressed gently against the cervix, then withdrawn slightly while the inoculum was slowly expelled. Then the pipet was inserted and withdrawn several times to simulate copulation.

Following the inoculation with FIV pathogens, the animals were allowed to recover and were left undisturbed for several weeks. The cats were housed individually and were observed for any behavioral or external signs of irritation by the inoculum or by the jelly; none was seen.

Detection of Infection

Infection was established by seropositivity to FIV. Also, specific pathogen-free cats were used to ensure that none was infected by this endemic disease, and all cats were found to be serologically negative at the time of the inoculation.

RESULTS

The experiment is ongoing, but the results to date merit reporting. Figure 1 shows the cumulative infections so far detected in the cats. To date, four of the five animals that were not treated with contraceptive jelly have become infected with FIV. In contrast, none of the five animals treated with jelly prior to inoculation has become infected. These results suggest that this animal model for vaginal transmission is efficient (80% transmission in the unprotected animals) and that a dose of contraceptive jelly comparable to a typical dose in humans blocks transmission ($P = 0.024$ by one-tailed Fisher's exact test). In one of the animals treated with jelly, the pipet tip was unintentionally driven too far into the vagina during delivery of the inoculum of infected cells, and the tip of the pipet was covered with blood when it was withdrawn from the vagina. (No blood was present on the pipet tip that had previously delivered the contraceptive jelly to this animal.) We expected this animal to become infected, but to date it has shown no sign of infection. Given the high rate of FIV transmission in the unprotected animals, we believe this unintentional experiment suggests that the contraceptive jelly helped protect the animal despite injury to the vaginal epithelium during delivery of the inoculum.

DISCUSSION

Since sufficient time has not elapsed to establish whether we have detected all infected animals, our results are preliminary but suggest that: 1) FIV can be transmitted vaginally with high efficiency and 2) a dose of contraceptive jelly with N-9, comparable in volume to a typical dose in humans, provides significant protection against vaginal transmission of this AIDS-like disease. The inoculations used in these animals contained free virus and infected T cells, two types of pathogens most likely to transmit AIDS in humans. Also, the T cells infected with FIV were delivered at very high concentrations, several orders of magnitude higher than the concentration of AIDS pathogens likely to be present in the ejaculates of seropositive men (see Chapter 14, this volume). Indeed, these inoculations transmitted infections with efficiencies several orders of magnitude greater than is estimated for heterosexual transmission of AIDS by a single episode of unprotected intercourse [2], 80% compared to about 0.1%, yet none of the five animals protected by jelly has yet become seropositive for FIV. Our preliminary results indicate that a detergent-based, vaginal method of contraception can provide significant protection against the transmission of AIDS in humans.

ACKNOWLEDGMENTS

We dedicate this report to B. Frank Polk for his early recognition of the urgent need for methods to prevent the transmission of AIDS.

We thank Clara J. Witt and Barbara Bishop for their help in developing the animal models. This investigation was supported by CONRAD project CSA-88-036, the Lalor Foundation, the Hopkins Population Center (grant HD-06268; to R.A.C. and K.J.W.), and NIAID (grant RO1 NS26646; to T.R.M.). The views expressed by the authors do not necessarily reflect the views of these funding agencies.

REFERENCES

1. **Olmsted R, Hirsch V, Barnes A, Purcell R, Johnson P:** Biochemical and molecular analysis of feline immunodeficiency virus (FIV). Conference on Animal Lentiviruses, San Antonio, Texas, November, 1988.

2. **Padian N, Wiley J, Winkelstein W:** Male-to-female transmission of human immunodeficiency virus (HIV). Abstract THP48: III International Conference on AIDS, Washington DC, June, 1987.

3. **Pederson NC, Ho EW, Brown ML, Yamamoto JK:** Isolation of a T-lymphotropic virus from domestic cats with an immunodeficiency-like syndrome. Science 235:790, 1987.

4. **Hicks DR, Martin LS, Getchell JP, et al.:** Inactivation of HTLV-III/LAV-infected cultures of normal lymphocytes by nonoxynol-9 in vitro. Lancet 2:1422, 1985.

5. **Malkovsky M, Newell A, Dalgleish AG:** Inactivation of HIV by nonoxynol-9. Lancet 1:645, 1988.

6. **Polsky B, Baron PA, Gold JWM, Smith JL, Jensen RH, Armstrong D:** In vitro inactivation of HIV-1 by contraceptive sponge containing nonoxynol-9. Lancet 1:1416, 1988.

DISCUSSION

DR. BERNSTEIN: I have one concern about this presentation, and it has to do with the passive model of putting semen into the vagina as opposed to what happens at the time of intercourse. We have done a lot of sperm transport studies using various types of vaginal barriers, and I do not know how much cervical transmission of HIV there is as opposed to vaginal or urethral transmission, but, in a subset of women, whatever barrier method is used whether it be jelly, cream, foam, or the sponge, sperm are not completely kept out of the cervix. If you compare postcoital testing before the application of a spermicide in one cycle and then with a spermicide in another cycle, the same number of sperm reach the cervix. I suspect that in these people the penis is very close to the cervical os at the time of the ejaculation, so that semen is basically injected into the cervix. I think that, without a solid, mechanical barrier, you are not going to get prevention in everyone.

DR. CONE: A small percentage of women will not be protected.

DR. BERNSTEIN: Do cats have strictly intravaginal ejaculation or is there intrauterine ejaculation?

DR. CONE: We do not know. In fact, there is a paucity of knowledge in animal models on the sexual transmission of anything, including sperm.

I want to go back to the point that there will simply be women who will not be protected by any given method. However, in the spermicidal suppository studies, there were 9,000 women-years with a 0.2–0.3% pregnancy rate.

DR. BERNSTEIN: That is not a realistic number. No barrier is that good.

DR. CONE: Throw in all the caveats you want about those studies, but you still get a very high level of protection. In fact, with the benzalkonium study, there were almost 200 women-years, with 7% lost to follow-up, and no pregnancies.

DR. BERNSTEIN: Yes, but we are conducting a study now with the benzalkonium sponge and, frankly, it is no better than the others.

DR. CONE: There are problems with the sponge. I do not think it is as good as a spermicidal suppository.

DR. BERNSTEIN: I am very suspicious. In any study where you get a pregnancy rate that low, there has to be a lot of bias in it.

DR. CONE: I am quite happy to look carefully at those studies, but I feel that, however you look at them, including the two large studies in Germany, the one in Spain, and the one in the United States, you have to conclude that those suppositories are giving high levels of protection.

DR. NORTH: There are a number of family planning experts here and we probably do not want to get into a debate on efficacy. I think the literature is very clear on the range of effectiveness for N-9 vaginal spermicides. Obviously, it is difficult to measure compliance. I hope the suppository to which you are referring is not the Encare Oval. Nevertheless, I think whether you are talking about a cream, a jelly, the N-9 sponge, or the benzalkonium sponge, the general consensus now is that they all have about the same effectiveness. It may be as high as 95% on an annual basis for highly motivated people, or, obviously, it may be much lower. I think it would be a mistake to suggest that a suppository is the only way.

DR. CONE: Dr. North, let me put the question this way. Would you not say that the efficacy is probably limited by user failure rather than by method failure?

DR. NORTH: Absolutely. And that is exactly why I am concerned.

MR. SPIELER: Let us curb the discussion on this particular issue.

I would like to ask Dr. Anderson to comment on the use of topical antibodies as an approach to effectively preventing the transmission of HIV.

DR. ANDERSON: Antibodies are a double-edged sword, as previously stated. They can neutralize HIV or can carry virus to macrophages having receptors for immune complexes. That could really exacerbate things, so you have to be careful.

DR. CONE: Of course, but I think, in general, antibodies help, and, if they are in the right place at the right time in the right doses, they are likely to be more of a help than a hindrance.

11

An Animal Model for Sexual Transmission of HIV

Preston A. Marx, Christopher J. Miller, Nancy J. Alexander, Suganto Sutjipto, Andrew A. Lackner, Agegnehu Gettie, Myra Jennings, and Andrew G. Hendrickx

The mechanism of heterosexual transmission of the human immunodeficiency virus (HIV) is not clearly defined [1]. Spermatozoa, white blood cells, and seminal plasma have been proposed as major cofactors in HIV transmission. Since these issues cannot be addressed effectively in human beings, an animal model for the heterosexual transmission of HIV provides a system to investigate this route of transmission and allows the study of the major cofactors involved in genital transmission.

This chapter summarizes studies that demonstrate that simian immunodeficiency virus (SIV) applied to the genital mucosa of mature male and female rhesus macaques results in the transmission of SIV and induction of disease [2].

ANIMAL MODELS OF ACQUIRED IMMUNE DEFICIENCY SYNDROME (AIDS)

The three major nonhuman primate models of AIDS are:

1 Infection of chimpanzees *(Pan troglodytes)* with HIV-1 [3];

2 Infection of rhesus macaques (MAC) *(Macaca mulatta)* with HIV-2 [4];

3 Infection of various macaque species (monkeys belonging to

Heterosexual Transmission of AIDS, pages 123–135

TABLE 1. Simian Immunodeficiency Viruses Found in Asian and African Monkeys

Old world monkey	Current name[a]	Infected animal location(s)	Natural range of monkeys
Asian species			
Rhesus macaque (*Macaca mulatta*)	SIV_{MAC}[b]	NIH Primate Colony, US	India and China
Cynomolgous macaque (*M. fascicularis*)	SIV_{CYN}	NIH Primate Colony, US	Southeast Asia
Pig-tailed macaque (*M. nemestrina*)	SIV_{Mne}	NIH Primate Colony, US	Indonesia and Southeast Asia
Stump-tailed macaque (*M. arctoides*)	SIV_{StM}	NIH Primate Colony, US	Indonesia and Southeast Asia
African species			
Sooty mangabey (*Cercocebus atys*)	SIV_{SM}	Primate Colonies and Zoo, US	West Africa
African green monkey (*Cercopithecus aethiops*) vervet subspecies	SIV_{AGM}	Primate Colony, Japan, and Primate Colony, Kenya	East Africa[c]

[a]A parenthetical identification is sometimes given to distinguish individual isolates (e.g., $SIV_{AGM(TYO)}$ and $SIV_{AGM(KEN)}$ distinguish the Tokyo and Kenyan isolates of SIV_{AGM}.
[b]Although rhesus, cynomolgous, pig-tailed, and stump-tailed monkeys are all macaques (members of the genus *Macaca*), by convention, the term SIV_{MAC} has been reserved for SIVs isolated from the rhesus macaque. SIVs from macaques other than the rhesus are identified by either a common or scientific name subscript (e.g., SIV_{StM} for SIV stump-tailed macaque and SIV_{Mne} for SIV *M. nemestrina*).
[c]AGMs are found throughout Africa, but thus far confirmed SIV isolates are from AGMs found in East Africa only [9].

the genus *Macaca*) with one of the SIVs isolated from Asian macaques, West African sooty mangabeys, or East African green monkeys (Table 1) [5–11].

HIV INFECTIONS OF ANIMALS

Although HIV-1 has been inoculated into numerous animal species [12], including macaques, only chimpanzees have become persistently viremic [1]. Thus the chimpanzee remains the only species naturally susceptible to HIV-1 infection. The HIV-1/chimpanzee model has been used for limited studies of the sexual transmission of HIV-1. HIV-1 inoculation of one chimpanzee via the vaginal mucosa has induced viremia [13]. In a second animal, the oral mucosa was not susceptible [13]. Although this chimpanzee and other HIV-1-infected chimpanzees have had prolonged systemic infections and HIV-antibody responses that are similar to those seen in infected humans, none has developed AIDS. The lack of disease in this model and the scarcity of chimpanzees for research have limited the usefulness of the HIV-1/chimpanzee model. However, a major use of the HIV-1/chimpanzee model will continue to be vaccine testing. Thus far, chimpanzees have been immunized with HIV-1 virion envelope preparations, recombinant expressed envelope, and vaccinia vectors expressing the HIV envelope. In one study, envelope gp120 expressed as a herpes virus fusion protein in Chinese hamster ovary cells induced neutralizing antibody and cell-mediated immunity but did not protect chimpanzees from an intravenous HIV-1 challenge [14].

HIV-2 also has been used to establish a nonhuman primate model in macaque monkeys. Several individual monkeys have become persistently infected, but the difficulty is that HIV-2 cannot be readily adapted to macaques because most inoculated animals have resisted infection (Lerche N, personal communication). The few rhesus macaques that are persistently infected with HIV-2 have not developed diseases (Lerche N, Fultz P, personal communications).

SIV IN NONHUMAN PRIMATES

An excellent animal model for sexual transmission of HIV is the SIV/rhesus macaque (SIV_{MAC}) model of AIDS. SIV_{MAC}, the initial isolate of SIV, came from a group of rhesus macaques with lymphomas and immunodeficiency [5]. Inoculation of SIV_{MAC} [15], SIV_{SM}, [8–10], or SIV_{MNE} (from pig-tailed macaques *(M. nemistrina)* [6] into various macaque species has consistently induced AIDS. In contrast, the pathogenesis of the SIV isolate from East African green monkeys (SIV/AGM) *(Cercopithecus aethiops)* [11] in macaques has not been established. The pathogenesis of SIV in the original African host is also unclear, but it appears that most infected AGMs and sooty mangabeys are inapparent carriers [8–11]. Seroepidemiologic surveys suggest that other species of African monkeys such as talapoins *(Miopithecus talapoin)*, De Brazza's monkeys *(C. neglectus)*, and Mandrills *(Mandrillus sphinx)* may have inapparent infections with SIV-related retroviruses [10]. Other isolates of SIV-like viruses such as simian

T-cell lymphotropic virus III_{AGM} (STLV-III_{AGM}) and human T-cell lymphotropic virus IV (HTLV-IV) are indistinguishable from SIV_{MAC} clone 251 [16] and probably resulted from laboratory contaminations.

Interest in the isolates of SIV is high because they are the closest known relatives to HIV [11,17–19] and because SIV from macaques and sooty mangabeys induces the full spectrum of clinical signs of AIDS when inoculated intravenously into Asian macaques [5–10,20]. However, the time of disease appearance and death varies greatly. Up to one-half die at 3 to 12 months postinoculation (PI) with three or more of the following clinical signs: generalized lymphadenopathy, maculopapular rash, adenovirus-associated colitis, retroviral encephalitis or pneumonia with giant cells, oral candidiasis, anemia, depressed T4/T8 ratio, wasting, cryptosporidiosis, trichomoniasis, and disseminated cytomegalovirus infection [5–10,15,20–23]. A similar immunodeficiency syndrome develops in animals 1 year or more postinfection, except that lymphomas may also occur [20]. Although the SIV group apparently is derived solely from several African monkey species [10,11], SIV infections with disease that were thought to be spontaneous have occurred in Asian macaques at North American primate centers. These SIV infections were probably from accidental or intentional exposure of macaques to SIV-containing African monkey tissue. Only one of these instances has been documented [7]. In some outbreaks of the disease of macaques, *Mycobacterium avium-intracellulare* infection and *Pneumocystis carinii* pneumonia have been observed [7]. No markers exist for predicting the emergence of a specific opportunist in SIV-infected macaques; however, the prognosis is poor for animals that fail to develop a strong antibody response by 4–6 weeks postexposure to SIV [20,21,23]. Immunohistochemical techniques show SIV antigens in multinucleated giant cells and macrophages of inoculated macaques [24].

MATERIALS AND METHODS

To determine whether transmission could take place via vaginal exposure, we mixed 1 ml of 15 $TCID_{50}$ (tissue culture infectious dose 50%) of cell-free SIV_{SM} [10] with SIV_{SM}-infected lymphocytes (approximately 5.25×10^2 infected cells). The suspension was infused into the vaginal vault of two anesthetized mature female rhesus through a soft plastic pediatric nasogastric feeding tube. The inoculations were repeated 10 times during a 4 week period (Fig. 1). Specimens of whole blood were taken at intervals to test for the presence of virus in the blood and serum antibodies. Another female (8063)

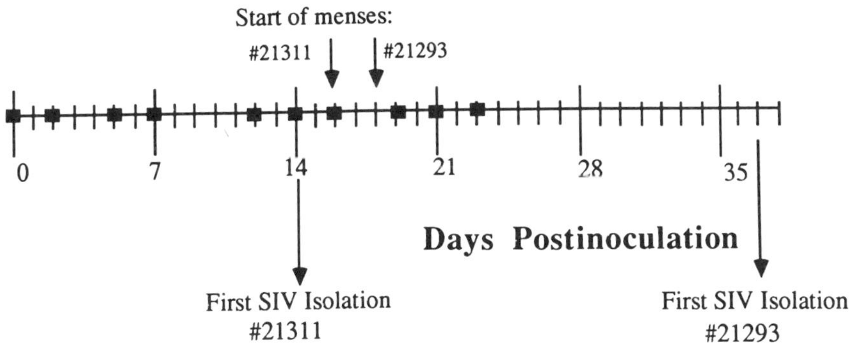

Fig. 1. Two mature female rhesus macaques were inoculated onto the vaginal mucosa with a mixture of cell-free SIV_{SM} (15 $TCID_{50}$) and cell-associated SIV_{SM} (5.25×10^2 SIV_{SM}-infected cells/ml). Each solid square represents one inoculation. Short black arrows show when menses began, and long black arrows indicate the first day when SIV was recovered from the peripheral blood mononuclear cells (PPMC) of the inoculated animals.

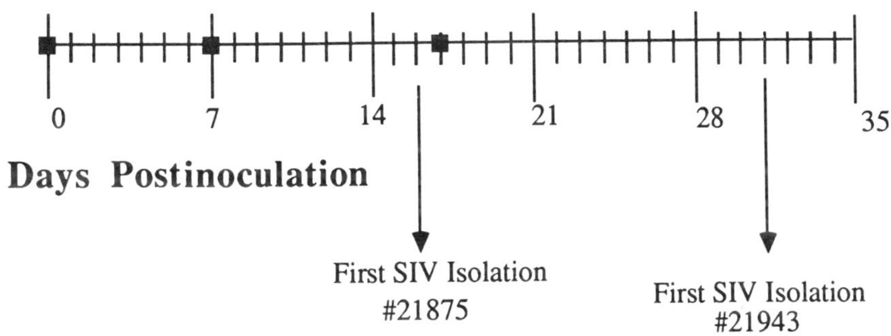

Fig. 2. The urethras of two mature male rhesus macaques were inoculated with 1 ml of human PBMC culture medium containing 25 $TCID_{50}$ of cell-free SIV_{MAC}. Solid squares represent one inoculation. Arrows show the first day when SIV_{MAC} was isolated from PBMC.

was inoculated with 1.0 ml of cell-free SIV_{SM} (15 $TCID_{50}$) twice in 1 week during the late follicular phase of the menstrual cycle.

To study genital transmission to males, two mature male rhesus monkeys were exposed to a 1 ml suspension containing 25 $TCID_{50}$ of cell-free SIV_{MAC} [5] three times during a 3 week period (Fig. 2). A pediatric nasogastric feeding tube was used to place the inoculum into the urethra of the males.

TABLE 2. Mucosal Transmission of Simian Immunodeficiency Virus (SIV) to Rhesus Macaques

Sex	Exposure route	SIV isolation days postinoculation	No. of inoculation prior to first SIV isolation	Antibody response to SIV	Clinical outcome
Female	Intravenous				
	22654	7	1	Weak	Died with SAIDS[a] Severe weight loss Diarrhea Adenoviral gastritis
	22659	14	1	Strong	Died with SAIDS Thrombosis right ventricle DIC, thrombocytopenia Lymphadenopathy
	Vaginal				
	21311	14	5	Strong	Euthanatized Mild interstitial pneumonia
	21293	37	10	Strong	Euthanatized Mild interstitial pneumonia
	8063	Negative	No infection	None	Alive

Male	Intravenous				
	23215	7	1	Weak	Euthanatized
	23225	7	1	Strong	Euthanatized with SAIDS Interstitial pneumonia
	21861	7	1	Strong	Euthanatized
	28191	7	1	Weak	Euthanatized with SAIDS Interstitial pneumonia
	Urethral mucosa				
	21875	16	2	Strong	Alive
	21943	31	3	Weak	Dead with SAIDS Interstitial pneumonia Severe weight loss Diarrhea

[a]SAIDS, simian AIDS.

RESULTS AND DISCUSSION

Both males and females seroconverted and became viremic during the study. Females were infected after six to ten inoculations; males were infected after as few as two or three inoculations. One of the females (8063) did not become viremic after two vaginal exposures of cell-free viruses; both males exhibited viremia, one at day 16 PI and one at day 31 PI (Table 2).

Table 2 shows that the clinical signs of disease that appeared in the animals that were exposed via the genital tract were identical to those produced by intravenous inoculation of SIV into rhesus macaques. The infected females were euthanatized 3 months after exposure, at which time they had early signs of simian AIDS, including generalized lymphadenopathy and splenomegaly. One male (21875) died of fulminant disease, with retroviral giant cell pneumonia and disseminated cytomegalovirus infection. This animal produced only a weak antibody response to the p55 and p66 SIV proteins and had no detectable antibody against any other SIV antigen.

These experiments showed that infection and fulminant disease can be produced by applying SIV to the surface of the genital mucosa of both male and female rhesus macaques. The experiment with the males further showed that animals with fulminant disease do not make a strong antibody response to SIV. Similar findings were observed in which intravenously inoculated animals also died with fulminant disease when they failed to make a strong antibody response to SIV [24].

To have a valid model, the inoculation procedure must not traumatize the genital epithelium. Trauma to the genital epithelium might allow the virus to enter the blood stream directly through a tear in the mucosal surface. Pertinent to this point is our finding that two doses of SIV_{SM}, each of which was four times the dose required for intravenous transmission, did not induce viremia or seroconversion in one female (8063) after 10 months of observation. If the inoculation procedure had been traumatic, this female would have become viremic from this dose of SIV.

The dose of virus required to produce infection in the male via the genital route appears to be much higher than the dose necessary to produce infection via the intravenous route. This finding suggests that the urethral inoculations of the male were not traumatic. Male 21943 received a urethral inoculation of SIV_{MAC} that was 500 times the required infectious dose by the intravenous route (0.05 $TCID_{50}$) but did not become viremic until 31 days PI. If the inoculation technique had been traumatic and caused SIV_{MAC} to be introduced directly into the blood stream, this rhesus monkey would have become infected and viremic 7–14 days PI, as was observed in intravenously inoculated animals.

The similarities in the reproductive biology between humans and macaques and the close relationship of HIV to SIV make this a valuable model for the heterosexual transmission of HIV. These studies show for the first time that SIV can be transmitted easily across the intact genital mucosa of both male and female rhesus macaques. Therefore, the transmission of SIV in the rhesus monkey provides a model to answer questions concerning prophylaxis, therapeutic agents, and mechanisms of transmission of HIV.

SUMMARY

The clinical signs and pathologic lesions of AIDS were produced in rhesus macaques by applying SIV to the genital mucosa of both male and female rhesus macaques. The disease that developed was identical to that produced by intravenous inoculations. Females were infected after five to ten exposures given throughout the menstrual cycle; males were infected with as few as two or three inoculations. Our data indicate that SIV, like HIV, can be transmitted via the genital mucosa. The use of the SIV/rhesus monkey model will allow identification of the cofactors important in the heterosexual transmission of lentiviruses.

ACKNOWLEDGMENTS

This work was supported by the Contraceptive Research and Development (CONRAD) Project, Eastern Virginia Medical School, under a Cooperative Agreement with the U.S. Agency for International Development (A.I.D.) (DPE-2044-A-00-6063-00); and by the base grant to the California Primate Research Center (RR-00169) from the Division of Research Resources, National Institutes of Health; by grant RO1-A120573 from the National Institute of Allergy and Infectious Diseases; and by NIAID-NIH grant NO1-AI-62559. The views expressed by the authors do not necessarily reflect the views of the A.I.D.

REFERENCES

1. **Peterman TA, Curran JW:** JAMA 256:2222, 1986. (also Peterman TA, et al.: JAMA 259:55, 1988).

2. **Miller CJ, Alexander NJ, Sutjipto S:** Genital mucosal transmission of simian immunodeficiency virus: An animal model for the heterosexual transmission of HIV. J Virol (in press).

3. **Alter HJ, Eichberg JW, Masur H, et al.:** Transmission of HTLV-III infection from human plasma to chimpanzees: An animal model for AIDS. Science 226:549–552, 1984.

4. **Fultz PN, Switzer W, McClure HM, Anderson D, Montagnier L:** Simian models for AIDS: SIV/SMM and HIV-2 infection of macaques. In Ginsburg H, Brown F, Lerner RA, Chanock RM (eds): Vaccines 88. New York: CSHL Publisher, 1988, pp 167–170.

5. **Daniel MD, Letvin NL, King NW, et al.:** Isolation of T-cell tropic HTLV-III-like retrovirus from macaques. Science 228:1201, 1985.

6. **Benveniste RE, Morton WR, Clark EA, et al.:** Inoculation of baboons and macaques with simian immunodeficiency virus/Mne, a primate lentivirus closely related to human immunodeficiency virus type 2. J Virol 62:2091–2101, 1988.

7. **Lowenstine L, Lerche N, Marx P, Gardner M, Pedersen N:** An epizootic of simian AIDS caused by SIV in captive macaques in the 1970s. In Girard M, Vallete L (eds): Pasteur Vaccines, Retroviruses of Human AIDS and Related Animal Viruses. 1987, pp 174–176.

8. **Murphey-Corb M, Martin LN, Rangan SRS, et al.:** Isolation of an HTLV-III related retrovirus from macaques with simian AIDS and its possible origin in asymptomatic mangabeys. Nature 321:435–437, 1986.

9. **Fultz PN, McClure HM, Anderson DC, Swenson RB, Anand R, Srinivasan A:** Isolation of a T-lymphotropic retrovirus from naturally infected sooty mangabey monkeys *(Cercocebus atys).* Proc Natl Acad Sci USA 83:5286–5290, 1986.

10. **Lowenstine LJ, Pedersen NC, Higgins J, et al.:** Seroepidemiologic survey of captive Old World primates for antibodies to human and simian retroviruses, and isolation of a lentivirus from sooty mangabeys *(Cercocebus atys).* Int J Cancer 38:563–575, 1986.

11. **Fukasawa M, Miura T, Hasegawa A, et al.:** Sequence of simian immunodeficiency virus from African green monkey, a new member of the HIV-SIV group. Nature 333: 457–461, 1988.

12. **Morrow WJW, Wharton M, Lau D, Levy JA:** Small animals species are not susceptible to HIV infection. J Gen Virol 68:2253–2257, 1987.

13. **Fultz P, McClure HM, Daugharty H, et al.:** Vaginal transmission of human immunodeficiency virus (HIV) to a chimpanzee. J Infect Dis 5:896–900, 1986.

14. **Berman PW, Groopman JE, Gregory T, et al.:** Human immunodeficiency virus type 1 challenge of chimpanzees immunized with recombinant envelope glycoprotein gp120. Proc Natl Acad Sci USA 85:5200–5204, 1988.

15. **Letvin NL, Daniel MD, Sehgal PK, et al.:** Induction of AIDS-like disease in macaque monkeys with T-cell tropic retrovirus STLV-III. Science 230:71–73, 1985.

16. **Kestler III HW, Yen L, Naidu YM, et al.:** Comparison of simian immunodeficiency virus isolates. Nature 331:619–620, 1988.

17. **Hirsch V, Riedel N, Mullins JI:** The genome organization of STLV-3 is similar to that of the AIDS virus except for a truncated transmembrane protein. Cell 49:307–319, 1987.

18. **Chakrabarti L, Guyader M, Alizon M, et al.:** Sequence of simian immunodeficiency virus from macaque and its relationship to other human and simian retroviruses. Nature 328:543–547, 1987.

19. **Franchini G, Gurgo C, Guo HG, et al.:** Sequence of simian immunodeficiency virus and its relationship to the human immunodeficiency viruses. Nature 328:539–543, 1987.

20. **Daniel MD, Letvin NL, Sehgal PK, et al.:** Long-term persistent infection of macaque monkeys with the simian immunodeficiency virus. J Gen Virol 68:3183–3189, 1987.

21. **Chalifoux LV, Ringler DJ, King NW, et al.:** Lymphadenopathy in macaques experimentally infected with the simian immunodeficiency virus (SIV). Am J Pathol 128:104–109, 1987.

22. **Baskin GB:** Disseminated cytomegalovirus infection in immunodeficient Rhesus monkeys. Am J Pathol 129:345–352, 1987.

23. **Kannagi M, Kiyotaki M, Desrosiers RC, et al.:** Humoral immune responses to T-cell tropic retrovirus simian T-lymphotropic virus type III in monkeys with experimentally induced acquired immune deficiency-like syndrome. J Clin Invest 78:1229–1236, 1986.

24. **Ward JM, O'Leary TJ, Baskin GB, et al.:** Immunohistochemical localization of human and simian immunodeficiency viral antigens in fixed tissue sections. Am J Pathol 127: 199–205, 1987.

DISCUSSION

DR. PETERMAN: I missed your evidence showing vaginal mucosa as a barrier. It looked as though you had achieved transmission with 5 $TCID_{50}$, so can you go over your evidence again showing it as a barrier?

DR. MARX: Yes. The 5 $TCID_{50}$ is the amount of virus that infects tissue culture cells. Intravenously, animal infectious doses are 100–200 times higher. So, if we titer a stock and get one $TCID_{50}$, it receives 200 animal infectious doses by the IV route. Therefore, the animal is more sensitive than the test we have in vitro.

DR. ADA: Have you made an attempt to estimate the number of virus particles compared to the in vivo infectious doses of, say, 10 virus particles per space, or 100?

DR. MARX: Live virus?

DR. ADA: Just virus particles per infectious dose. You can do that by electron microscopy, right?

DR. MARX: No, we have not.

DR. ADA: It would be of some interest to know how good a model it really is for picking up the virus.

DR. MARX: Really? I do not see why.

DR. ADA: Is the monkey resistant to the infection?

DR. MARX: Well, the important question is how much live virus is present, and if we have the 1,000 animal infectious doses, meaning that we have 1,000 doses by the IV route, and an animal can resist that much, then I think that is the important question. You want to know how much live virus is present, not how many particles are present.

DR. WITKIN: Have you compared the infectivity of virus in the presence or absence of sperm or seminal plasma?

DR. MARX: No. We could do this in vitro, and we have talked about it. In vivo we would like to see if seminal plasma, which is immunosuppressive, is a cofactor in transmission, whether it would increase the animal infectious dose or lower it.

DR. WITKIN: Well, I think it would lower it.

DR. ALEXANDER: We are planning to use human seminal plasma for these studies, because monkey seminal plasma is such a plug that we will not be able to place it into the monkey vagina and then add the viral dose. Because we were trying to develop a model that mimics the human situation as closely as possible, we thought that the use of human seminal plasma was appropriate.

DR. WITKIN: If the seminal plasma is antigenic in monkeys, it would then counteract any naturally suppressive effects.

DR. MARX: It would not be a problem because we will only give one inoculation, and the animals would be naive as far as the seminal plasma is concerned.

DR. RESNICK: What is your experimental design when you are testing the spermicide? How long after you put spermicide in do you add virus?

DR. MARX: We are going to add it immediately. We modeled our studies after those of Larry Zaneveld, who did the original work at the University of Chicago showing that spermicides were effective in preventing fertilization in Macaques. That is the level of effectiveness we want to reach with the spermicides. Use 1 cc of spermicide, and then the inoculum is infused. We are not using the 8 French tube, but a narrow polished glass tube that is mounted on the end of a syringe and that goes about three-quarters of the way into the vagina. This is our best estimate for the average placement of semen. The amount we will use should cause 100% transmission.

DR. SCOFIELD: I would be very curious to know whether you have a dose dependence with sperm number inoculated intravaginally with a constant dose of virus? We have reason to believe that there may be a cofactoring role.

DR. MARX: We certainly could do that when we get our ID_{50} straightened out.

DR. SCOFIELD: Yes. I think that is critically important for reasons that you know.

DR. MARX: Yes, it is something that we want to do. We cannot do it now because we have 100% transmission, so if this model is going to work for those questions, we have to raise a reliable 50%, 70%, 20%. I would like about 20%.

General Discussion: The Most Appropriate Animal Model for the Study of HIV Sexual Transmission

Murray B. Gardner, Moderator

DR. ARCHER: I would like to ask this question of Dr. Marx, but perhaps Dr. Whaley could answer it for me also. If an animal is infected, is the viremia persistent or is it intermittent? In other words, are there shedders and nonshedders as there are in humans with herpes virus?

DR. MARX: In many isolations, 50 or 100, I think I could count on one hand the number of times we failed to isolate the virus from antibody-positive animal.

For example, the last culture from the animal that received the mucosal transmission (the male), which has been alive for one and one-half years, was not positive. It is one of the first in my memory. All of those preceding it were positive. So the animals are consistently viremic. Occasionally there will be a negative culture, but, then, if you look a month later, it is positive again.

DR. ARCHER: Do you know if there is shedding into the saliva?

DR. MARX: We have not investigated it. Murray, has anybody in your group carried out saliva isolations on SIV?

DR. GARDNER: Yes, on a few animals. It is not as consistent as in the white cells.

DR. MARX: It is clearly not in semen all the time.

DR. SCOFIELD: Are you discounting the REV model in chickens altogether from the candidate models here? And the reason I ask is that this is an avian retrovirus that causes a marked AIDS-like syndrome in birds, and the REV agent's relationship to the Mason Pfizer monkey virus was introduced to me by you 2 years ago.

A Kaposi's Sarcoma (KS)-like syndrome developed in these birds. They developed marked and irreversible hemorrhagic lesions in the skin and organs.

Heterosexual Transmission of AIDS, pages 137–145

DR. GARDNER: REV might be an undiscovered model waiting to be employed. It certainly is an important retrovirus, and it was this model in which Howard Temin first showed retroviruses to be cytopathic. It is an interesting virus that has a primate-like envelope related to RD114 and baboon endogenous virus and an avian-like core. It is one of these peculiar recombinants that comes along in nature. It produces outbreaks of lymphoma-like disease in turkeys. When you pass it experimentally, it makes vascular neoplasms similar to those induced by certain other avian leukosis viruses. It is a marvelous virus for studying the cytopathic effect of retroviruses.

DR. SCOFIELD: You may remember from my own work from the 1970s that it is also rapidly immunosuppressive.

DR. GARDNER: In fact, Ed Boce in Texas and yourself were the people who first showed that phenomenon.

DR. RESNICK: Do these animals get antigen to p27 and lose their antibody response as do humans?

DR. MARX: Well, antibody has a positive correlation to clinical outcome; the stronger the antibody response, the longer the animals live. Failure to make antibody early results in early death.

Murray, in some of those animals you used, did you look at p27?

DR. GARDNER: Yes. The animals that survived longest are those that make the most vigorous immune response, but before death they sometimes lose the p27 antibody, just as humans lose core antibodies shortly before decline. At that time, antigenemia increases, the CD4 comes down, and the animal is put to sleep.

Every animal in our primate center that has become infected with either SIV_{MAC} or SIV_{SM} has eventually died. Once they are infected, the die is cast, but it may take anywhere from 2 months in the poor responders to as long as 2 years in those that make good antibody responses. The mean survival is about 8 months. This has the advantage of quicker results in terms of prevention or therapy, but it also has a disadvantage in that you are accelerating the course of events. The incubation period is shorter, and virus soon overwhelms the animal, leading to fatal immunodeficiency.

DR. RESNICK: What if you specifically give them antibody? Do you increase their life span?

DR. GARDNER: You mean by passive immunity can you prolong life? This has not been done. We have not given them back their cytotoxic T cells yet, either, but we would like to try that.

DR. MARX: Post-exposure vaccination did not do anything.

DR. GARDNER: We gave an inactivated whole SIV immunogen to SIV-infected seropositive monkeys 4 months after infection. These monkeys were the counterpart of an HIV-infected human with progressive generalized lymphadenopathy (PGL). By giving those animals an immunogenic dose of a whole inactivated SIV of the same type they are infected with, we asked the question, can we boost humoral immunity, lower virus levels, and prolong the life span? The immunogen apparently had no effect whatsoever on the infected monkeys. It did not hurt the animals; it did not help them; nor did it boost humoral immunity; and it did not lower the amount of virus or alter the disease course. So we saw no plus or minus effects, no benefit whatsoever.

DR. POTTS: When we visited the primate center in Franceville, Gabon, last year, they said they had isolated HIV from wild-caught chimpanzees, and they were going to be sequenced. Clearly a chimpanzee, it seems to me, is a relevant animal from the point of view of the evolution of the virus. Does anybody know what has happened there?

DR. MARX: It is one animal, and, yes, the animals apparently are HIV-infected. It was done by a competent laboratory.

DR. JOHN: Do we know the cell tropism of the simian retrovirus and the simian immunodeficiency virus? Are they the T cells?

DR. GARDNER: You asked about both type D and SIV, is that correct?

DR. JOHN: Yes.

DR. GARDNER: The type D virus was the first immunosuppressive retrovirus to be discovered in the macaques. It does not use the CD4 receptor. It has a wide cellular tropism and will infect fibroblasts, epithelial cells, both T4 and T8 lymphocytes, and B cells. You can easily find virus in the salivary gland, gastrointestinal epithelial cells, and lymph node follicular centers. We do not know the cellular receptor.

SIV uses the same receptors as HIV. The rhesus CD4 receptor has been cloned and sequenced and is very much the same as that of the human.

DR. JOHN: My second question: a lot of people have reported antibody response in people to something like the P24 of HIV as false-positive response in western blots. Has anybody determined what the actual antigen is for this?

DR. GARDNER: This one band alone is considered to be false-positive, but I do not believe that the nature of the fortuitous cross-reactive antigen has been identified.

DR. WITKIN: In the case of HIV, the evidence is pretty good that it is sexually transmitted by infected cells and not by free virus and that these infected cells are resistant to spermicides.

DR. MARX: You are right. And we would need to look at infected cells as well. And to do both, we started with cell-free virus, and, if we can show that it is effective against cell-free virus, we would look at cell-associated virus next.

DR. ALEXANDER: If you use a detergent, it will break up cells as well.

DR. MARX: They may be a little more resistant.

DR. ALEXANDER: I cannot imagine that they would be more resistant, and so it would seem to me that, in either case, you may really be dealing with free virus whether you have cells there or not. They may be little depots from which the virus is released.

DR. WHALEY: Tomorrow, Dr. Cone will be presenting data on human white blood cells in semen, showing that it exhibits the same killing concentration for sperm HIV as white blood cells.

DR. STEVENS: Do you see any advantage in your murine model, Dr. Whaley, in using infected macrophages vs. free virus vs. lymphocytes infecting the lymphocytes?

DR. WHALEY: We would like actually to define which one is the appropriate pathogen. We are not sure it is free virus. Our suspicion is that it is an infected macrophage or an infected T cell, but we have to demonstrate that, and we want to pursue it to see which of those three is the pathogen, or are all three the pathogens?

DR. STEVEN: Is the inoculum that you are using (100,000 cells I think) appropriate for what is delivered in a seminal package?

DR. WHALEY: No, I do not think it is. We came to this meeting hoping to talk to a number of other people and get a feel for the actual concentration found in AIDS patients so that we can then lower the titer, which is definitely what we want to do. We think it is too high at this point.

DR. RESNICK: I can sympathize with the development of these animal models in trying to determine dose size and standardize your virus input dose. That is quite relevant, because we have had similar problems with our in vitro systems in spite of having a lot more control. But the question I have for Dr. Marx is, with AZT, which is one of the drugs you have been using, can you actually halt the infection if you give AZT prior to the onset of the infection, the infectious particles?

DR. MARX: We have been approached to develop that model. We have begun calling it the needle-stick model and Julie Gerberding at UCSF and Murray and I have started work in which we would first need to define a model best suited to the human situation, and establish the antibody conversion rate. One in 100, one in 200 from needle sticks? It is quite low. So the very first thing we have to do is establish 100% transmission, because we cannot do experiments with a 1% or 2% positive rate. We would never get any data. We can employ a trancutaneous injection of a defined amount of the virus to establish 100% infection and then use AZT and almost certainly gammagobulin in combination to see if we can mitigate 100% transmission.

DR. RESNICK: But I am speaking about sexual transmission now, not intravenous. I am asking, can you actually set up your system so you have a dose of virus with which you already can get 100%. Can you go ahead and give AZT prior to the input of the virus and prevent infection, not delay disease?

DR. MARX: You really think it has a practical use? I mean, it is interesting scientifically but prophylactic AZT for sexually transmitted HIV? What do you think of that?

DR. RESNICK: But the realities are that if you believe that AZT does work in the reverse transcriptase step, meaning it is actually a preventive measure rather than working in a chronically infected situation, then this would be the optimum way of really seeing if indeed that would be the case.

DR. MARX: It certainly has value. I think it's practical application is occupational exposure and needle sticks in the hospital and clinical care. Those are the people who are likely to take AZT and who would want to know what conditions are going to work. Of course, you know of the Burroughs Wellcome study, in which they are signing up people for placebos and AZT after needle sticks; because the seroconversion rate is so low, it is going to take 20 years to finish the study. And we can do it much more quickly.

DR. ALEXANDER: What animal model would you think has the greatest potential for giving us meaningful data as far as sexual transmission?

DR. GARDNER: I have tried to organize my thoughts by making a list of all the so-called animal models of AIDS. Let me go through them very quickly. I think the answer to your question is probably FIV in cats and SIV in macaques. The viruses are of the same lentivirus family as HIV, with similar pathogenesis and immune response mechanisms and latency.

The wild mouse type C oncovirus model is good for sexual transmission and for trying to use drugs against milk spread of virus or against spread across the blood–brain barrier. However, this oncovirus does not really produce immune depression.

Friend MuLV has been somewhat forgotten. Its immunosuppressive nature was studied by Keglowski and Freidman in the early 1970s. The virus caused a B-cell proliferation and dysregulation of the immune system with immunosuppression.

Another MuLV model of immunosuppression is the so-called

MAIDS model. This is a nonneoplastic lymphoproliferative disease in C57BL/6 mice infected with the Laterjet-Duplan strain of MuLV, which was isolated from a radiation-induced leukemia in C57 mice. This virus, now called LP-BM5, is a recombinant of a defective and a helper MuLV. It induces a tremendous B-cell polyclonal hyperactivity, hypergammagobulinemia, lymphadenopathy, and immunosuppression. This model may resemble early AIDS in that T-cell dysregulation seems to be due to the retrovirus induced B-lymphocyte activation. However, the mice do not show a T4 numerical depression or profound lymphoid depletion as with AIDS in humans. Nor is the virus spread sexually, as far as I know. The SCID mouse is going to be useful because you can indeed transplant into them the human immune tissues and cells, which then carry out some of their normal differentiation and function. The in vivo explanted human immune cells give those mice back their immune competence, and they get rid of their PCP. The human lymphoid tissues are susceptible to HIV infection. As yet, we do not know whether the reconstituted SCID/HN mice will get an AIDS-like disease. No one has yet shown that HIV is transmitted genetically in SCID/HN mice. It remains to be seen how useful this will be as an AIDS model.

HIV transgenic mice may prove to be useful models. The HIV-1 TAT gene expressed in the skin of transgenic mice causes a Kaposi's sarcoma-like tumor in the adjacent dermis. The tumor does not express the TAT gene but is thought to be responding to growth factors released by epidermal Langerhans cells in which the TAT gene is expressed. Of course, this is not a model for sexual transmission of a whole retrovirus.

HIV-1 will infect rabbit monocytes and macrophages at low level and can be found in vivo for over 1 year. However, the infection has not caused any disease as yet and there has been no evidence of sexual transmission.

FeLV spreads through saliva of cats, not sexually. FIV seems to be spread primarily by saliva and fighting, and sexual transmission has not been shown as yet.

In the case of lentivirus of sheep (visna virus), goats (CAEV), and horses (EIAV), the animals do not transmit the viruses sexually, and they do not develop an immune deficiency syndrome, but the viruses are marvelous models for retrovirus latency and the role of cofactors in pathogenesis.

The type D retrovirus of macaques causes a fetal immunodeficiency syndrome, but the virus is not closely related to HIV and is not spread sexually.

DR. MARX: The SIV is probably potentially the best model for sexual transmission, but we do not know yet how the virus is spread in nature. It is not confirmed in African green monkeys and sooty monkeys that SIV is spread through sex. We see them seroconvert around puberty, but maybe that is for other reasons such as fighting. We have shown that SIV can be transmitted experimentally across the whole genital mucosa, but we do not know how if this happens in nature.

So we are left with the mouse (MuLV) as the only proved example of sexual transmission of retrovirus, but the cat (FIV) and, especially, the macaque (SIV) are potentially the best models for sexual transmission.

DR. BERNSTEIN: I have a technical question. In these vaginal models that you are using, particularly with the cat and the mouse, have you precluded the possibility of oral ingestion of some of the virus?

DR. WHALEY: I do not think we can rule it out totally. We observed them for an hour or two after we inoculated them to check for licking. We did not observe any licking. We did put nonoxynol-9 on the external genitalia, but we certainly cannot rule it out, no.

DR. PORTIS: We have actually fed the virus to mice, and they are really quite resistant to retrovirus infection by the oral route.

DR. GARDNER: We could never transmit MuLV orally. We fed MuLV-infected lymphomas to mice and mouse lymphomas to cats. It is not possible to find these viruses spread horizontally other than by the very routes we have been talking about.

DR. CONE: My question is just Nancy's question repeated, and that is, this is a conference on sexual transmission, heterosexual transmission of AIDS, and so looking at the animal models, what do you think will be—and this would be to all of the speakers of the session—what are going to be the best models for studying methods for preventing transmission, for preventing the exchange of pathogens? In other words, curing the disease is a big deal and the course of the disease is a big deal, but it strikes me as a very important question for this conference to pick out the mechanism of transmission in the cat and monkey models.

DR. ALEXANDER: FIV and SIV.

DR. HODGEN: If the virus is introduced in an intrauterine fashion or an intraperitoneal fashion vs. a vaginal fashion, you may begin to look at issues that were discussed a few minutes ago about the load or presentation that is given and therefore the potential potency it would have at inducing the response in the recipient, the efficiency of infectivity? Have any of the animal models looked at those loads of presentation, then, the same amount presented intraperitoneally, intrauterine, and intravaginally?

DR. GARDNER: No.

DR. MARX: We have not done exactly that. We have done intravenous challenge as compared to vaginal mucosa, and it is along the lines of Tom's question earlier, 1 to 1,000 dilution of a stock infects 100% of animals by the intravenous route. With one inoculation, by 14 days later, the animal is positive in the blood.

Eight inoculations of a 1 to 10 dilution into the vagina of the same stock induced infection in only one of two animals. So it is resisting many, many thousand times the challenge dose, but, on each individual dose, it is about 100 to 200.

DR. HODGEN: But the case of one of two may not be enough to say very much? If one is not an experiment, two is not much more.

DR. MARX: I agree, but we have done many intravenous inoculations, and all the animals become infected at 7–14 days or they never become infected. The nice thing about this model is that you can deal in terms of 100% infection. And there is no difficulty whatsoever. All this is done with SIV to infect 100% of animals.

MR. SPIELER: This is actually a follow-up of that question I wanted to raise with you, Preston, or anybody else. When you are using a model to determine whether, for instance, a new spermicide is effective, and you have a 100% model and you are going to see by how much you are going to reduce transmission, or if you are using the model as you said before, Preston, where you get a 50% infection rate and then you want to see what cofactors might be responsible or what may facilitate transmission to increase the rate, the question comes down ultimately to size also. If you are looking at a 100% response, and you treat 10 animals and you get all 10 to convert, if all respond in the manner you want, you can have a small sample size, but if you are looking only at three or four animals and one or two animals respond, I do not know if you can say anything.

DR. MARX: I agree.

MR. SPIELER: You are going to have a real dilemma when it comes to predicting whether something is going to be efficacious in human trials.

DR. MARX: That is why it has to be 100%, because we are dealing with six to eight, group size of six to eight, and if you find large differences, large observed differences between 100% of an effect and 10 or 20 or even zero, then you have data that can serve as a guide, but, short of that, twofold differences are not going to be meaningful with small sizes like this. That is why we aim for a 100% effect and then try to back off from that. It is a difficult question. It is one we deal with with monkeys, and it is even worse with chimpanzees. As far as the reviewers are concerned, when you send papers in, if you work with chimpanzees, one animal is statistically significant. In macaques it is two, and in mice it is 100, I hear. So there are practical questions, and we have only practical approaches. Murray and I insist on large differences. Twofold means nothing to us. If you had your salary increase twofold, it would make a very significant difference to you, so that is a real change at twofold, but it is not a real change in the context of the way we carry out our experiments. We are looking for tenfold changes, and we think we can do work that can serve as a basis for future experiments when we are looking at those large differences with small groups. So, the summary is, large differences and small groups, yet we believe we are doing real science.

12

Transfer of HIV by Semen: Role of Sperm

Veronica E. Miller and Virginia L. Scofield

The transfer of pathogens during sexual intercourse potentially can occur through skin lesions or by direct contact with body fluids such as semen or vaginal secretions. In the United States, transfer of the human immunodeficiency virus (HIV) by semen is a major mechanism for the sexual transmission of acquired immune deficiency syndrome (AIDS). This conclusion is based on the predominantly unidirectional (male-to-female) transfer in heterosexuals [1], the high seroconversion risk associated with semen receptivity in the male homosexual population [2], and the seroconversion of three artificial insemination recipients inseminated with semen from the same infected donor [3].

Normal semen consists of seminal fluid, small numbers of leukocytes, and spermatozoa, each of which is a potential vehicle for HIV transport. HIV has been identified in cell-free seminal fluid [4] and in seminal leukocytes [5,6]. Recently, our experiments and those of others [7] suggested that HIV particles can bind to normal spermatozoa. The identification of the semen component(s) involved in virus transmission is important since the sperm, seminal leukocytes, and seminal fluid differ substantially in the degree to which they have access to the recipient's systemic environment.

Of the three semen components listed above, sperm are unique in several ways. First, sperm greatly outnumber leukocytes in the ejaculate [8]. Second, their motility allows them extensive access to the recipient's interior tissues. For example, after normal heterosexual intercourse, sperm are found in the peritoneal cavity, where they are phagocytosed by macrophages [9,10]. Third, the possibility that virus-transporting sperm may infect the fetus by germline incorpora-

Heterosexual Transmission of AIDS, pages 147–154

tion at fertilization or subsequently before blastocyst implantation has not been ruled out [11]. In spite of these important considerations, it has been assumed that the sexual spread of HIV is due to infected seminal leukocytes, or cell-free virus, or both. Infection by either of these routes would require the presence of susceptible target cells at the point of entry as well as survival of cell-free virus in the latter case, two conditions not required by sperm.

The notion that spermatozoa could function to transport surface-bound pathogens has been reported previously, as in *Chlamydia trachomatis* [12], *Neisseria gonorrhoeae* [13], and the mycoplasma *Ureaplasma urealyticum* [14]. In mice, retrovirus particle association with sperm has been reported [15,16]. In the above examples, the pathogens or virus particles were bound and were detectable on the sperm cell surface, presumably via nonspecific sticking. In the case of HIV, however, where CD4 has been identified as a specific receptor on target cell surfaces, binding of HIV to CD4 leads to fusion with the cell surface membrane and internalization of the virus [17,18]. Assuming the presence of an appropriate virus receptor on the sperm surface (see below), infectious HIV particles could conceivably be carried either on the sperm cell surface or inside the sperm membrane, in which case they would not be as easily detectable.

The nature of sperm–HIV interaction would depend on whether the interaction is specific (through a CD4-like receptor), in which case internalization would follow binding, or nonspecific, in which case internalization would not be expected. The two mechanisms (specific vs. nonspecific binding) are not mutually exclusive, however. The sperm surface is quite sticky, and many proteins are added externally as the sperm cells mature and travel through the epididymis [19–21]. Because of the extensive membrane changes in sperm during differentiation, maturation, and capacitation, the stage at which sperm come in contact with virus particles may significantly affect the nature of specific or nonspecific interactions. However, at this time, little is known about where in the male reproductive tract, and by which cells, the virus is secreted or carried into the semen. Spermatogenesis in AIDS patients is affected during the progression of disease; a decrease in sperm number and motility is accompanied by an increase in immature germ cells, and many patients are azoospermic at the time of death (Miller VE and Scofield VL, unpublished observations; Staszcewski S, personal communication). Whether this is a direct effect of HIV infection of the testes is not known, but the possibility that the virus affects spermatogenesis by infection of immature cells should not be ruled out at this time.

Although a model of sperm-mediated HIV transport does not de-

TABLE 1. Normal Human Sperm Binding to T and B Cells and Monocytes and Cells Lines[a]

Cell type	HLA-DR	Cells with sperm bound/penetrated (%)
T cells (resting)	Neg	4.5 ± 1.3[b]
CEM	Neg	4.5 ± 1.7
JM	Neg	8.0 ± 1.0
B cells	Pos	28.3 ± 6.5
729 Neo	Pos	32.5 ± 3.2
MT2	Pos	41.5 ± 5.1
Monocytes	Pos	30.2 ± 2.2
U937	Neg	8.5 ± 1.1
I937	Pos	38.6 ± 2.7

[a]T and B cells and monocytes were isolated from normal peripheral blood. Origin of cell lines has been described by Ashida and Schofield [22].
[b]Values are mean ± SEM.

pend absolutely on a specific HIV–target cell receptor interaction, this possibility should be considered. In AIDS, target cell CD4 is responsible for HIV binding, fusion, and cell entry [17,18]. Specific HIV–sperm interaction would require the presence of CD4, or, minimally, the epitopes of CD4 responsible for virus binding to be present on the sperm surface, at some stage of differentiation. In our studies [22] (also, Scofield et al., submitted for publication), we have shown that normal, ejaculated sperm specifically bind to HLA-DR- and -DQ-positive cells (Table 1, Fig. 1A,B), and this event is followed by sperm-target cell fusion and internalization of sperm (Fig. 1). Since these molecules are natural ligands for CD4, this finding leads to prediction of a CD4-like epitope on sperm; we have found CD4 epitopes on a small subpopulation of sperm [22]. The lack of replication of this result by other investigators appears to be due to differences in sperm isolation and fixation procedures, which have substantial and unpredictable effects on the serological detection of sperm surface markers. We are investigating this matter in our laboratory.

Sperm-transported HIV, to be infectious, must enter susceptible target cells. This could occur in several ways: 1) by phagocytosis by macrophages, 2) through antibody-mediated enhanced phagocytosis, 3) by endocytosis, or 4) by direct membrane fusion and entry. Data exist to support each of these proposed mechanisms. First, sperm phagocytosis by macrophages is a normal physiological event [9,10]. Second, antibody enhancement of sperm phagocytosis, although undocumented, is possible, especially in individuals with

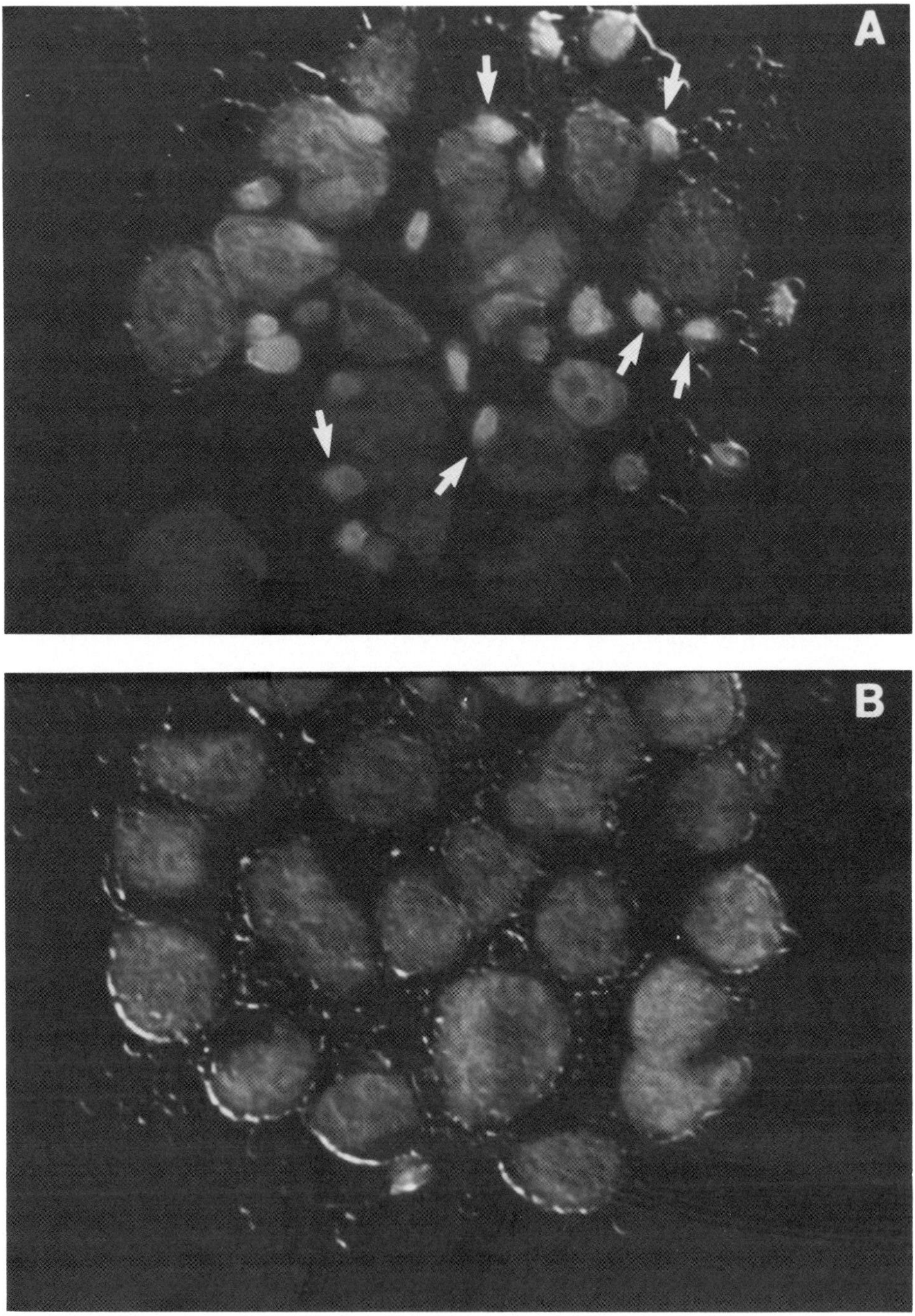

Figs. 1A and 1B.

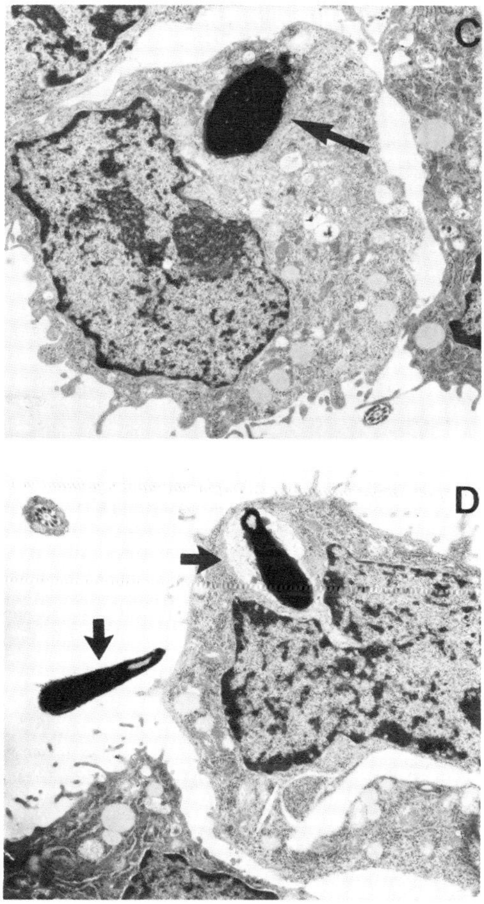

Fig. 1. Interaction of normal human sperm with HLA-DR-positive cells. **A, B:** Sperm were incubated with T5.1, an HLA-DR-positive B lymphoblastoid cell line (A), or the 6.1.6 HLA-DR-negative mutant (B) derived from the parental T5.1. Aliquots were fixed and stained with DAPI as described [22]. Only the DR-positive cells bind sperm (arrows). (The T5.1 and 6.1.6 cell lines were received from P. Gladstone, Seattle, Washington.) **C, D:** Sperm entry into HLA-DR-transfected murine fibroblasts (cell surface DR-positive) occurs by direct fusion (C) or endocytosis (D). Cells were incubated with sperm, fixed, and processed for electron microscopy as described. (A and B, courtesy of ER Ashida; C and D, courtesy of R Raghupathy.)

high circulating titers of antisperm antibodies. Furthermore, antibody-enhanced viral uptake has been documented [23]. Therefore, anti-HIV antibody-mediated uptake of virus-coated sperm may be an additional factor in virus transfer by sperm. Finally, normal sperm entry into DR-positive target cells can occur via endocytosis or by direct fusion with the cells [22] (Fig. 1); both these pathways resemble described modes of entry of HIV into cells through CD4 [17,18,24]. We suggest that sperm enter cells by either HLA-DR or CD4 in vivo, since we have found that exposed HIV particles or gp120 on the sperm surface allow sperm fusion with, and uptake by, CD4-positive DR cells.

Our model for sperm transport of HIV predicts the direct infection of target cells at the portal of entry, without prior systemic infection. That entrechromaffin cells at the base of the bowel crypts can be productively infected supports this notion [25].

Experimental support for sperm-mediated venereal transmission of HIV will require evidence that purified sperm from AIDS patients can infect target cells in vitro. Our preliminary results with leukocyte-free AIDS patient sperm preparations and normal sperm incubated with HIV isolates indicate that sperm-mediated transmission does occur. We are establishing which variables are important for the in vitro studies, toward defining conditions that may operate in vivo. Until the infectious status of spermatozoa in vivo is established or refuted, reports that sperm from HIV-positive donors are safe for insemination should be viewed with caution [26].

REFERENCES

1. **Padian N, Marquia L, Francis DP, et al.:** Male to female transmission of human immunodeficiency virus. JAMA 258:788–790, 1987.

2. **Kingsley LA, Kaslow R, Tinaldo DR, et al.:** Risk factors for seroconversion to human immunodeficiency virus among male homosexuals. Lancet 1:345–349, 1987.

3. **Stewart GJ, Cunningham AL, Driscoll GL, Tyler JPP, Barr JA, Gold J:** Transmission of human T-cell lymphotropic virus type III (HTLV-III) by artificial insemination by donor. Lancet 2:581–584, 1985.

4. **Borzy MS, Connell RS, Kiessling AA:** Detection of human immunodeficiency virus in cell-free seminal fluid. J AIDS 1:419, 1988.

5. **Zagury D, Bernard J, Leibowitch J, et al.:** HTLV-III in cells cultured from semen of two patients with AIDS. Science 226:449–451, 1984.

6. **Ho DD, Schooley RT, Rota TR, Kaplan JC, Flynn T:** HTLV-III in semen and blood of a healthy homosexual man. Science 226:451–453, 1984.

7. **Bagasra O, Freund M, Weldmann J, Harley G:** Interaction of human immunodeficiency virus with human sperm in vitro. J AIDS 1:431, 1988.

8. **Wolff H, Anderson DJ:** Immunohistologic characterization and quantitation of leukocyte subpopulations in human semen. Fertil Steril 49:497–504, 1988.

9. **Haney AF, Misokonis MA, Weinberg JB:** Macrophages and infertility: Oviductal macrophages as potential mediators of infertility. Fertil Steril 39:310–315, 1983.

10. **Syrop CH, Halme J:** Peritoneal fluid environment and infertility. Fertil Steril 48:1–9, 1987.

11. **Park CL, Streicher H, Rothenberg R:** Transmission of human immunodeficiency virus from parents to only one dizygotic twin. J Clin Microbiol 25:1119–1121, 1987.

12. **Wolner-Hanssen P, Mardh PA:** In vitro tests of the adherence of *Chlamydia trachomatis* to human spermatozoa. Fertil Steril 42:102, 1984.

13. **Gomez CI, Stenback WA, James AN, Criswell BS, Williams RP:** Attachment of *Neisseria gonorrhoeae* to human sperm. Microscopical study of effect of trypsin and iron. Br J Venereal Dis 55:245–255, 1979.

14. **Barwin BN:** Transmission of *Ureaplasma urealyticum* by artificial insemination by donor. Fertil Steril 41:326–327, 1984.

15. **Portis JL, McAttee FJ, Hayes SF:** Horizontal transmission of murine retroviruses. J Virol 61:1037–1044, 1987.

16. **Kiessling AA, Crowell RC, Connell RS:** Sperm-associated retroviruses in the mouse epididymis. Proc Natl Acad Sci USA 84:8667–8671, 1987.

17. **Stein BS, Gowda SD, Lifson JD, Penhallow RC, Bensch KG, Engleman EG:** pH-independent HIV entry into CD4-positive T cells via virus envelope fusion to the plasma membrane. Cell 49:659–668, 1987.

18. **Maddon PJ, McDougal JS, Clapham PR, et al.:** HIV infection does not require endocytosis of its receptor, CD4. Cell 54:865–874, 1988.

19. **Eddy EM, Vernon RB, Muller CH, Hahnel AC, Fenderson BA:** Immunodissection of sperm surface modifications during epididymal maturation. Am J Anat 174:225–237, 1985.

20. **Saxena NK, Russell LD, Sasena N, Peterson RN:** Immunofluorescence antigen localization on boar sperm plasma membranes: Monoclonal antibodies reveal apparent new domains and apparent redistribution of surface antigens during sperm maturation and at ejaculation. Anat Rec 214:238–252, 1986.

21. **Yanagimachi R:** Mechanisms of fertilization in mammals. In Mastrioani L, Biggers JD (eds): Fertilization and Embryonic Development In Vitro. New York: Plenum Press, 1981, pp 81–182.

22. **Ashida ER, Scofield VL:** Lymphocyte major histocompatibility complex-encoded class II structures may act as sperm receptors. Proc Natl Acad Sci USA 84:3395–3399, 1987.

23. **Robinson WE, Montefiori DC, Mitchell WM:** Antibody dependent enhancement of human immunodeficiency virus type 1 infection. Lancet 1:790–794, 1988.

24. **Maddon PJ, Dalgleisch AC, McDougal JS, Clapham PR, Weiss RA, Axel R:** The T4 gene encodes the AIDS virus receptor and is expressed in the immune system and the brain. Cell 47:333–348, 1986.

25. **Nelson JA, Reynolds Kohler C, Margaretten W, Wiley CA, Reese CE, Levy JA:**

Human immunodeficiency virus detected in bowel epithelium from patients with gastrointestinal symptoms. Lancet 2:259–262, 1988.

26. **Kolata G:** Discovery on AIDS virus raises a possibility of safe fatherhood. *New York Times,* October 12, 1988, p 1.

DISCUSSION

DR. ANDERSON: You did not show the data with the percoll sperm pellets, did you?

DR. MILLER: No, I did not show those here, but the results were strongly positive.

DR. ANDERSON: How many patients did you use?

DR. MILLER: We have not had positive results with all of the patients we tried. Actually, we have had difficulty getting all the semen from the patients lately. We have tested a lot of seropositive men who are not AIDS patients, and we have had negative results with one of them, but we have had some positive results with AIDS patients. We find a lot of round cells in patient semen.

DR. ANDERSON: And what is your evidence that HIV binds to sperm other than the sperm that have been incubated with HIV?

DR. MILLER: We are addressing that question using other techniques, such as PCR. These results are not ready to be reported at this time. I think Dr. Freund's paper will address some of that.

13

In Vitro and In Vivo Studies of HIV-1 and Human Sperm

Omar Bagasra and Matthew Freund

Epidemiological studies have shown that the human immunodeficiency virus (HIV) can be transmitted venereally by either heterosexual or homosexual intercourse and that infected semen plays a role in the process [1–5]. Follow-up rates of seroconversion among seronegative partners in monogamous heterosexual couples, in which the other partner was seropositive, demonstrated the heterosexual transmission of HIV and the protective effect of condoms [6–13]. The role of infected semen in heterosexual transmission was documented by a clinical report that four of eight recipients became seropositive after artificial insemination with semen from an HIV-positive donor [14].

The presence of an endogenous DNA-synthesizing complex sensitive to ribonuclease in purified preparations of human sperm heads from pooled semen was reported in 1975 [15]. This reverse transcriptase-like activity was also found in cell-free seminal fluid. A similarity of the sperm DNA polymerase to viral RNA-dependent DNA polymerase was shown, suggesting the presence of retrovirus in the sperm DNA. This work was confirmed and extended in 1988 to demonstrate the presence of HIV by an assay of reverse transcriptase in cell-free seminal fluid from men with acquired immune deficiency syndrome (AIDS) [16]. Virus concentrations in the range of 10^8 particles/ml semen were reported.

Studies reported in 1984 and 1985 [17–19] using coculture methods demonstrated the presence of HIV in the mononuclear cell fraction of human semen from one HIV-positive and two AIDS donors. HIV was not detected in the sperm of the HIV-positive donor by the coculture method used. Only small numbers of monocytes/macro-

Heterosexual Transmission of AIDS, pages 155–166

phages or CD4-positive T lymphocytes have been reported for human semen [20–22]; that this was the only basis for the role of semen in the sexual transmission of HIV seemed improbable.

Moreover, the 1975 work cited above also found reverse transcriptase-like activity in murine sperm [15]. More recently, a well-documented system for the venereal transmission of murine retroviruses from infected males to females has been shown. The presence of retrovirus particles associated with mouse sperm and the presence of retroviral reverse transcriptase activity in mouse epididymal fluids have been demonstrated [23–26].

The presence of OKT4 and OKT4A antigens [27] and of a CD4 ligand [28] on normal human sperm has been documented recently. However, the inability to find CD4 antigen on sperm or on testicular germ cells has also been reported [29]. Taken together, these findings suggest the hypothesis that human sperm are involved in the venereal transmission of HIV.

MATERIALS AND METHODS

In Vitro Studies

Cell-free HIV-1 (IIIB) was incubated for 5 hr at 37°C with aliquots of washed sperm from seronegative donors; other sperm aliquots were used as controls. At the end of the incubation period, the sperm were washed four times and processed for analysis. Half of each sperm sample was fixed in 2.5% gluteraldehyde for electron microscopy, and the other half was used for indirect immunofluorescence microscopy and for immunofluorescence flow cytometry. Details of materials and methods were reported in a recent paper from this laboratory [30].

In Vivo Studies

Each of three HIV-seropositive patients (one of whom was diagnosed with AIDS by criteria of the Centers for Disease Control [CDC]) collected three semen specimens by masturbation at weekly intervals, for a total of nine specimens. The sperm were separated from the seminal plasma by centrifugation and washing and were resuspended in RPMI-1640 with interleukin-2 (IL-2). Aliquots of sperm were prepared for electron microscopy (EM), immunogold labeling, and DNA hybridization. EM preparation was standard and included fixing in 2.5% glutaraldehyde and postfixing in 1% osmiumtetroxide, dehydration in ethanol, embedding in Spurr resin, and sectioning followed by staining with lead citrate and uranyl acetate. Immunogold labeling preparation included short pulsing with methanol, incubation with a mixture of five HIV-1 antigen-specific monoclonal antibodies, washing, incubation with gold-conjugated goat antimouse IgG, and preparation for EM. A blinded research design was used in which the senior author performed the immunogold labeling work (five specimens from HIV-infected men, five negative controls, and one positive control [an HIV-infected H9 cell line]), and the junior author and a technician prepared the sperm for EM and examined and classified them. For DNA hybridization preparation, we used the DuPont HIV-SNAP hybridization kit described in the SNAP manual (DuPont) and by others [31,32]. Control sperm samples were treated similarly but without the HIV probes, to detect nonspecific background (Bagasra et al., submitted for publication).

RESULTS

In Vitro Studies

Viral particles were present on and inside the cell membrane of many sperm from the aliquots that had been incubated with HIV, but viral particles were not seen in the controls. Viral particles were characterized by the presence of centrally located electron-dense cores and appeared to be penetrating the intact plasma membrane. Viral particles within the sperm gave the appearance of disassembly of the viral envelope and decondensation of the viral central core.

Immunofluorescence microscopy of sperm incubated with HIV and then with anti-HIV polyvalent sera yielded many small patches of fluorescence on the heads of 5% to 10% of the sperm, whereas fluorescence was not observed in control specimens. The presence of positive binding by sperm with epitope-specific anti-CD4 monoclonal antibodies (mAbs) was demonstrated by fluorescence microscopy and by flow cytometry. Using fluorescence microscopy, 1% to 11% of sperm expressed surface antigens, as follows: OKT4 = 5% to 8%, OKT4A = 6% to 11%, OKT4B = 5% to 7%, OKT4C = 1% to 2%, OKT4D = 3% to 4%, OKT4E = 0, and OKT4F = 6% to 9%, with negative control = 0. Using immunofluorescence analysis by flow cytometry, values were: OKT4A = 9.9%, OKT3 = 14.0%, OKT6 = 28.1%, OKT8 = 8.0%, with negative control = 1.0%.

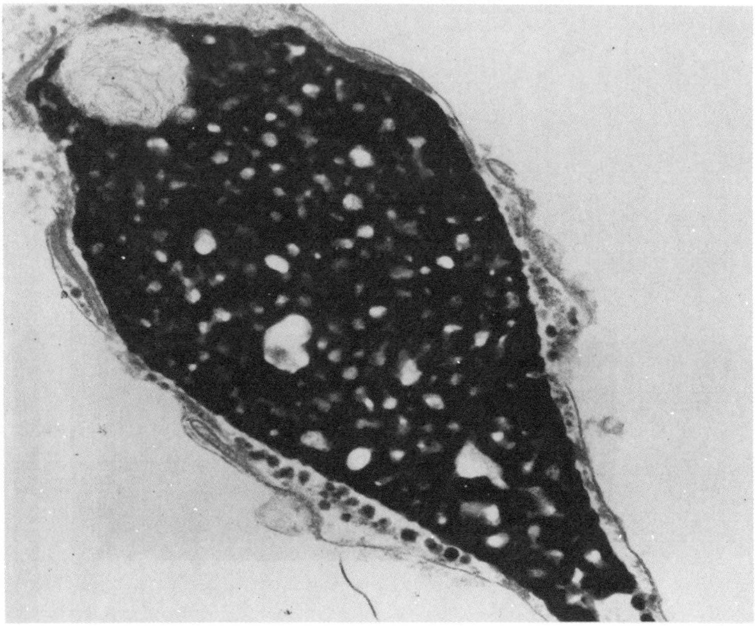

Fig. 1. Electron micrograph of viral particles in a sperm from an HIV-positive donor. ×18,000.

In Vivo Studies

HIV-like particles were observed by EM in sperm from all nine semen specimens of the three HIV-positive patients (Fig. 1). Virus particles were observed in both sagittal and cross sections of many sperm and appeared to be aligned primarily in rows in the space between the nucleus and the cell membrane.

Using HIV-specific mAbs and immunogold labeling in a blinded design as described above, five specimens from HIV-infected men, five negative controls, and one positive control (HIV-infected H9 cell line) were correctly identified and differentiated by the presence of aggregations of gold particles on and outside the sperm cell membrane in the infected specimens (Fig. 2). The negative controls were characterized by the absence of either specific or nonspecific gold particles.

The degree of HIV DNA hybridization in sperm from HIV-positive men (Fig. 3) was significant compared to controls. The percentage of positive sperm in nine specimens from HIV-positive donors ranged from 5% to 28% (mean = 13.4%), whereas in the six controls (HIV-

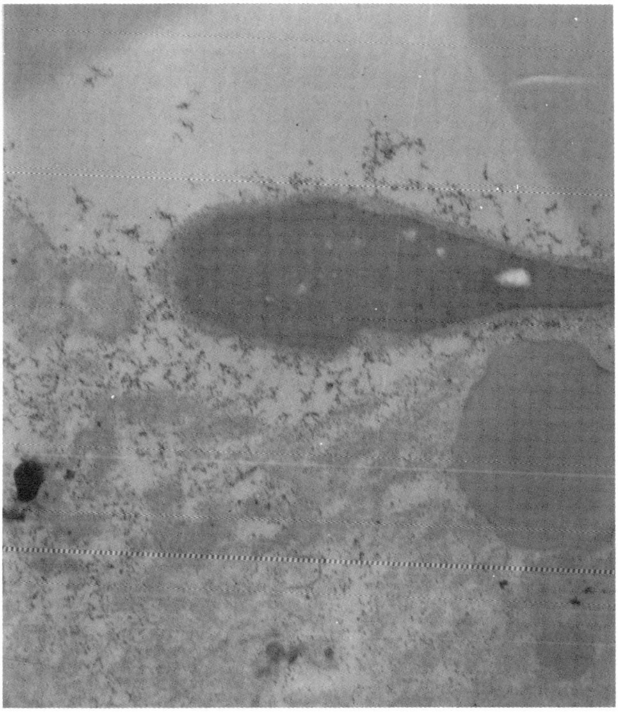

Fig. 2. Electron micrograph: presence of immunogold aggregates on and outside the sperm membrane from an HIV-positive donor. ×17,000.

negative donors) the range was 1% to 5% (mean = 2.5%, $P < .001$ by the unpaired t test). Aliquots of all 15 specimens were run without probes as additional controls, and the percentage of positive sperm ranged from 0% to 3% (mean = 0.39%), with 11 of 15 specimens showing no positive sperm.

DISCUSSION

Substantial evidence shows that infected semen from an HIV-seropositive man or from a male AIDS patient is an important vector in the venereal transmission of HIV by either the vaginal or the anal route [1–13] Additionally, the male-to-female transmission of murine retroviruses and the role of mouse sperm in this process have been shown [15,23–26]. Evidence has begun to accumulate that human sperm play a key role in the venereal transmission of HIV from the insertor to the insertee.

Well before the discovery of AIDS, a report in 1975 [15] documented the presence of reverse transcriptase-like activity in both

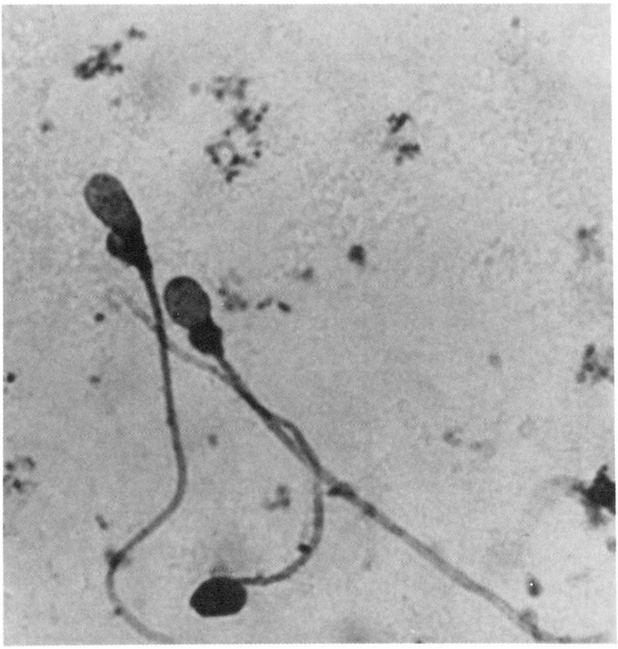

Fig. 3. Presence of HIV DNA hybridization in sperm from an HIV-positive donor.

human and mouse sperm heads and in human cell-free seminal fluid. Moreover, this important work demonstrated the similarity of human sperm DNA polymerase to viral RNA-dependent DNA polymerase and provided a possible link to the concept of human sperm-associated retroviruses. Part of this early work was confirmed in 1988 [16] by the assay of reverse transcriptase in cell-free seminal fluid from men with AIDS. The assay indicated high virus concentrations in the range of 10^8 particles/ml semen. Although the presence of reverse transcriptase in mouse epididymal fluid and the chronic retroviral infection of mouse epididymal cells have been demonstrated by the same group [24,33], these investigators were unable to detect the CD4 antigen in normal human epididymal tissue by immunofluorescence staining. In their cell-free preparations, technical efforts were made to prevent cell disruption, although this could not be excluded. Moreover, nothing in this report indicated that sperm were considered to contain reverse transcriptase (as previously shown) [15] or the possibility that sperm from AIDS patients might be infected and shedding virus. However, finding high concentrations of HIV in cell-free seminal fluid led the authors to suggest that mononuclear cells may not be the only cell type involved in HIV transmission in human semen.

The role of the mononuclear cell fraction of human semen as the sole cell type infected with HIV rests on evidence from two 1984 reports that apparently were based solely on coculture methods [17–19]. In one study [18], in which HIV was cocultured from the mononuclear cells of two AIDS patients, coculture trials with sperm were not mentioned. Another study [17], in which HIV was cocultured from the mononuclear cells of one HIV-positive man, reported that "attempts to find virus in the spermatozoa fraction of semen from 11 individuals have yielded negative results." It seems improbable that the small number of monocytes/macrophages or lymphocytes reported for human semen [20–22] could be the sole basis either for the relatively high concentrations of HIV reported for human seminal fluid or for the venereal transmission of HIV.

Demonstration of the presence of OKT4 and OKT4A antigens on normal human sperm and of a CD4-like ligand on normal sperm coincubated with HIV [27,28] supports the work reported from this laboratory [30]. One abstract does report a failure to find the CD4 antigen on sperm from healthy men by immunoperoxidase or radioimmunoassay (RIA) techniques [29]. However, several questions may be raised about the techniques described in that report. Acetone, used to fix smears of washed sperm for the immunoperoxidase technique, has been reported to destroy CD4 antigen [34]. The anti-Leu-3a + b antibodies that were used have been reported to be weakly binding compared to OKT4A and OKT4F [35,36], which were used in similar work by this laboratory [30] (also, Bagasra et al., submitted for publication) and by others [20,28,36]. In the RIA technique, "fresh motile spermatozoa, obtained by swim-up . . ." were used, which means that only a small percentage (probably 5% to 10%) of the sperm were selected on the basis of motility and velocity. This separation procedure may have selected against the CD4-positive sperm.

Our data show an association between HIV and human sperm in vitro and in vivo and provide evidence for the mechanisms involved. In vitro after 5 hr of incubation with HIV, 5% to 10% of sperm from normal men showed signs of infection with HIV by EM, by immunofluorescence microscopy after incubation with anti-HIV polyvalent antibodies, and by fluorescence microscopy or immunofluorescence flow cytometry using epitope-specific anti-CD4 mABs [30]. In vivo HIV was identified in sperm from HIV-positive men by EM, by immunogold labeling using HIV antigen-specific mAbs, and by HIV-specific DNA probes with in situ hybridization (Bagasra et al., submitted for publication). These data provide the basis for proposing a potential mechanism for the venereal transmission of HIV by human sperm from HIV/AIDS patients, as has been demonstrated in the mouse for murine retroviruses [15,23–26].

In an HIV-seropositive man, only one in 10,000 circulating lymphocytes were shown to produce HIV [37]. In this work, 5% to 28% (mean = 13.4%) of sperm in nine semen specimens from HIV-positive men produced HIV. One explanation for this difference may be that the testis and male reproductive tract are a "privileged site" in immunological terms, in that they may be protected to some degree against normal immune surveillance. Elsewhere in the body, normal anti-HIV immune defenses are active and both humoral and cell-mediated immunity against HIV have been documented [33,38,39]. In the testis and male reproductive tract, lack of or a reduction in such immunity might provide a site for a greater degree of infection of sperm cells by HIV.

During the DNA hybridization procedures in this study, more than 90% of the midpieces, in those sperm that showed positive staining with HIV DNA probes, were significantly enlarged. Many of these enlarged midpieces were approximately four to ten times greater in diameter than normal sperm midpieces. In addition, the HIV DNA probes appeared to be more concentrated in the midpiece than in the head in terms of relative intensity of staining (Fig. 3). Moreover, in the immunogold work, aggregations of gold particles were also seen in association with sperm mitochondria. Finally, in a few cases, using EM, HIV-like particles in mitochondria were directly observed. Some of these mitochondria resembled pods with HIV-like particles bursting out of them like spores. These observations suggest that HIV in sperm may be replicating in the mitochondria, using mitochondrial DNA as a replicating device. In human sperm, where the DNA is condensed and tightly packaged in the nucleus relative to that in other cells, the random integration of the HIV provirus DNA into open frames of cellular DNA may take place in the mitochondria as well as, or instead of, in the nucleus.

REFERENCES

1. **Quinn TC, Mann JM, Curran JW, Piot P:** AIDS in Africa: An epidemiologic paradigm. Science 234:955–963, 1986.

2. **Piot P, Plummer FA, Mhalu FS, Lamboray J-L, Chin J, Mann MM:** AIDS: An international perspective. Science 239:573–579, 1988.

3. **Castro KG, Lieb S, Jaffe HW, et al.:** The Belle Glade Field-Study Group. Transmission of HIV in Belle Glade, Florida: Lessons for other communities in the United States. Science 239:193–197, 1988.

4. **Curran JW, Jaffe HW, Hardy AM, Morgan WM, Selik RM, Dondero TJ:** Epidemiology of HIV infection and AIDS in the United States. Science 239:610–616, 1988.

5. **Padian NS:** Heterosexual transmission of acquired immunodeficiency syndrome: International perspectives and national projections. Rev Infect Dis 9:947–960, 1987.

6. **Kreiss JK, Kitchen LW, Prince HE, Kasper CK, Essex M:** Antibody to human T-lymphotropic virus type III in wives of hemophiliacs: Evidence for heterosexual transmission. Ann Intern Med 102:623, 1985.

7. **Redfield WR, Markham PD, Salahuddin SZ, et al.:** Frequent transmission of HTLV-III among spouses of patients with AIDS-related complex and the acquired immunodeficiency syndrome. JAMA 253:1571–1573, 1985.

8. **Fischl MA, Dickinson GM, Scott GB, Klimas N, Fletcher MA, Parks W:** Evaluation of heterosexual partners, children, and household contacts of adults with AIDS. JAMA 257: 640–644, 1987.

9. **Goedert JJ, Eyster ME, Biggar RJ, Blattner WP:** Heterosexual transmission of human immunodeficiency virus: Association with severe depletion of T-helper lymphocytes in men with hemophilia. AIDS Res Hum Retroviruses 3:355–361, 1987.

10. **Padian N, Marquis L, Francis DP, et al.:** Male-to-female transmission of human immunodeficiency virus. JAMA 258:788–790, 1987.

11. **Peterman TA, Stoneburner RL, Allen JR, Jaffe HW, Curran JW:** Risk of human immunodeficiency virus transmission from heterosexual adults with transfusion-associated infections. JAMA 259:55–58, 1988.

12. **Ragni MV, Gupta P, Rinaldo CR, Kingsley LA, Spero JA, Lewis JH:** HIV transmission to female sexual partners of HIV antibody-positive hemophiliacs. Public Health Rep 103:54–58, 1988.

13. **Smiley ML, White GD, Becherer P, et al.:** Transmission of human immunodeficiency virus to sexual partners of hemophiliacs. Am J Hematol 28:27–32, 1988.

14. **Stewart GJ, Tyler JPP, Cunningham AL, et al.:** Transmission of human T-cell Lymphotropic Virus Type III (HTLV-III) by artificial insemination by donor. Lancet 2:581–584, 1985.

15. **Witkin SS, Korngold GG, Bendich A:** Ribonuclease sensitive DNA-synthesizing complex in human sperm heads and seminal fluid. Proc Natl Acad Sci USA 72:3295–3299, 1975.

16. **Borzy MS, Connell RS, Kiessling AA:** Detection of human immunodeficiency virus in cell-free seminal fluid. J AIDS 1:419–424, 1988.

17. **Ho DD, Schooley RT, Rota TR, et al.:** HTLV-III in the semen and blood of a healthy homosexual man. Science 226:451–453, 1984.

18. **Zagury D, Bernard J, Leibowitch J, et al.:** HTLV-III in cells cultured from semen of two patients with AIDS. Science 226:449–451, 1984.

19. **Zagury D, Fouchard M, Cheynier R, et al.:** Evidence for HTLV-III in T cells from semen of AIDS patients: Expression in primary cell culture, long-term mitogen-stimulated cultures, and coculture with a permissive T-cell line. Cancer Res 45 [Suppl]: 4595s–4597s, 1985.

20. **Anderson DJ, Hill JA:** Letter to the Editor: CD4(T4+) lymphocytes in semen of healthy heterosexual men: Implications for the transmission of AIDS. Fertil Steril 48: 703–704, 1987.

21. **Wolff H, Anderson DJ:** Letter to the Editor: Potential human immunodeficiency virus-host cells in human semen. AIDS Res Hum Retroviruses 4:1–2, 1988.

22. **Wolff H, Anderson DJ:** Immunohistologic characterization and quantitation of leukocyte subpopulations in human semen. Fertil Steril 49:497–504, 1988.

23. **Levy JA, Joyner J, Borenfreund E:** Mouse sperm can horizontally transmit type C viruses. J Gen Virol 51:439–443, 1980.

24. **Kiessling AA:** Evidence that reverse transcriptase is a component of murine epididymal fluid. Proc Soc Exp Biol Med 176:175–182, 1984.

25. **Kiessling AA, Crowell RC, Connell RS:** Sperm-associated retrovirus in the mouse epididymis. Proc Natl Acad Sci USA 84:8667–8671, 1987.

26. **Portis JL, McAtee FJ, Hayes SF:** Horizontal transmission of murine retroviruses. J Virol 61:1037–1044, 1987.

27. **Ashida EE, Scofield VL:** Lymphocyte major histocompatibility complex-encoded class II structures may act as sperm receptors. Proc Natl Acad Sci USA 84:3395–3399, 1987.

28. **Miller VE, Scofield VL:** Role of spermatozoa in sexual transmission of AIDS. Abstract 2550: IV International Conference on AIDS, Stockholm, June, 1988.

29. **Wolff H, Zhang WH, Anderson DJ:** The CD4 antigen (HIV-Receptor) is not detectable on human testicular germ cells or spermatozoa. Abstract 2547: IV International Conference on AIDS, Stockholm, June, 1988.

30. **Bagasra O, Freund M, Weidmann J, Harley G:** Interaction of human immunodeficiency virus with human sperm in vitro. J AIDS 1:431–435, 1988.

31. **Suggs S, Wallace RB:** Use of synthetic oligonucleotides as hybridization probes: Isolation of cloned DNA sequence for human B_2-microglobulin. Proc Natl Acad Sci USA 78:6613–6617, 1981.

32. **Jablonski E, Moomaw EW:** Preparation of oligodeoxynucleotide-alkaline phosphatase conjugates and their use as hybridization with DNA immobilized on a membrane. J Mol Biol 12:829–842, 1986.

33. **Kannagi M, Chahfour LV, Lord CI, Letvin NL:** Suppression of simian immunodeficiency virus replication in vitro by $CD8^+$ lymphocytes. J Immunol 140:2237–2292, 1988.

34. **Lifler J:** Methodologies for enumerating peripheral T lymphocytes. J Clin Immunol 2 [July Suppl]:20–26, 1982.

35. **Sattentau GJ, Dalgleish AG, Weiss RA, Beverley PL:** Epitopes of the CD4 antigen and HIV infection. Science 234:1120–1123, 1986.

36. **Bagasra O, Lischner HW:** Activity of dextran sulfate and other polyanionic polysaccharides against human immunodeficiency virus. J Infect Dis 158:1084–1087, 1988.

37. **Harper ME, Marselle LM, Gallo RC, Wong-Staal F:** Detection of lymphocyte expressing human T-lymphotropic virus type III in lymph nodes and peripheral blood from infected individuals by in situ hybridization. Proc Natl Acad Sci USA 83:772–776, 1986.

38. **Rook AH, Lane C, Folks T, McCoy S, Alter H, Fauci AS:** Sera from HTLVIII/LAV antibody-positive individuals mediate antibody-dependent cellular cytotoxicity against HTLVIII/LAV-infected T cells. J Immunol 138:1064–1067, 1986.

39. **Walker CM, Moody DJ, Stites DP, Levy JA:** $CD8^+$ lymphocytes can control HIV infection in vitro by suppressing virus replication. Science 234:1563–1566, 1986.

DISCUSSION

DR. WITKIN: To show activity, you first need controlled experiments to show that if you carry out the incubation at 4°C or with dead sperm or dead virus nothing happens.

DR. FREUND: I agree. We need to do that.

DR. KAPLAN: Did you conduct any additional research to determine whether an HIV-impregnated spermatozoa is still motile and is capable of penetrating an ova? You can use a hamster cell ova model if possible.

DR. FREUND: No, we have not. I might add one afterthought. We considered the issue of whether a human sperm could fertilize an ovum, and we searched the literature on pediatric AIDS. We also called three of the people most active in pediatric AIDS. We were looking for fraternal twins among whom one was positive and one was negative. There are six such fraternal twins described in the literature. It does not prove very much, but, much to my surprise, I found one report on monozygotic twins among whom one child was, at the time of the report, up to 3 years seronegative and the other was seropositive. We have been thinking along those lines, about that possibility.

DR. PUDNEY: I have some trouble interpreting your in vitro results where you show what you consider to be a virus binding. You have a virus that you assume is binding to the spermatozoa. Then you had in the same picture a virus within the cytoplasm of the sperm. Are you saying that the virus is reassembled in the cytoplasm, because, if you are, that goes against all accepted tenets of how retroviruses are assembled and secreted. How does the intact virus cross the plasma membrane of the sperm cell?

DR. FREUND: I do not know the answer to that question. It apparently crosses it, because we see virus particles in cytoplasm between the membrane and the nucleus in many different sperm. In most of our preparations, the virus penetration is after the fact. How it got through, I do not know.

DR. PUDNEY: Well, the accepted idea of how retroviruses infect is that they bind to the plasma membrane, the core is injected, then the genetic material directs the assembly of the virus within the cytoplasm. I find it difficult to envision that such a large virus could pass intact across the cell membrane. The sperm are not undergoing any endocytosis. If you are assuming that the virus is disassembled and the core is injected, then it would not necessarily be assembled within the cytoplasm. It would have to go into the nucleus first.

DR. FREUND: I do understand your question. None of the electron microscopy pictures that we looked at sheds any light on that particular issue. We have shown in the in vitro incubation work that HIV can penetrate the intact sperm cell membrane, as has been shown for certain $CD4^+$-positive cell lines (see Marsh M, Dalgleish A: How do immunodeficiency viruses enter cells? Immunol Today 8:369–371, 1987).

DR. PUDNEY: I propose two potential questions about the immunogold because I am very interested in that. Was that preimbedding or postimbedding?

DR. FREUND: They were incubated first, fixed, and then processed.

DR. PUDNEY: What was the primary antibody?

DR. FREUND: We used a mixture of five primary monoclonal antibodies, anti-HIV gp120, the anti-HIV p24, an anti-gp120a, an anti-gag55, and an anti-envelope9.

DR. ANDERSON: I am intrigued by your immunofluorescence data localizing CD4 on sperm. We have used the same antibodies that you have used and do not see the subpopulation of positive cells that you report. I was wondering if you know anything more about this subpopulation? Are they acrosome-reacted, or are they physiologically different from the sperm in general?

DR. FREUND: The answer I will give you is speculative. We think it is associated with sperm mitochondria, and we have four lines of evidence to indicate that. We are even speculating that it may be associated with mitochondrial DNA.

14

Presence of HIV in Semen

Deborah J. Anderson, Hans Wolff,
Jeffrey Pudney, Zhang Wenhao,
Adriana Martinez, and Kenneth Mayer

The human immunodeficiency virus type 1 (HIV-1) is acquired sexually through semen, yet little is known about the mechanisms underlying this route of transmission. Furthermore, epidemiologic studies [1,2] indicate that transmission of HIV via semen to sexual partners occurs with varying efficiency, indicating that as yet undefined cofactors may be involved. In this chapter, we review current literature on HIV in semen and present new findings from our laboratory concerning: 1) the localization of HIV in semen, 2) the incidence of infectious HIV in seropositive homosexual men, and 3) genital tract inflammation as a potential cofactor underlying the infectious potential of semen.

LITERATURE REVIEW AND COMMENTARY

HIV-1 has been cultured from the "round cell" fraction of semen [3–5], which consists of a mixture of immature germ cells, granulocytes, lymphocytes, and macrophages [6]. Furthermore, HIV-infected cells of lymphocytic/monocytic appearance have been detected in low numbers in semen smears of seropositive men by in situ hybridization [7]. Infectious HIV has also been cultured from cell-free seminal plasma from seropositive men at frequencies ranging from 11% [8] to 30% [7,9]. Our experience with HIV detection in semen, described below, confirms and extends these published reports.

Recently published data suggest that HIV can attach with high affinity to motile spermatozoa. Ashida and Scofield [10] and more recently Bagasra and coauthors [11] reported results of immunoflu-

Heterosexual Transmission of AIDS, pages 167–180

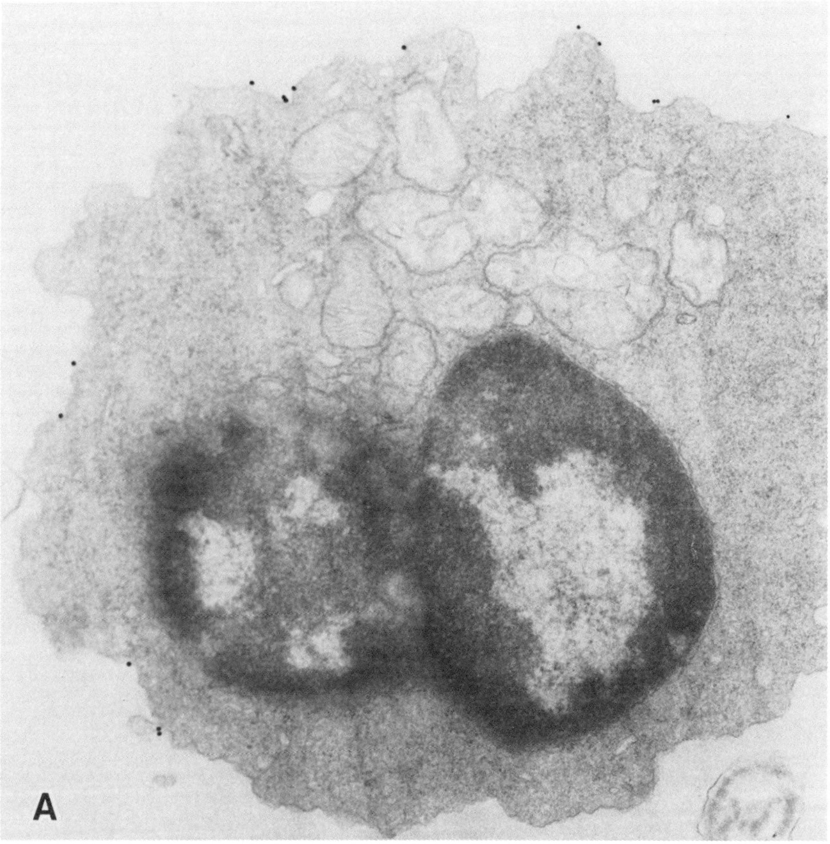

Fig. 1. Electron micrograph of a semen lymphocyte **(A)** and spermatozoon **(B)** that were incubated with a monoclonal antibody specific for the CD4 antigen (HIV receptor) and subsequently processed for immunogold visualization of antigen. Numerous gold particles could be seen on the surface of lymphocytes in this preparation, whereas spermatozoa were negative. A, ×52,000. B, ×56,000.

orescence and cell-interaction studies indicating that CD4-like antigens (HIV receptors) may be expressed on the surface of human sperm. The levels of CD4 antigens on sperm, if present, are exceedingly low. Using a variety of anti-CD4 monoclonal antibodies in radioimmunoassay, immunogold transmission electron microscopy

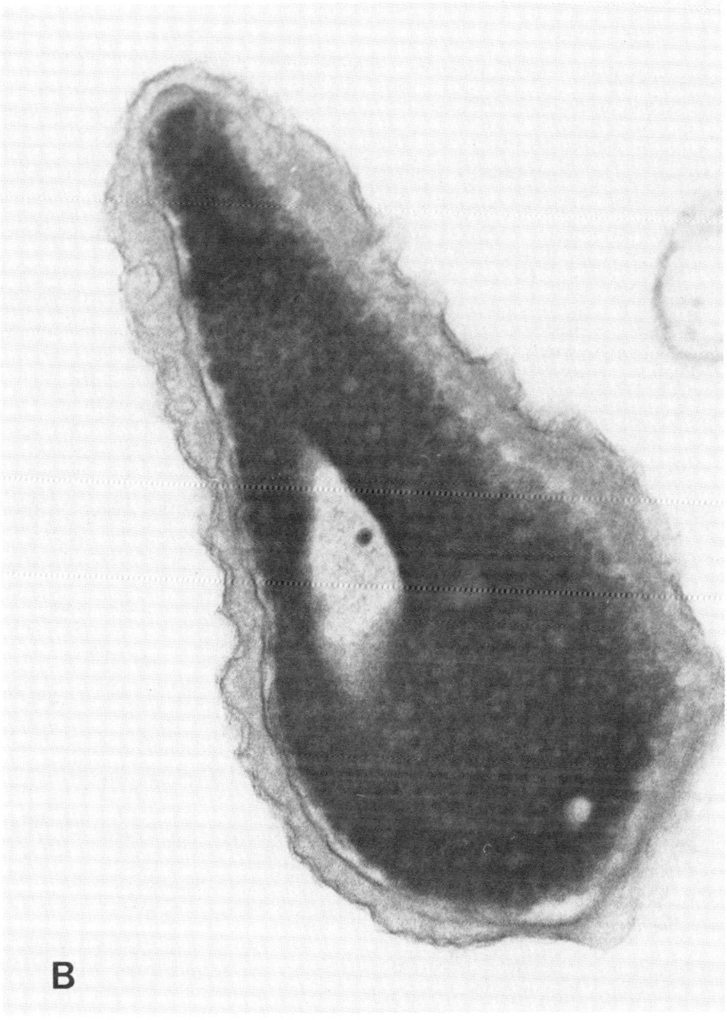

Fig. 1B.

(TEM; Fig. 1), and other immunohistologic assays, we have consistently failed to detect CD4 antigens on human sperm or testicular germ cells [6,12]. Other investigators who have used antibodies to CD4 epitopes to characterize lymphocyte subpopulations in male reproductive tissues and semen also have not commented on CD4 antigen expression by sperm or germ cells [13,14]. However, if CD4 antigens are expressed on the sperm surface, these receptors may enable HIV to bind to sperm and to be carried directly to susceptible host cells, such as T lymphocytes and macrophages [15].

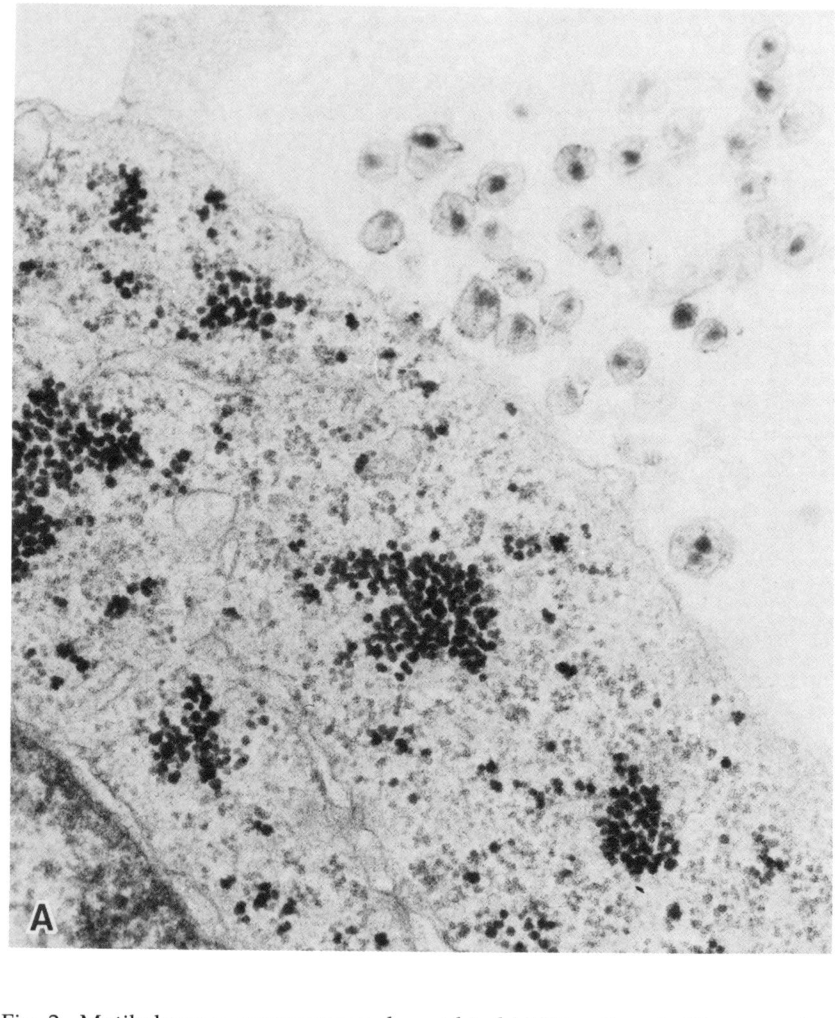

Fig. 2. Motile human spermatozoa do not bind HIV in vitro. **A:** Electron micrograph of HIV-infected Jurkatt cell line used as a source of HIV for sperm coincubation studies. **B:** Electron micrograph of motile spermatozoa recovered from supernatant of HIV-infected cell culture. No attachment of HIV to the sperm surface was observed A, ×31,000. B, ×32,000.

Borzy, Connell, and Kiessling [16] published a TEM picture showing an HIV-like viral particle near a sperm tail in semen from an HIV-seropositive man, and Basgara and coauthors [11] reported nu-

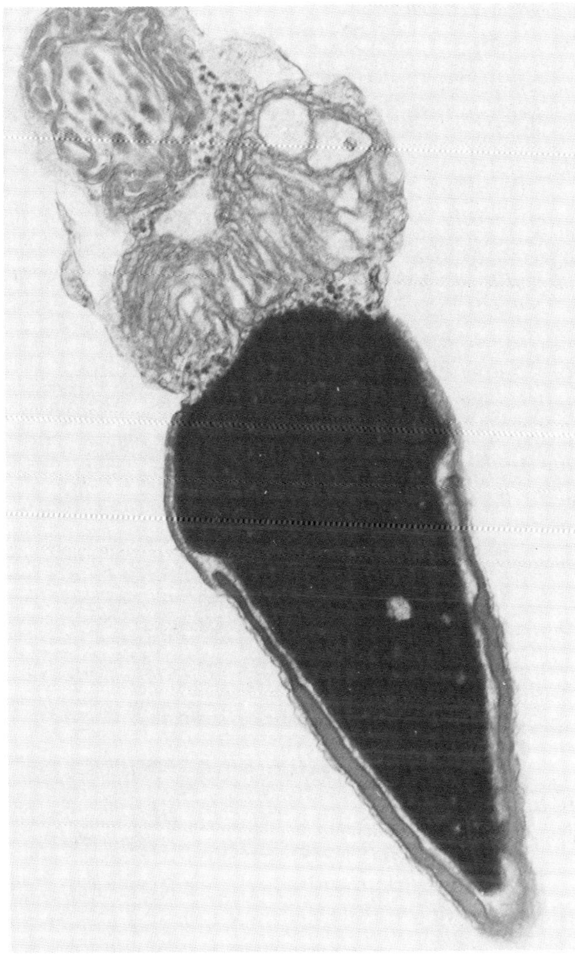

Fig. 2B.

merous virus-like particles associated with the acrosomal membrane in sperm that had been coincubated with supernatants of HIV-infected cell lines. However, additional studies are needed to clarify this issue, since many types of particles, vesicles, and other viruses (including endogenous retroviruses in semen) can resemble HIV (see Chapter 16, this volume). Immunogold techniques with anti-HIV antibodies should be applied to confirm that virus-like particles are indeed HIV. Studies from our laboratory, using a variety of sperm/HIV coculture conditions in combination with TEM immunogold

TABLE 1. In Vitro Coincubation Experiments of Cultured HIV-1 With Human Sperm From HIV-1 Seronegative Donors[a]

Sperm–HIV-1 interaction	HIV-1 on sperm (TEM)[b]	HIV + Culture[c]
HIV added to fresh ejaculate	None seen	Sperm − SP + WBC/germ cells +
HIV added to mixture of fresh ejaculate + vaginal secretions	None seen	N.A.[d]
Washed motile sperm added to HIV-infected Jurkatt cell culture	None seen	N.A.
Washed sperm incubated with HIV in the time course at:		
37°C	None seen	Sperm −
4°C	None seen	Sperm −

[a]The HIV-1_{IIIb} substrain was cultured in Jurkatt cells. Supernatants contained 200 × 10^3 cpm/ml reverse transcriptase units.
[b]Aliquots of semen were removed from 37°C incubator at 30 min and 1 and 4 hr. The cellular fraction was pelleted by centrifugation and either fixed immediately in glutaraldehyde for direct TEM visualization of virus or reacted with antibodies directed against the gp120 HIV envelope antigen and processed for immunogold detection of virus.
[c]After 4 hr of incubation with HIV at 37°C, components of semen were separated on a percoll gradient and washed 3 times. Forty lambdas of cell-free seminal fluid, 2 × 10^6 "round cells" (white blood cells and immature germ cells), or 2 × 10^6 motile spermatozoa were added to 2 × 10^6 PHA-activated PBL target cells in 24 well plates. Culture supernatants were assayed biweekly for 4 weeks for p24 HIV antigen.
[d]N.A., not available.

procedures, have not detected a physical association between HIV and sperm (Table 1, Fig. 2). However, our studies have been subject to the limitations of the TEM approach.

In TEM studies, 100–1,000 sperm cross sections have been examined per specimen. Since HIV is very small (120 nm in diameter) in relation to sperm (head 3–5 μm in diameter), the TEM approach would not detect a small number of HIV particles attached to sperm. For this reason, we have also used the more sensitive technique of culturing purified motile sperm that had been coincubated with HIV on phytohemagglutinin (PHA)-activated lymphocyte target cells. When the motile sperm fraction is isolated carefully from contaminating white blood cells (WBCs), free virus, and bacterial contaminants on Percoll gradients [17,18], sperm do not serve as vectors for HIV transmission in this model system (Table 1). Furthermore, Percoll-purified sperm from semen of 12 seropositive men did not convey infectious HIV to target cells, although infectious virus was recovered from seminal plasma from seven of these samples (as described below). Poiesz [19] tested more than 200 sperm fractions from semen of seropositive men by polymerase chain reaction (PCR) assay for HIV DNA and reported preliminary evidence that all samples were negative. His study provides the first evidence that integration of HIV DNA into germ line (sperm) DNA is unlikely to be a primary mechanism of transmission of HIV to sexual partner or offspring.

In summary, few laboratories have published studies on HIV detection and localization in semen; the limited data are conflicting and must be considered preliminary. Evidence is mounting that HIV is produced by mononuclear cells in semen and can be present in free form in seminal fluid. Data indicating a biologically relevant association between HIV and spermatozoa are more controversial and await confirmation.

HIV CULTURE FROM COMPONENTS OF SEMEN

Human semen contains seminal plasma (cell-free fluid) and various cell types in addition to spermatozoa (Table 2). To identify semen components that transmit HIV and to describe other variables in semen that may be influenced by HIV infection, we evaluated semen from 49 HIV-seropositive homosexual men; 152 HIV-seronegative homosexual men; and 17 healthy, low-risk heterosexual men. The methods used were: TEM, enzyme-linked immunosorbent assay (ELISA), immunohistology, in situ hybridization, and, when possible, peripheral blood leukocytes (PBL) coculture.

Semen specimens are diluted 1:1 in sterile phosphate-buffered saline (PBS) and centrifuged at 400*g* for 10 min, and the seminal plasma is removed and filter-sterilized (0.45 μm). Aliquots of seminal plasma are reserved for p24 antigen ELISA, anti-HIV antibody ELISA, and HIV culture. Aliquots of the semen cell pellet are processed for TEM and immunohistology. The remaining cells are resuspended in sterile Tyrode's/3% bovine serum albumin (BSA) medium, layered onto a 47%/90% Percoll gradient, and centrifuged for 30 min at 400*g* [8]. The top layer at the 47% interface contains most of the WBCs and immature germ cells; the middle layer at the 90% interface contains a few WBCs and a mixture of motile and immotile sperm; the pellet below the 90% layer is composed almost exclusively of motile sperm (Fig. 3). We place 40 μl of seminal plasma, and a maximum of 1×10^6 cells from the top interface and 2×10^6 sperm from the Percoll pellet each into individual wells (24 plate) containing 2×10^6 PHA-acti-

TABLE 2. Cellular Components of Semen in Healthy Heterosexual Donors (N = 17)

Cell type	Median	Range
Sperm	224×10^6	14×10^6–348×10^6
Immature germ cells[a]	58,000	N.D.[b]–16×10^6
WBCs (total)[c]	170,000	8,970–20×10^6
Granulocytes	100,000	6,250–19×10^6
Macrophages	51,900	2,800–997,000
Lymphocytes		
$CD4^+$	4,140	N.D.–51,900
$CD8^+$	2,243	N.D.–56,666
B cells	N.D.	N.D.–25,200
Sertoli cells	Occasional	
Epithelial cells	Occasional	

[a]Estimate based on the number of nonepithelial "round cells" in semen that were not positive in immunoperoxidase assay for the common leukocyte marker (HLe-1).
[b]N.D., not detectable.
[c]From Wolff and Anderson [24].

vated PBLs, and monitor supernatants for p24 HIV antigen by Du Pont ELISA biweekly for 4 weeks.

Seminal plasma specimens from seropositive men were uniformly negative for p24 antigen in the Du Pont ELISA, except for one symptomatic (AIDS) patient, whose semen contained more than 30×10^6 WBCs/ml (dramatic leukocytospermia). Seminal plasma from this sample contained p24 antigen levels comparable to more than 10,000 infectious units/ml. When 1 ml aliquots of representative p24-negative seminal plasma from seropositive men were centrifuged at 10,000*g* for 1 hr, two of 13 pellets were positive in the p24 assay, indicating that low levels of virus were present in at least some of the ELISA-negative samples. Twelve of 21 seminal plasma samples were HIV-positive by coculture on PHA-activated PBLs. Significant numbers of HIV-infected WBCs were not detected in semen smears by immunohistology, in situ hybridization, or TEM, but HIV was cultured from six of 14 WBC-enriched fractions of semen [20]. In contrast, motile sperm, isolated by Percoll gradient centrifugation from 12 samples (seven of which were positive for HIV in the seminal plasma fraction), were HIV-negative by virus culture on activated PBLs. Furthermore, no physical association between sperm and HIV was observed in 20 semen samples from seropositive men that have been studied to date by TEM [21,22]. Data from these studies indicate that semen from HIV-infected men can contain cell-free infectious

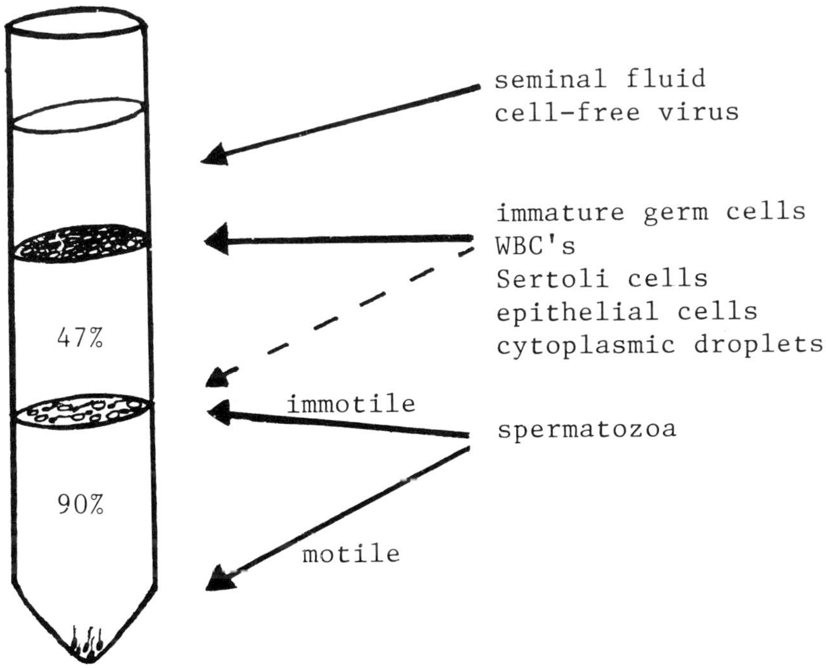

Fig. 3. Separation of components of human semen on percoll gradients.

virus as well as HIV-infected WBCs and provide further evidence that HIV does not bind in large quantities to sperm.

GENITAL TRACT INFLAMMATION AS A COFACTOR IN HIV TRANSMISSION

Our studies of WBCs have focused on WBCs in semen. We recently adapted immunohistology and ELISA techniques to quantify WBC subpopulations in semen [6,23] and to assess genital tract inflammation biochemically [24]. We used these methods to enumerate total WBCs and WBC subpopulations in every semen sample processed. In a study of infertility patients, we noted that genital tract inflammation, detected by significant elevations of the granulocyte elastase enzyme in seminal plasma (>1,000 ng/ml) or total WBCs ($>1 \times 10^6$ ml) occurred in approximately 20% of the patients studied and was accompanied by dramatic increases in levels of CD4-positive lymphocytes and macrophages (potential HIV host cells) [25]. These data led us to speculate that genital tract inflammation may be a significant cofactor in semen HIV infectivity [25,26].

TABLE 3. White Blood Cell Parameters (median numbers) in Semen of Heterosexual Laboratory Volunteers (LV), HIV-Seronegative Homosexual (HS) Men, and HIV-Seropositive HS Men

	HIV^- LV (N = 17)	HIV^- HS (N = 20)	HIV^+ HS asymptomatic (N = 12)	HIV^+ HS symptomatic (N = 7)
Total WBC/ml	48,571	163,800	431,620	1,067,000
Macrophages/ml	14,828	32,535	65,427	101,000
$CD4^+$ lymphocytes/ml	1,182	684	2,450	14,000
$CD8^+$ lymphocytes/ml	640	2,012	10,500	50,000
Sperm/ml ($\times 10^6$)	94.1	35	51	22.3

In our studies of WBC numbers and subpopulations in HIV-seronegative and HIV-seropositive homosexual men, we noted that 1) semen from seronegative homosexual men contains significantly higher numbers of total WBCs and potential HIV host cells than semen from heterosexual men at low risk and 2) semen from symptomatic seropositive men contains significantly more WBCs and CD4-positive cells than semen from either seronegative men or asymptomatic HIV-positive men (Table 3). This significant increase in WBC number is contrary to significant decreases in levels of WBCs and CD4-positive cells in the peripheral blood of these patients [27], and probably is a result of increased levels of genital tract infections due to the severely immunosuppressed status of these patients. Currently, we are investigating potential associations between levels of infectious virus and levels of total WBCs, CD4-positive lymphocytes, and macrophages in semen. The possibility that semen from patients with advanced-stage disease is more infectious than that of asymptomatic HIV-positive men is also under study.

SUMMARY AND CONCLUSIONS

We detected infectious HIV by coculture technique in semen from approximately 50% of homosexual HIV-seropositive men participating in this study. Infectious virus was most frequently recovered from seminal fluid and was frequently isolated from the WBC-enriched fraction of semen. Our studies failed to detect infectious virus in association with highly purified motile sperm. Our findings support the concept that WBCs are primary producers of HIV in male reproductive tract secretions and may themselves be vectors of HIV transmission [28]. The incidence of leukocytospermia was 27% in

HIV-seropositive men, and semen from men with symptomatic disease contained significantly higher levels of total WBCs, CD4-positive lymphocytes, and macrophages than semen from seronegative and asymptomatic seropositive men. This finding could indicate that semen has the potential to be more infectious in advanced-stage disease. In support of this concept, one patient with AIDS had marked leukocytospermia and extremely high levels of infectious free HIV and HIV-infected WBC in his semen. By laboratory criteria, this individual could be classified as a supertransmitter.

The studies reported here have not addressed other cofactors that may influence the sexual transmission of HIV through semen. The competency of physical barriers and the presence of immunosuppressive factors in the male reproductive tract may influence host immune defense mechanisms and levels of HIV in the male reproductive tract [29,30]. Antisperm autoimmunity or concomitant genital tract infections with other viruses [i.e., cytomegalovirus (CMV), Epstein-Barr virus (EBV), herpes simplex virus (HSV), human papilloma virus (HPV)] or microorganisms could not only attract HIV host cells to the reproductive tissues but may induce latent-infected cells to actively produce virus [31]. Anti-HIV antibodies in sexual secretions could have viral-neutralizing effects or, conversely, could promote HIV infection by directing HIV–immune complexes to macrophages, which are natural host cells of HIV [29]. Genetic factors may also determine levels of HIV in reproductive tissues and susceptibility of sexual partners to HIV infection. Different strains of HIV may have different infectivity patterns. Insight into such mechanisms may suggest new approaches to preventing HIV transmission and treating HIV-infected individuals.

ACKNOWLEDGMENTS

This research was supported by contract CSA-88-020 from the Contraceptive Research and Development (CONRAD) Program, Eastern Virginia Medical School, under a cooperative agreement with the United States Agency of International Development (U.S.A.I.D.), which in turn receives funds for AIDS research from an interagency agreement with the National Institute of Child Health and Human Development (NICHD). The views expressed by the authors do not necessarily reflect the views of the U.S.A.I.D. or CONRAD.

REFERENCES

1. **Padian N, Marquis L, Francis DP, et al.:** Male-to-female transmission of human immunodeficiency virus. JAMA 258:788, 1987.

2. **Peterman TA, Stoneburtner RL, Allen JR, Jaffe HE, Curran JW:** Risk of immunodeficiency virus transmission from heterosexual adults with transfusion-associated infections. JAMA 259:55–58, 1988.

3. **Ho DD:** HTLV-III in the semen and blood of a healthy homosexual man. Science 226:451–453, 1984.

4. **Zagury D:** Evidence for HTLV-III in T cells from semen of AIDS patients. Cancer Res 45[Suppl]:4595s–4597s, 1985.

5. **Zagury D:** HTLV-III in cells cultured from semen of two patients with AIDS. Science 226:449, 1984.

6. **Wolff H, Anderson DJ:** Immunohistologic characterization and quantitation of leukocyte subpopulations in human semen. Fertil Steril 49:497–504, 1988.

7. **Levy JA:** The transmission of AIDS:The case of the infected cell. JAMA 259:3037, 1988.

8. **Coombs RW, Collier A, Nikora B, et al.:** Recovery of HIV from semen and plasma following chronic oral zidovudine therapy (Abstract). ICAAC, 1988.

9. **Sannerud K:** Culture of HIV-1 from semen fractions using a p24 antigen EIA. Abstract 2548: IV International Conference on AIDS, Stockholm, June, 1988.

10. **Ashida ER, Scofield VL:** Lymphocyte major histocompatibility complex-encoded Class II structures may act as sperm receptors. Proc Natl Acad Sci USA 84:3395, 1987.

11. **Bagasra O, Freund M, Weidmann J, Harley G:** Interaction of human immunodeficiency virus with human sperm in vitro. J AIDS 1:431–436, 1988.

12. **Wolff H, Zhang W, Anderson DJ:** The CD4 antigen (HIV receptor) is not detectable on human testicular germ cells or spermatozoa. Abstract 2547: IV International Conference on AIDS, Stockholm, June, 1988.

13. **El-Demiry MIM, Hargreave TB, Busuttil A, James K, Ritchie AWS, Chisholm GD:** Lymphocyte subpopulations in the male genital tract. Br J Urol 57:769–778, 1985.

14. **Ritchie AWS, Hargreave TB, James K, Chisholm GD:** Intrepithelial lymphocytes in the normal epididymis. A mechanism for tolerance to sperm antoantigens? Br J Urol 56:79–83, 1984.

15. **Miller VE, Scofield VL:** Role of spermatozoa in sexual transmission of AIDS. Abstract 2550: IV International Conference on AIDS, Stockholm, June, 1988.

16. **Borzy MS, Connell RS, Kiessling AA:** Detection of human immunodeficiency virus in cell-free seminal fluid. J AIDS 1:419–424, 1988.

17. **Berger T, Marrs R, Moyer D:** Comparison of techniques for selection of motile spermatozoa. Fertil Steril 43:268–273, 1985.

18. **Sun L, Gastaldi C, Peterson E, De La Maza L, Stone S:** Comparison of techniques for the selection of bacteria-free sperm preparations. Fertil Steril 48:659–663, 1987.

19. **Poiesz B:** HIV detection by polymerase chain reaction assay. Seminar presented at Harvard School of Public Health, December, 1988.

20. **Anderson DJ, Wolff H, Wenhao Z, et al.:** Human immunodeficiency virus (HIV) in semen from seropositive men. Abstract: American Society of Andrology Annual Meeting, New Orleans, April, 1989.

21. **Anderson DJ, Wolff H, Zhang W, Pudney J, Dorfman T, Mayer K:** Localization of HIV-1 in semen: Evidence against HIV-1 attachment to human spermatozoa (submitted).

22. **Anderson DJ, Wolff H, Zhang W, Pudney J, Dorfman T, Mayer K:** No evidence of HIV-1 attachment to motile sperm. Abstract 19: Society for Gynecologic Investigations, San Diego, March, 1989.

23. **Anderson DJ, Hill JA:** CD4 ($T4^+$) lymphocytes in semen: Implications for the transmission of AIDS. Fertil Steril 48:703, 1987.

24. **Wolff H, Anderson DJ:** Evaluation of granulocyte elastase as a seminal plasma marker for leukocytospermia. Fertil Steril 50:129–132, 1988.

25. **Wolff H, Anderson DJ:** Male genital tract inflammation is associated with increased numbers of potential human immunodeficiency virus host cells in semen. Andrologia 20:404–405, 1988.

26. **Wolff H, Anderson DJ:** Male genital tract inflammation is associated with increased numbers of $CD4^+$ lymphocytes and monocytes/macrophages in semen. Abstract 2546: IV International Conference on AIDS, Stockholm, June, 1988.

27. **Mayer KH, Wolff H, Martinez A, Saltzman S, Anderson DJ:** Increased seminal leukocytes with progression of HIV-1 infection in homosexual males (Abstract). Am Soc Clin Invest (submitted).

28. **Anderson DJ, Yunis EJ:** "Trojan horse" leukocytes in acquired immunodeficiency syndrome (AIDS). N Engl J Med 309:984, 1983.

29. **Anderson DJ, Wolff H, Zhang W, Pudney J:** Immunology of the male reproductive tract: Implications for the sexual transmission of human immunodeficiency virus. In Voeller B, (ed): Fourth Kinsey Symposium on AIDS and Sex: An Integrated Biomedical and Behavioral Approach. New York: Oxford University Press (in press).

30. **Zhang W, Anderson DJ:** Effects of human seminal plasma (HSP) on mechanisms of HIV infection. Abstract 2549: IV Conference on AIDS, Stockholm, June, 1988.

31. **Anderson DJ:** Transmission of AIDS. Immunol Today 8(6):170, 1987.

DISCUSSION

DR. SCOFIELD: Are these motile sperm?

DR. ANDERSON: Yes. Motile sperm are the only ones that go through the 90% gradient, so they would be motile sperm.

DR. CATES: Did you correlate the higher levels of the type of abnormalities in your normal sperm? I wonder, did you look for gonorrhea, chlamydia, any of the mycoplasma, ureaplasma in forcing the white blood cell count up higher in the non-HIV sperm?

DR. ANDERSON: We would very much like to look at those variables, but we are not really set up to do that right now. We want to explore another dimension.

DR. HESS: I would like to ask the question in another way. Have you had an opportunity to look at hemophiliacs who are HIV-positive and have AIDS, and would you expect a different profile? I would also ask the obvious question for your sperm on the percoll gradient. Did you find any evidence of virus, or did you do any of those studies?

DR. ANDERSON: In hemophiliacs?

DR. HESS: No, in the study you just presented. I mean, you had a little pellet of sperm. Did you say it was negative?

DR. ANDERSON: Yes. One problem with semen culture is that you can get bacteria, so not all of our semen cultures have been successful. We have attempted to culture every sample we get, and for 28 days we successfully cultured eight sperm pellets and 14 white blood cell fractions. In no case, including the superinfected individual, did we find conversion with the sperm pellet, and we have found it in a majority of white blood cell layers.

15

Structure of the Male Reproductive Tract in AIDS Patients

Martin Dym and Jan Orenstein

Semen is a body fluid responsible for the sexual transmission of the human immunodeficiency virus (HIV). However, it is not clear how HIV is transported from an infected man's blood stream across his reproductive tract endothelium and epithelium to reach his semen. Nor is the precise site in the male reproductive tract of this viral transport known. It is generally believed that blood-borne lymphocytes, or macrophages, or both transport the virus, although this view is not supported by direct evidence. Clearly, the virus-infected cell (or free virus) must exit the small blood vessels in the genital area and enter the interstitial spaces surrounding the reproductive tract epithelium. Then, the virus or the virus-infected cell must traverse the reproductive tract epithelium to reach the semen compartment. A blood–testis barrier has been described that normally prevents serum proteins and cells from entering the lumen of the seminiferous tubules [1]. Other physiological barriers in the male reproductive tract [2] also may be important in determining the exact site and the mechanism by which HIV crosses from the blood vessels through the epithelium into semen. This basic cell biological problem of HIV transport across endothelia and epithelia has not been addressed.

The male reproductive tract consists of a series of ducts, starting with the seminiferous epithelium and culminating in the urethra. Sperm, produced in the seminiferous epithelium, pass through these ducts (rete testis, ductuli efferentes, epididymis, vas deferens, and urethra) as they acquire their fertilizing ability and await ejaculation. Two secretory glands (prostate and seminal vesicle) produce the bulk of seminal fluid. Figure 1 is a schematic drawing of

Heterosexual Transmission of AIDS, pages 181–196

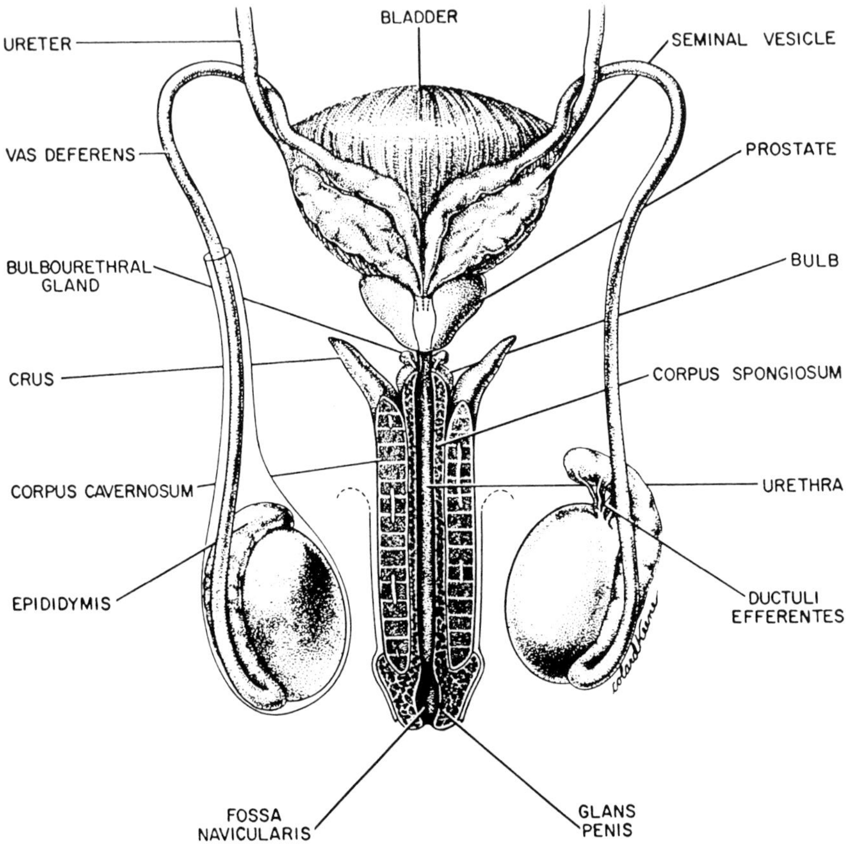

Fig. 1. Schematic drawing showing a posterior view of the human male reproductive system. (Reproduced from Dym [14], with permission of the publisher.)

the posterior aspect of the component parts of the human male reproductive tract. As the schematic drawing in Figure 2 emphasizes, for the purposes of HIV transmission from blood to semen, the entire male reproductive tract may be depicted as a single epithelial duct. Sperm and seminal fluid are located inside the lumen of this duct (shaded areas), whereas blood vessels and lymphatic vessels (not shown) are located outside, not unlike all epithelial ducts in the body.

METHODS

In a retrospective study, we examined the male reproductive tract in 25 men who died of acquired immune deficiency syndrome

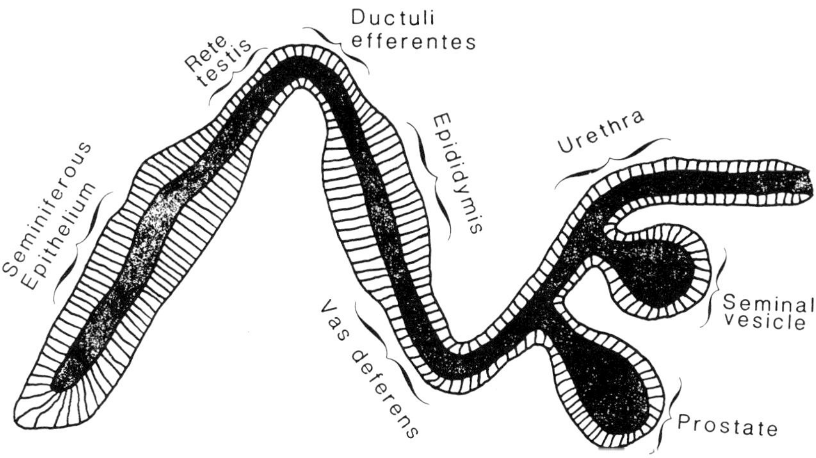

Fig. 2. Simplified outline of the male reproductive tract. The shaded area represents the lumen of the tract. Blood vessels, lymphatics, interstitial connective tissue, fibrocytes, lymphocytes, and macrophages are located outside the duct (not shown).

(AIDS). The men, most of whom were homosexuals, ranged in age from 22 to 48 years. Most of the men were not taking therapeutic drugs for their disease, nor were they drug addicts. At autopsy, the entire male reproductive tract was dissected and divided into the following parts: testis, epididymis (head, body, tail), vas deferens, prostate, and seminal vesicle. The tissue was fixed in 10% formalin and embedded in paraffin. In a number of patients, the tissue was prepared for electron microscopic examination. One millimeter cubes of tissue were prepared for each portion of the male reproductive tract and fixed in 2.5% paraformaldehyde in cacodylate buffer. After postfixation in osmium, the tissue was embedded in Epon.

Testis

Figure 3 illustrates the six stages of the cycle of the seminiferous epithelium in normal men. The seminiferous epithelium consists of two populations of cells, the tall columnar supporting elements, the Sertoli cells, and the more numerous differentiating elements, the germ cells. The various germ cell types (spermatogonia, spermatocytes, and spermatids) are easily distinguished in the seminiferous tubules of normal men. In addition, the tunica propria consists of several layers of contractile cells surrounding the seminiferous tubules. In a loose, connective tissue framework, the interstitial area of

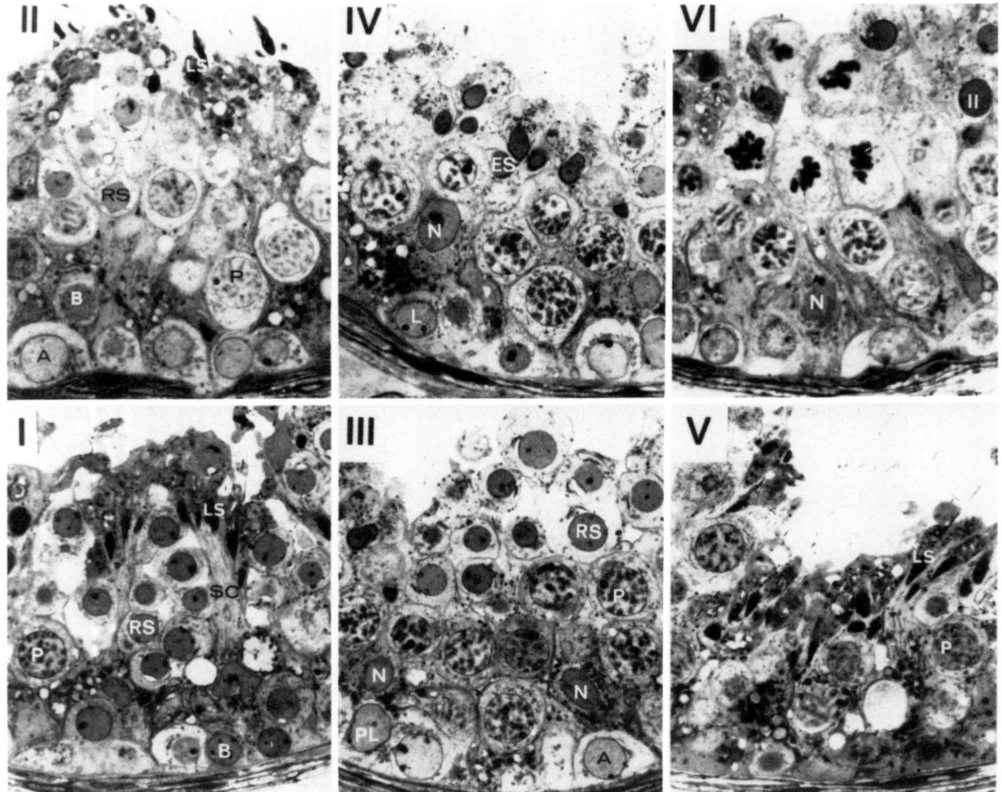
II
LS
RS
P
B
A
IV
ES
N
L
VI
II
N
Z
I
LS
SC
RS
P
B
III
RS
P
N
N
PL
A
V
LS
P

the testis contains the blood vessels, lymphatics, fibrocytes, macrophages, lymphocytes, mast cells, and Leydig cells.

In the testis of the AIDS patients that we examined, we noted only Sertoli cells, some spermatogonia, and other early germ cells in the seminiferous epithelium (Fig. 4). The lack of normal spermatogenesis in each patient was a surprisingly consistent result. Although the tunica propria of the seminiferous tubule appeared normal in most of the cases we examined, in several men there was the characteristic thickening (Fig. 4A) that is commonly present in a number of testicular disorders. There also appeared to be a modest increase in interstitial fibrosis in a number of cases, and in some of the men the Leydig cells appeared hypoplastic. The number of interstitial leukocytes did not appear to have increased, nor did we detect intraepithelial lymphocytes or macrophages in the seminiferous epithelium.

We also recently examined the testis of a 2-year-old boy who died of AIDS. Initial observations revealed an infiltration of small cells, apparently lymphocytes, in all areas of the testis (Fig. 5A). Testis tissue from a 2-year-old boy who died an accidental death (non-AIDS control) did not demonstrate a similar lymphocytic invasion (Fig. 5B).

Ductuli Efferents, Epididymis, Vas Deferens

The epididymis in men is a highly sinuous single tube, 4–5 m in length. The epithelium is pseudostratified and columnar and rests on a thin basement membrane deep to which is found smooth muscle cells, with the fibers oriented circularly. For descriptive purposes, the epididymis may be divided into three portions: the head, body, and tail. Sperm and fluid produced in the seminiferous tubules exit the testis via the rete testis, a collecting chamber lined with simple cuboidal epithelium at the posterior portion of the testis. From the rete, the sperm and fluid reach the epididymis through 10–15 ductuli efferentes. The vas deferens connects the epididymis to the prostatic urethra (Fig. 1). The ductuli efferentes, epididymis, and vas deferens in the AIDS patients appeared to be normal (Fig. 6). The pseudostratified columnar epithelium remained intact, and the intertubular connective tissue also appeared normal. Apparently, leukocytes did not infiltrate any part of the ductuli, epididymis, or vas.

Fig. 3. Testis from a normal man. The six stages of the cycle of the seminiferous epithelium are shown (I–VI). Note the tall columnar Sertoli cells (SC) and the various classes of germ cells. B, type B spermatogonium; P, pachytene spermatocyte; RS, round spermatid; LS, late spermatid; L, leptotene spermatocyte; N, Sertoli cell nucleus; ES, early spermatid; II, secondary spermatocyte; PL, preleptotene spermatocyte; Z, zygotene spermatocyte. ×900. Courtesy of A.F. Holstein.

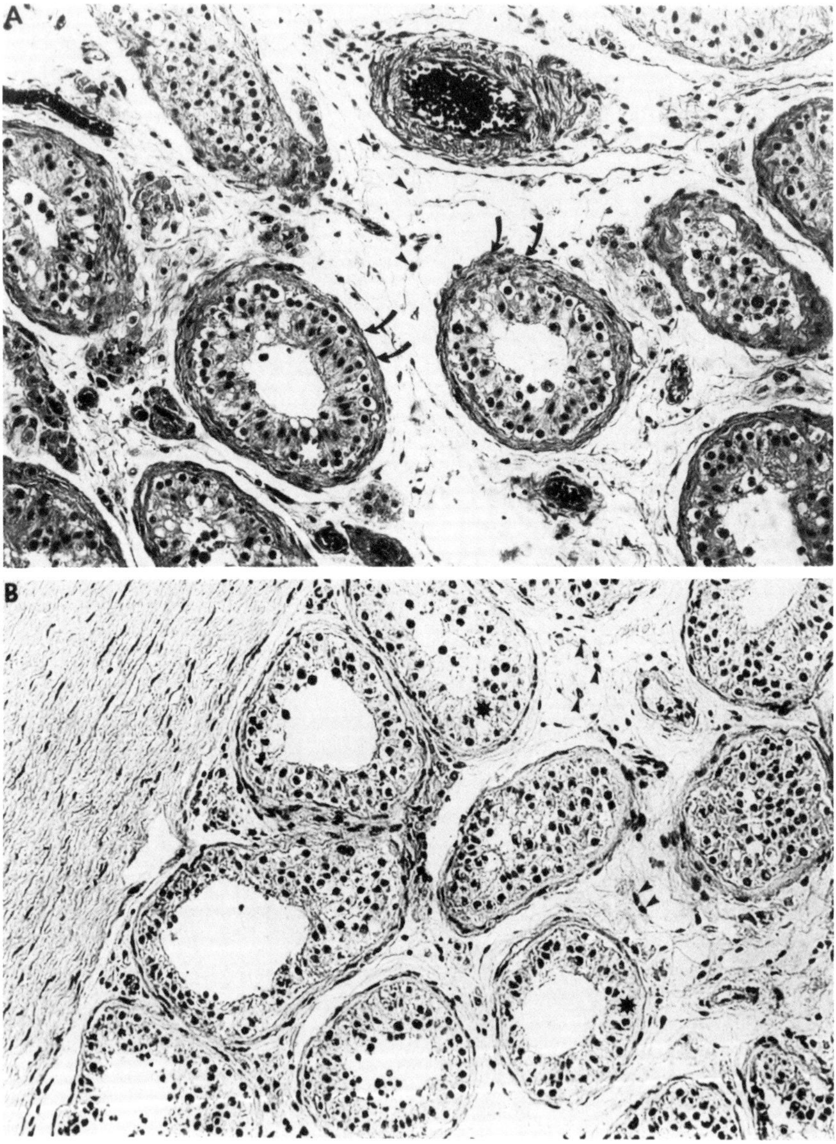

Fig. 4. **A–B:** Testis from an AIDS patient. The seminiferous epithelium (arrows) consists only of Sertoli cells and early germ cells (asterisks). There is a lack of normal spermatogenesis. Note the thickened basement membrane in A (arrows). The Leydig cells also appear to be hypoplastic (arrows). A, ×250. B, ×300.

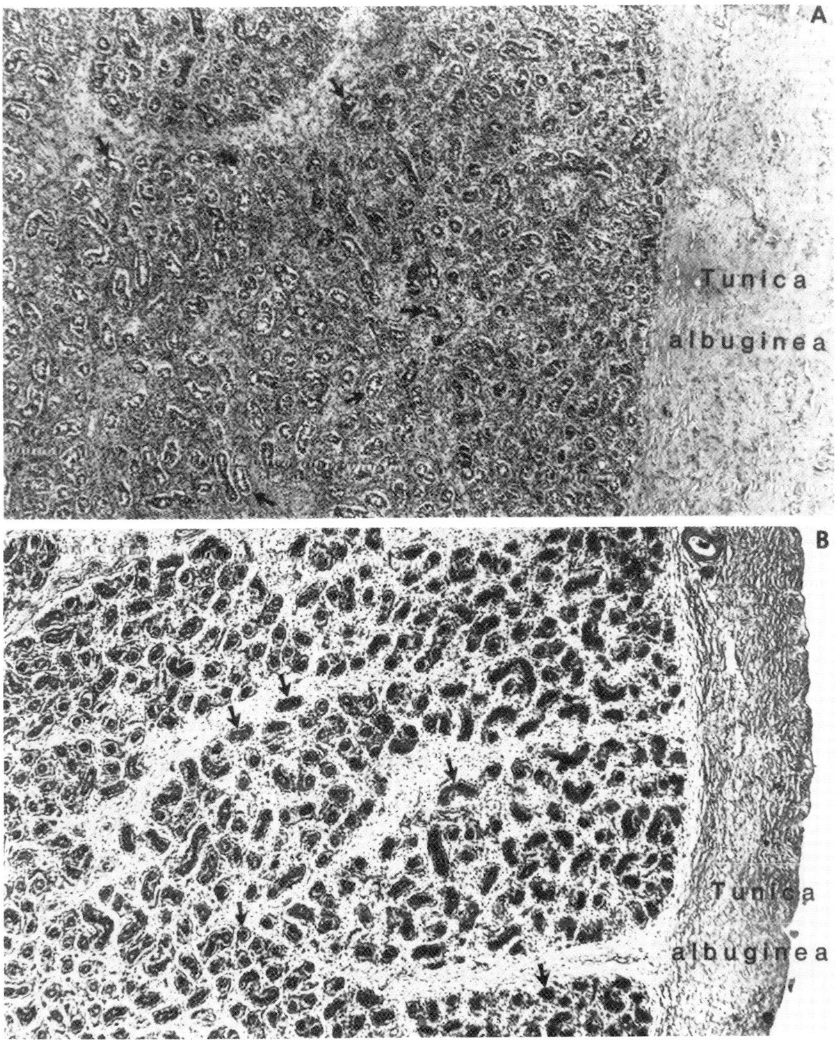

Fig. 5. **A:** Testis from a 2-year old boy who died of AIDS. The seminiferous tubules (cords) are indicated by arrows. Note the numerous small nuclei (black dots) between the cords. They are the apparent lymphocytes. **B:** Testis from a 2-year-old boy who died of an accidental death (non-AIDS control). The seminiferous cords are indicated by the arrows. Note the few cell between the cords compared to A. Both ×55.

Seminal Vesicles

The seminal vesicles are glandular outgrowths from the vas deferens distal to the ampulla at the posterior aspect of the bladder

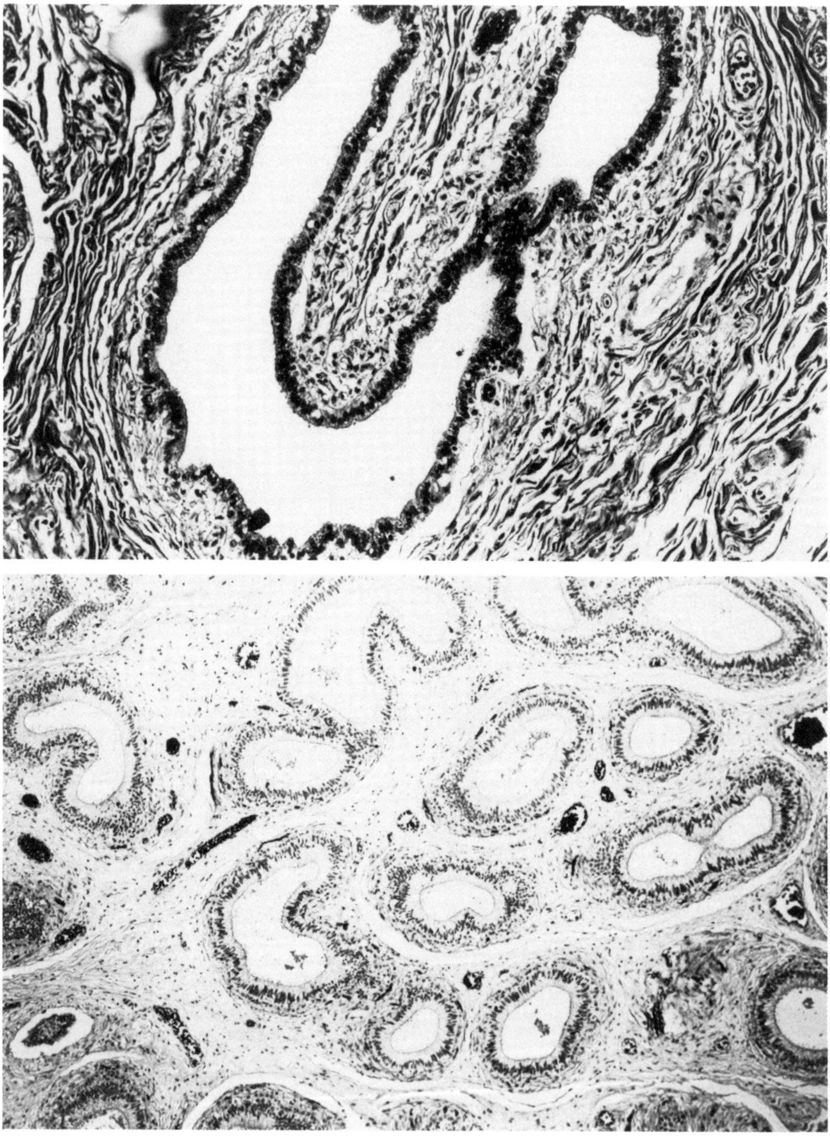

Fig. 6. Ductuli efferentes **(top)** and epididymis **(bottom)** from an AIDS patient. The epithelium and the intertubular tissue appear normal.

(Fig. 1). The proximal extremity of the seminal vesicle joins with the terminal portion of the vas deferens to form the ejaculatory duct, which empties into the prostatic urethra. The gland is lined by a pseudostratified columnar epithelium and its secretions form a substantial portion of the seminal fluid. We could not detect any abnormalities in the seminal vesicles in the AIDS patients.

Prostate

The prostate gland, like the seminal vesicle, is a major contributor to semen. The glandular epithelium is composed of simple cuboidal to pseudostratified columnar cells. In most of the men with AIDS whom we examined, the prostate appeared to be generally normal (Fig. 7). The tubule lumens were devoid of leukocytes, and the epithelium seemed to be intact and normal. In some of the men, the lumens of the gland and the duct system were filled with a very large number of cells (Fig. 8). These luminal cells seemed to be sloughed lining epithelial cells; in a few instances, there appeared to be an increase in the number of leukocytes in the lumen, similar to what is found in a prostatitis. In two of the patients, the lumens of the gland were filled with enormous eosinophilic, flocculent cells, with a frothy cytoplasm (Fig. 9). Many of the nuclei within the cells contained large inclusions, which were separated from the nuclear envelope by a halo. Cytoplasmic inclusions were also common in these cells. Collectively, these features are consistent with cytomegalovirus-infected cells.

DISCUSSION

As was pointed out by Henry [3], few publications have addressed the issue of where in the reproductive tract HIV enters the semen, nor has the structure of the male reproductive tract been described adequately in patients with AIDS, although two relevant abstracts have recently been published [4,5]. High numbers of unusual forms of germ cells have been found in semen obtained from AIDS patients at various stages of the disease (Anderson DJ, et al., personal communication). This observation alone strongly suggests that the presence of HIV in the male reproductive tract has a primary effect in the seminiferous epithelium. In this report, we show depleted seminiferous tubules containing only Sertoli cells and early germ cells, thus supporting this view. The abnormalities in the testis suggest that an early response to HIV may be a breakdown of the normal barriers in the seminiferous epithelium, allowing circulating virus to enter the seminal compartment. The tight junctions between Sertoli cells, which form the morphological basis of the blood–testis barrier [6], may become leaky, permitting viral entry. In accord with this hy-

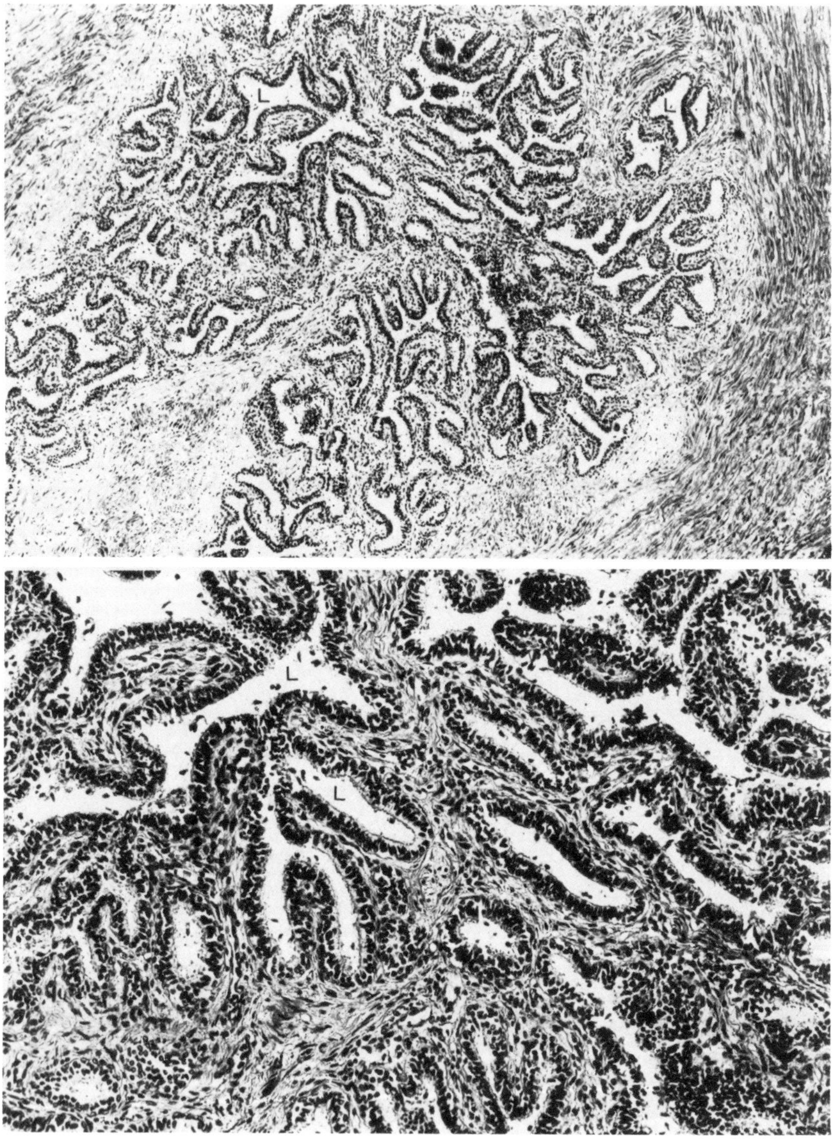

Fig. 7. Prostate gland from an AIDS patient. The epithelium and the intertubular tissue appear normal in about one-half the men whom we examined, as demonstrated in these two photographs. The lumina (L) of the glands and ducts appear empty, as in normal control prostates.

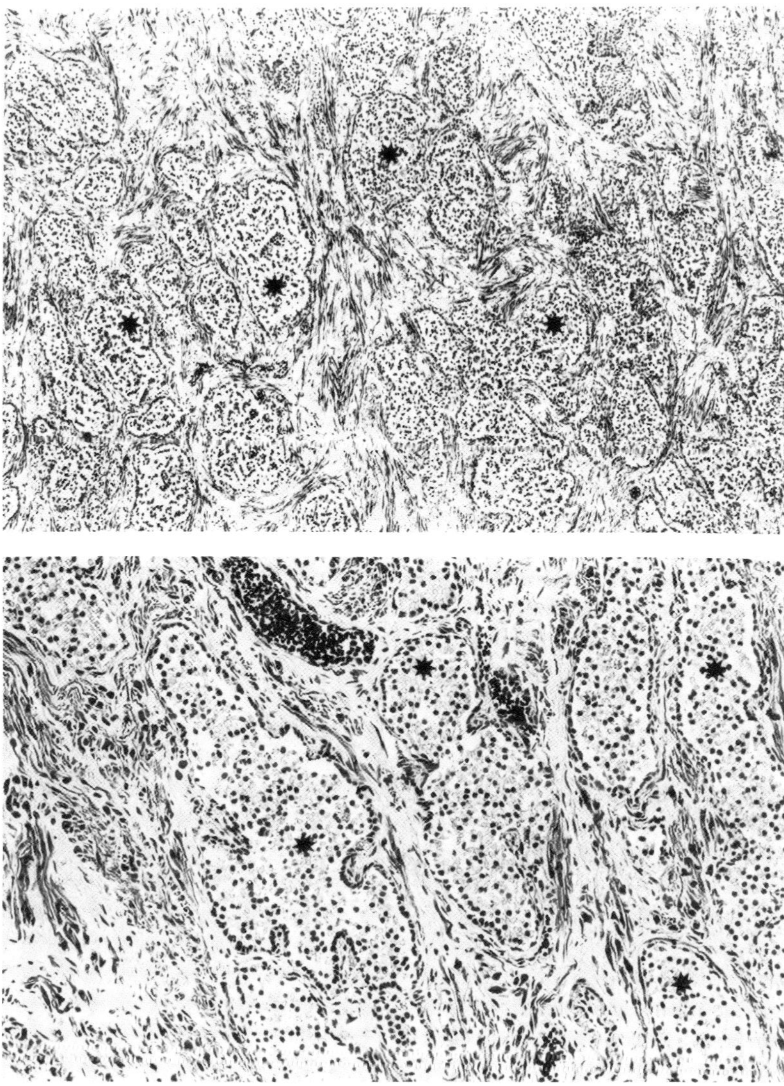

Fig. 8. Prostate gland from an AIDS patient. Numerous small cells are present in the lumen of the gland and ducts. Many of the cells look like sloughed epithelial cells. In some instances, lymphocytes were noted in the lumina, typical of prostatitis. A typical inflammatory response was not noted.

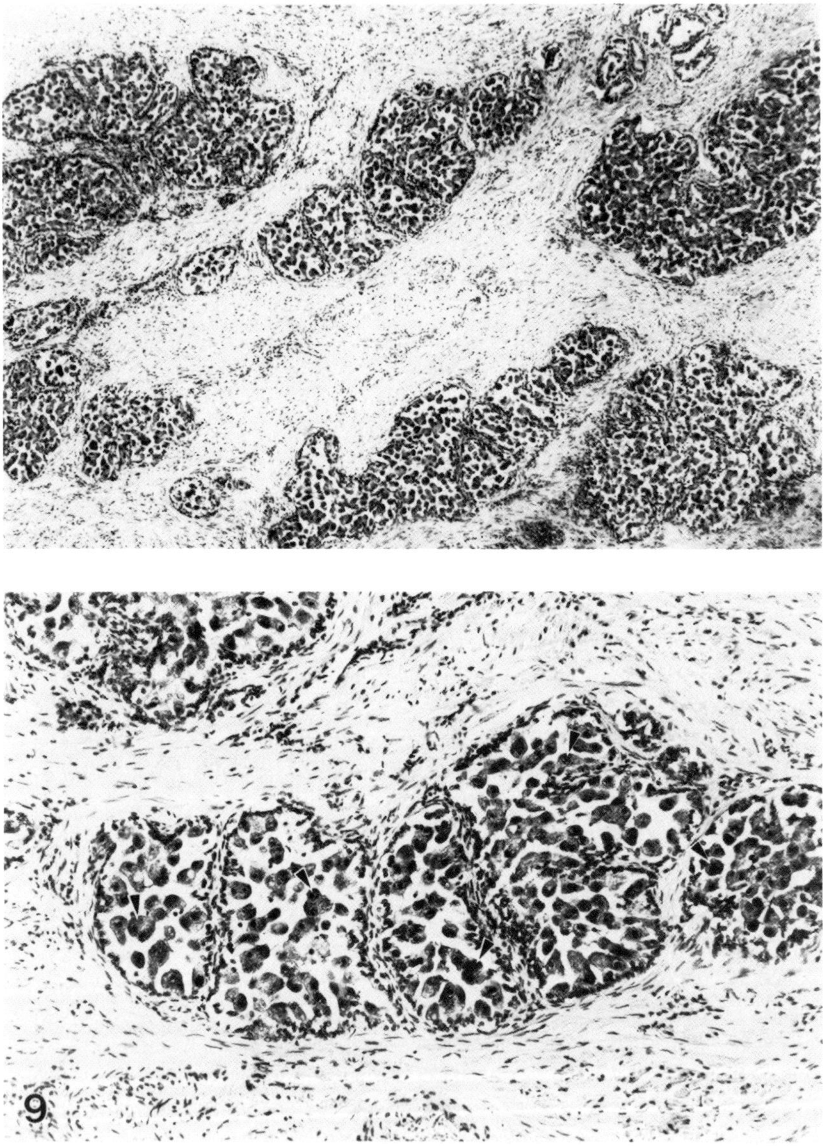

Fig. 9. We found numerous, very large eosinophilic-staining cells in the lumen of the prostate (arrowheads) in two patients. They resemble typical cytomegalovirus-infected cells.

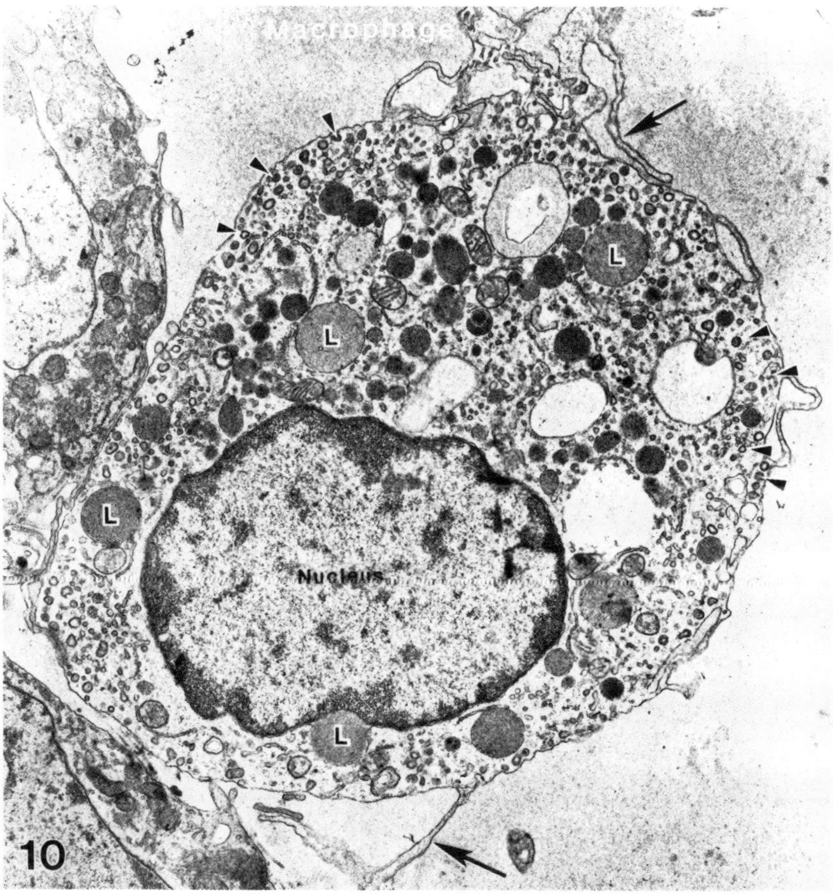

Fig. 10. Electron micrograph of a macrophage in the interstitial area of a normal human testis. Note the pseudopodia (arrows), lysosomes (L), and numerous small subsurface vesicles (arrowheads) typical of this cell type. ×4,765.

pothesis, Borzy and coauthors [7] recently demonstrated the presence of free virus in semen, although they suggested that epithelial cells of the epididymis may productively be infected with the virus and that budding of free virus into the lumen may occur.

An alternate hypothesis that remains to be tested is that CD4-positive lymphocytes transport the virus across the epithelium. Intraepithelial lymphocytes are generally located in most epithelia of the body, including the epididymis. Indeed, we and others have reported that a resident population of immunocompetent lymphocytes in the epididymis made up between 5% to 10% of the epithelial cells [6,8]. Macrophages are often found in the interstitial areas of the male reproductive tract (Fig. 10). This resident leukocyte population must be important in HIV transmission. Furthermore, lymphocytes including CD4-positive cells and macrophages are found in significant but variable numbers in semen from normal individuals; they may enter the seminal compartment through the epididymis (or in more proximal regions of the tract) [9–11], since the number of leukocytes in semen of vasectomized men is greatly reduced [12,13].

Knowledge of the precise site of entry of the virus into the male reproductive tract may be important in limiting the sexual spread of the disease. A vasectomy in patients with AIDS could help to limit the sexual spread of the disease if the virus enters the lumen of the male reproductive tract in regions that are proximal to the site of a vasectomy (i.e., in the seminiferous tubules, rete testis, ductuli efferentes, epididymis, or proximal vas deferens). However, if prostatitis develops, permitting leukocyte invasion into the prostate lumen, a vasectomy is not an option.

REFERENCES

1. **Dym M, Fawcett DW:** The blood-testis barrier in the rat and the physiological compartmentation of the seminiferous epithelium. Biol Reprod 3:308–326, 1970.

2. **Hoffer AP, Hinton BT:** Morphological evidence for blood-epididymis barrier and the effects of gossypol on its integrity. Biol Reprod 30:991–1004, 1984.

3. **Henry K:** Setting AIDS priorities: The need for a closer alliance of public health and clinical approaches toward the control of AIDS. Am J Public Health 78:1210–1212, 1988.

4. **Hilton MS, Fourcroy JL, Allen J, Amorosa JK:** J Androl 9:39, 1988 (Abstract).

5. **Lefrere JJ, Laplanche JL, Vittecoq D, et al.:** Hypogonadism in AIDS. AIDS 2:135–143, 1988.

6. **Dym M, Romrell LJ:** Intraepithelial lymphocytes in the male reproductive tract of rats and rhesus monkeys. J Reprod Fertil 42:1–7, 1975.

7. **Borzy MS, Connell RS, Kiessling AA:** Detection of human immunodeficiency virus in cell-free seminal fluid. J AIDS 1:1–6, 1989.

8. **Ritchie AWS, Hargreave TB, James K, Chisholm GD:** Intraepithelial lymphocytes in the normal epididymis. A mechanism for tolerance to sperm auto-antigens? Br J Urol 56:79–83, 1984.

9. **Taylor-Emery S, Battaile A, Anderson D:** An immunohistological study of lymphoid cells in the human male reproductive tract. J Reprod Immunol [Suppl]:71, 1986.

10. **Anderson DJ, Hill JA:** CD4 ($T4^+$) lymphocytes in semen of healthy heterosexual men: Implications for the transmission of AIDS. Fertil Steril 48:703, 1987.

11. **Wolff H, Anderson DJ:** Immunohistologic characterization and quantitation of leukocyte subpopulations in human semen. Fertil Steril 49:497–504, 1988.

12. **Olsen GP, Shields JW:** Seminal lymphocytes, plasma and AIDS. Nature 309:116–117, 1984.

13. **Anderson DJ, Wolff H, Zhang W, Pudney J:** Immunology of the male reproductive tract: Implications for the sexual transmission of human immunodeficiency virus. In Voeller B (ed): Fourth Kinsey Symposium on AIDS and Sex: An Integrated Biomedical and Behavioral Approach (in press).

14. **Dym M:** The male reproductive system. In Weiss L (ed): Cell and Tissue Biology: A Textbook of Histology, Sixth Edition. Urban and Schwarzenberg, 1988, pp 929–972.

DISCUSSION

DR. WITKIN: Are you saying that the major difference between HIV-positive and HIV-negative men is the absence of sperm in the tract?

DR. DYM: There is an absence of normal spermatogenesis. These men, who had frank AIDS, died of the disease. Obviously, in earlier stages, there were sperm. Yes, this is the only difference we have seen so far. We have not gone into detailed electron microscopic evaluation. So far, the only thing that we have seen is a major change in the seminiferous epithelium. I have to add, though, that I cannot say this is primary damage due to AIDS. It could be secondary to something else, but it is a fact that the seminiferous epithelium in these 25 men is abnormal.

DR. LAWRENCE: I am interested in the 2-year-old child you described who died of AIDS and had all those lymphocytes. In view of the fact that, essentially, this child would not have had a sexual disease, do you have any idea what chemoattractant may have brought those lymphocytes, which are probably already in scarce supply throughout the body, to such a specific place. Would you also speculate that either a microbial antigen or the derepression perhaps of an endogenous, normally tolerant antigen is the cause?

DR. DYM: There has been some interesting work from a group in Europe showing that the seminiferous epithelium actually produces a chemoattractant for lymphocytes, and it is possible that there is a barrier in the adult. Of course, this barrier develops at puberty. Sperm are foreign to the body; they will elicit an autoantigenic response. Normally, in a man, this forms a barrier to proteins and lymphocytes. The chemoattractant may well be present in a child when there is no barrier, so lymphocytes or macrophages come in. These are speculations.

We have tried a few experiments with dual compartment chambers, or bicameral culture chambers, where we have put Sertoli cells and epididymal cells on one side and added lymphocytes and/or macrophages on the other side, with or without a chemoattractant. We are trying to address the issue of lymphocyte transport across the epithelium with or without a chemoattractant.

DR. PUDNEY: I would like just to concur with your findings concerning the testes. I have looked at the testes of 33 deceased AIDS patients, and, regardless of age at death, duration of infection, or cause of death, the consistent finding is that they are azoospermic. I have also looked at the whole reproductive tract in four cadavers, including the rete testes, and again found no real evidence for any inflammatory response that could account for increased numbers of leukocytes probably in the semen. I have also looked at semen from HIV-seropositive donors, and I found a consistent pattern of gradually decreasing concentrations of spermatozoa down to a leukospermia, and maybe even azoospermia, with a concomitant increase in round cells. In four cases, the semen consisted of immature abnormal germ cells, anuclear cytopathic fragments, or a vast number of leukocytes, presumably lymphocytes and macrophages. There seems to be a trend about the time that overt AIDS symptoms appear. Among the four cases I looked at, three were symptomatic for AIDS. Somewhere in the progression of that disease there is a lesion either primarily in the testes or secondarily between the pituitary and gonadal axis that affects spermatogenesis. It would be of interest to look at endocrine profiles, testosterone levels, follicle-stimulating hormone (FSH), and luteinizing hormone (LH) in a longitudinal study of people who are HIV-positive. Perhaps one of these hormones could act as a marker for the progression of the disease. The consistent finding that these testes are azoospermic is indirect evidence against transmission of HIV by spermatozoa as a prime vector.

DR. JOHNSON: In view of the comment you made about vasectomy and where virus might enter the system, is there any work being done on the lymphocytosis and leukocyte counts of vasectomized and nonvasectomized men? Second, has anybody looked at viral isolation in vasectomized men who are HIV-positive?

DR. DYM: I should let Dr. Anderson answer that question because she has carried out work on vasectomized men.

DR. ANDERSON: We have not had any seropositive vasectomized men, but we have done a study on 18 vasectomized men, and in one case we found leukocytospermia. In every other case we found virtually no white cells, so we think that in uninfected individuals most of the white cells enter at the level of the epididymis, or at least upstream of the vasectomy site, but, in an occasional man, perhaps with prostatitis, you will find white cells in the semen.

16

Caveats Associated With Identifying HIV Using Transmission Electron Microscopy

Jeffrey Pudney

Transmission electron microscopy (TEM) has been used extensively for detecting the human immunodeficiency virus (HIV) in infected tissues [1,2]. However, problems associated with this procedure and with using morphological criteria alone to identify HIV limit the usefulness of TEM as a diagnostic tool for locating HIV in tissues without the use of other confirmatory tests. A major limitation inherent in TEM is the poor sampling size, which results from examining ultrathin sections (50–80 nm) that represent only a small fraction of the tissue specimen being analyzed. Sampling size is not a serious concern if the tissue is fairly homogeneous, since the sections will represent the total morphological appearance of the sample. However, sampling size is crucial when either the tissue is heterogeneous or small particles, such as HIV (100–120 nm), are sought in a tissue specimen, especially if they are scarce.

TEM, however, is widely and successfully used to confirm the presence of HIV in experimentally infected cell cultures [3,4]. Under these conditions, the abundance and characteristic appearance of HIV facilitate the recognition of viral particles. HIV is a retrovirus, consisting of an outer envelope (or caspid) and an elongated, centrally located electron-dense core (Fig. 1). This structural simplicity of HIV, however, can preclude its positive identification in sectioned tissue, due to the presence of a large array of structures that resemble viral particles in both size and appearance.

Heterosexual Transmission of AIDS, pages 197–204

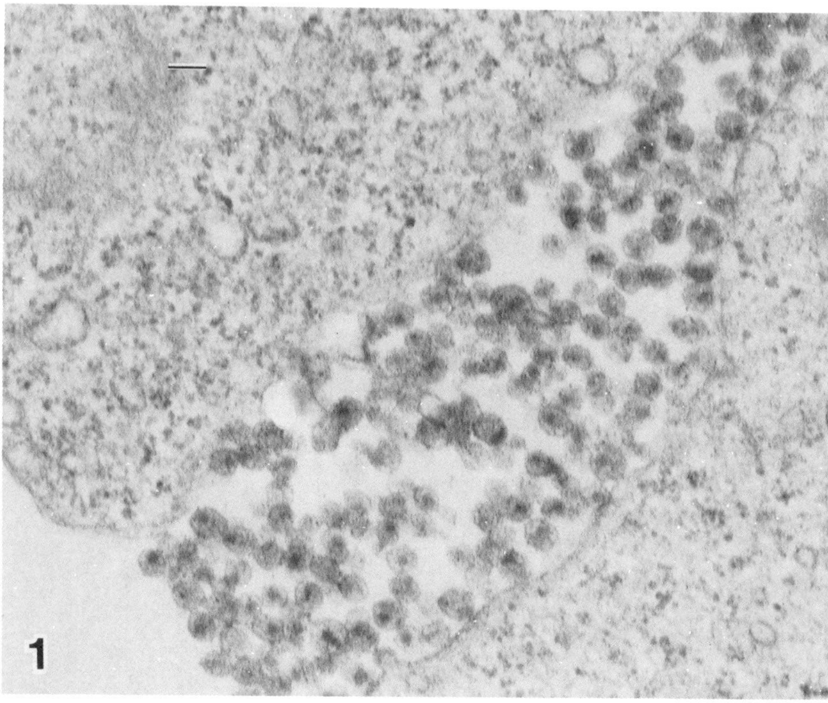

Fig. 1. HIV from an infected cell line showing, in sectioned tissue, the characteristic appearance of viral particles that consist of an outer envelope and inner electron-dense core. Bar = 100 nm. ×60,000.

Several recent publications have demonstrated the need for caution in relying on TEM alone to detect HIV in infected tissue. In one study, an ultrastructural analysis of lymph nodes from patients with acquired immune deficiency syndrome (AIDS)-related persistent generalized lymphadenopathy (PGL) and non-HIV-related reactive lymph nodes was carried out [5]. In both cases, TEM revealed the presence of viral particles that were morphologically indistinguishable from each other. However, when an immunocytochemical test was applied to these lymph nodes, using an antibody to the HIV core protein p24, HIV could be identified only in the PGL lymph nodes. The conclusion was that the viral particles seen in non-HIV-related reactive lymph nodes may represent a species of human endogenous retrovirus.

Two other reports describe the presence of HIV in semen. As yet, the mechanisms responsible for the sexual transmission of HIV have not been established. Which cell type acts as the primary host for HIV in seminal plasma is controversial. In one study, whole semen from HIV-seropositive donors was examined by TEM [6]. A micrograph was presented depicting a viral-like particle that was thought to be HIV. Although the size and structural appearance of this particle resembled those of HIV, immunocytochemical analysis for viral antigens specific for HIV was not carried out; therefore, positive identification of this structure was not possible. Semen from HIV-seropositive donors is usually obtained from persons who are also at risk for other viral infections. Cytomegalovirus, herpes simplex virus, hepatitis B virus, and possibly endogenous retrovirus, along with HIV, could all populate the semen from these donors [7]. In sectioned material, transverse profiles of these virions may appear so similar that they preclude exact identification based purely on their structural appearance. Since often no specialized morphological criteria distinguish viruses (particularly retroviruses) using routine TEM analysis, other techniques that demonstrate the presence of specific viral antigens (or viral RNA) are required before the presence of HIV can be confirmed in a tissue. Confirmation can be achieved by means of immunocytochemical procedures, using antibodies of proved specificity against HIV proteins (e.g., gp120) or using HIV-positive human sera followed by immunogold TEM (Fig. 2).

Another study adopted an in vitro approach and incubated spermatozoa (from HIV-seronegative donors) with cell-free HIV [8]. From TEM examination, data were presented purporting to show HIV not only bound to the plasma membrane of spermatozoa but also located within these cells. Unfortunately, the micrographs offered as evidence for these events were not convincing, since the particles portrayed did not resemble HIV. An electron-dense central core was not apparent in any sectioned profile of these structures, the presence of which would have identified them as HIV. Semen consists of a heterogeneous collection of cell types, many of which possess various granules and vacuoles (Fig. 3). As a result of physical or chemical trauma, these cells often are disrupted during the processing of semen for TEM. Specimen preparation liberates many membrane-bound structures into the seminal plasma. These granules and vacuoles could be mistaken for viral particles, particularly if they became associated with a putative cell host (e.g., spermatozoa) or a potential cell host (e.g., lymphocytes).

Spermatozoa have also been reported to contain HIV [8], a finding that is difficult to understand. HIV is a retrovirus; following binding to the host cell surface, viral RNA enters the cell, where it is converted to viral DNA that is integrated into the host cell genome. Viral copies are then produced that are secreted by a process of budding from the host cell membrane. Therefore, how fully assem-

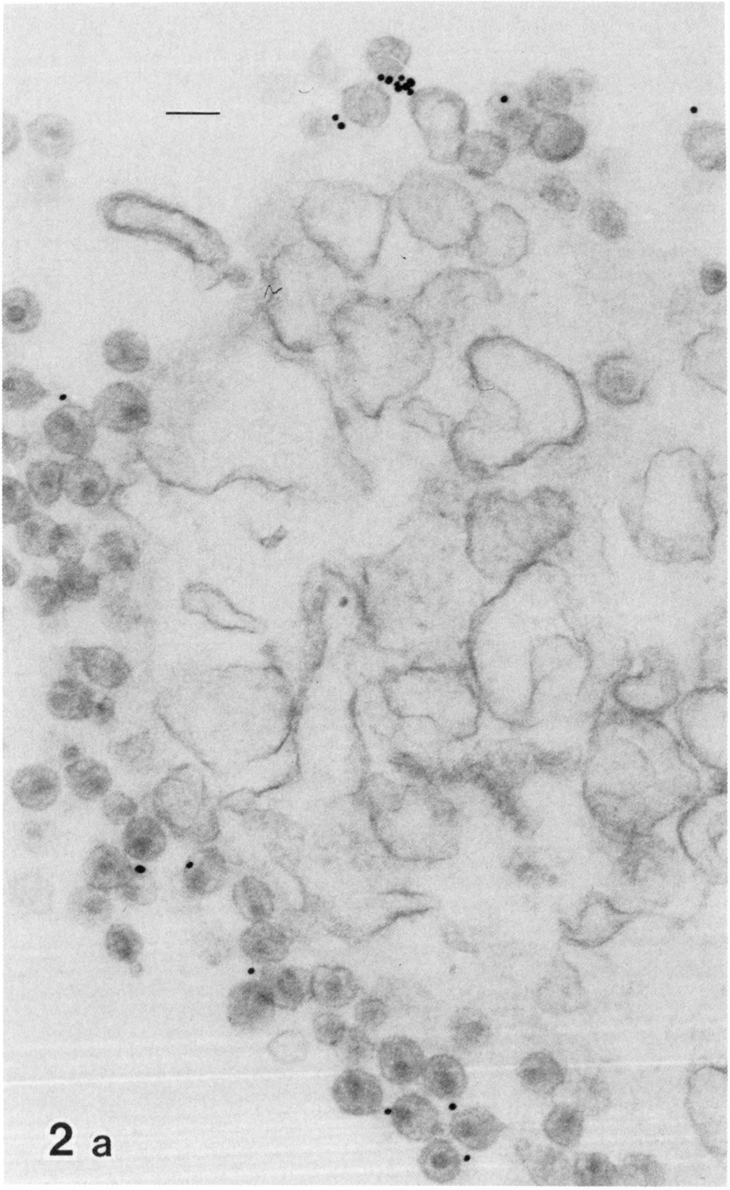

Fig. 2. Immunocytochemical detection of HIV in an infected cell line using a monoclonal antibody directed against gp120, followed by GAM-IgG linked to colloidal gold 15 nm in diameter **(a)** and HIV-positive human sera followed by GAH-IgG linked to colloidal gold 5 nm in diameter **(b).** Unstained sections. Bar = 100 nm. a, ×70,000. b, ×84,000.

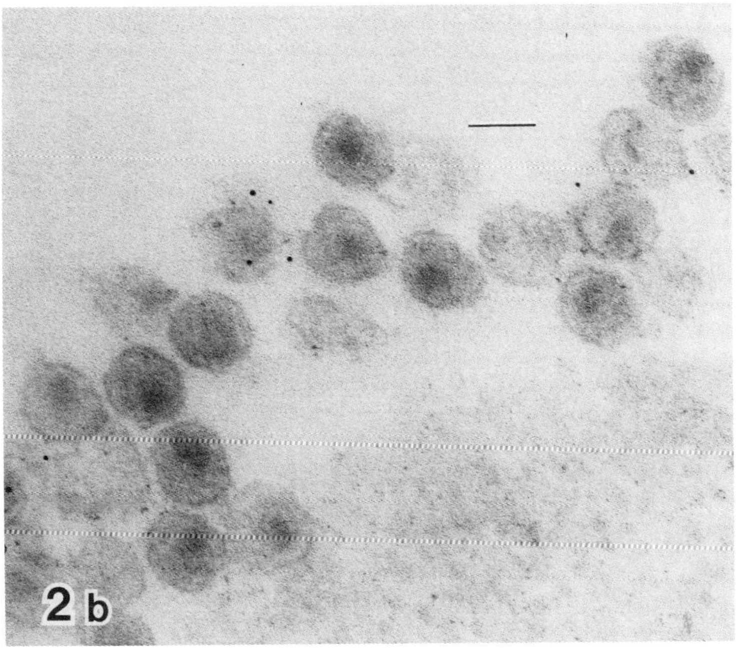

Fig. 2b.

bled HIV could exist in the cytoplasm of spermatozoa is inexplicable. Mechanisms of entry that could involve uptake of whole HIV, such as receptor-mediated endocytosis or phagocytosis, are not processes carried out by mature spermatozoa. The cytoplasmic assembly of HIV within host cells has not been documented [9,10]. A more likely explanation of these findings is that the particles assumed to be HIV actually represented either granules resulting from an incipient acrosome reaction (Fig. 4a,b) or one of the several structures, variously called "scattered densities" or "fibrillar structures," located between the nucleus and the acrosome of human spermatozoa [11]. Furthermore, the genome of mature spermatozoa is composed of highly condensed chromatin, capable of limited, if any, transcriptional activity. Therefore, it is unlikely that HIV DNA could be integrated into the DNA of spermatozoa, let alone undergo transcription for the viral proteins and RNA needed to synthesize whole viral particles.

Which cell types host HIV in infected semen is an important and

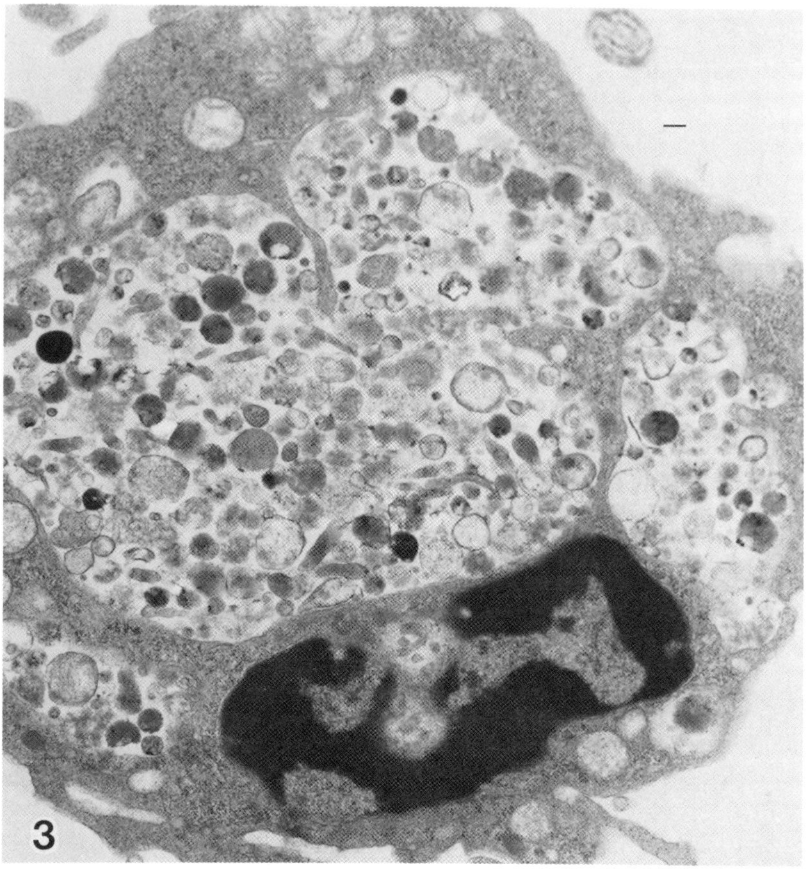

Fig. 3. Round cell (possibly granulocyte) containing many vacuoles and membrane-bound granules observed in semen from an HIV-seronegative donor. From their size and appearance, these structures could be mistaken for viral particles if they were released, due to disruption of this cell, into the seminal plasma. Bar = 160 nm. ×20,000.

controversial issue that could affect the management of acquired immune deficiency syndrome (AIDS) and the prevention of the sexual transmission of HIV. Any pronouncement about the cellular mechanisms involved in the sexual transmission of HIV should therefore be supported by irrefutable data. This caution is especially important if the findings rely on TEM as the sole means of analysis, since the positive identification of HIV in infected tissue can be extremely difficult and can lead to erroneous conclusions if unconfirmed by other analytical methods.

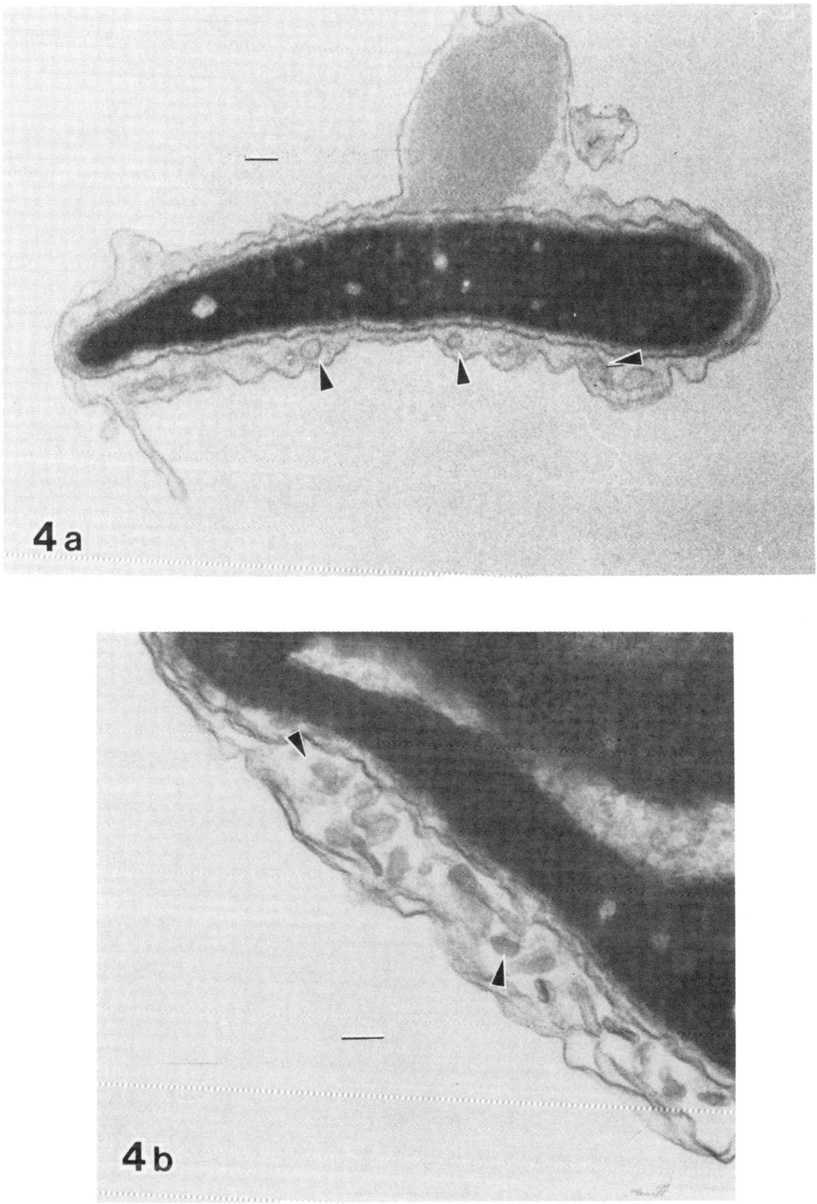

Fig. 4. Spermatozoa from HIV-seronegative donors. Granules and vacuoles (arrowheads) in these cells could be mistaken for HIV. These structures probably result from the acrosome reaction occurring in these spermatozoa. Bar = 100 nm. a, ×40,000. b, ×72,000.

ACKNOWLEDGMENTS

This work was supported by contract CSA-88-020 from the Contraceptive Research and Development (CONRAD) Program, Eastern Virginia Medical School, under a cooperative agreement with the United States Agency of International Development (U.S.A.I.D.), which in turn receives funds for AIDS research from an interagency agreement with the National Institute of Child Health and Human Development (NICHD). The views expressed by the authors do not necessarily reflect the views of U.S.A.I.D. or CONRAD.

REFERENCES

1. **Sharer IR, Cho E-S, Epstein LG:** Multinucleated giant cells and HTLV-III in AIDS encephalopathy. Hum Pathol 16:760, 1985.

2. **Wiley CA, Schrier RD, Nelson JA:** Cellular localization of human immunodeficiency virus infection within the brains of acquired immune deficiency syndrome patients. Proc Natl Acad Sci USA 83:7089, 1986.

3. **Popovic M, Sarngadharan MG, Read E, Gallo RC:** Detection, isolation, and continuous production of cytopathic retroviruses (HTLV-III) from patients with AIDS and pre-AIDS. Science 224:497, 1984.

4. **Orenstein JM, Meltzer MS, Phipps T, Gendelman HE:** Cytoplasmic assembly and accumulation of human immunodeficiency virus Types 1 and 2 in recombinant human colony-stimulating factor-1-treated human monocytes: An ultrastructural study. J Virol 62:2578, 1988.

5. **O'Hara JC, Groopman JE, Federman M:** The ultrastructural and immunocytochemical demonstration of viral particles in lymph nodes from human immunodeficiency virus-related and non-human immunodeficiency virus-related lymphadenopathy syndromes. Hum Pathol 19:545, 1988.

6. **Borzy MS, Connell RS, Kiessling A:** Detection of human immunodeficiency virus in cell-free seminal fluid. J AIDS 1:419, 1988.

7. **Greenblatt RM, Handsfield HH, Sayers MH, Holmes KK:** Screening therapeutic insemination donors for sexually transmitted diseases: Overview and recommendations. Fertil Steril 46:351, 1986.

8. **Bagasra O, Freund M, Weidman J, Harley G:** Interaction of human immunodeficiency virus with human sperm in vitro. J AIDS 1:431, 1988.

9. **Hoxie JA, Haggerty BS, Rackowski JL, Pilsbury N, Levy JA:** Persistent noncytopathic infection of normal human T lymphocytes with AIDS-associated retrovirus. Science 229: 1400, 1985.

10. **Palmer E, Sporborg C, Harrison A, Martin ML, Feorino P:** Morphology and immunoelectron microscopy of AIDS virus. Arch Virol 85:189, 1985.

11. **Bernstein MH, Teichman RJ:** Regional differentiation in the heads of spermatozoa of rabbit, man and bull. Am J Anat 133:165, 1972.

17

Sensitization to Sperm as a Risk Factor for the Heterosexual Transmission of HIV

Steven S. Witkin

The human immunodeficiency virus (HIV), the causative agent of acquired immune deficiency syndrome (AIDS), is transmitted by sexual contact or by exposure to infected blood or blood products. The heterosexual transmission of HIV by coitus is apparently much more efficient from man to woman than from woman to man. Undoubtedly, this difference is due to the unilateral (male-to-female) transfer of ejaculated fluids. However, the cofactors in the semen donor or in the female recipient that influence the probability that an HIV-negative woman will become infected with the virus following coitus with an HIV-positive man remain largely unknown.

To address this issue, a study of 110 female drug abusers in New York City, many of whom were prostitutes or exchanged sex for drugs, was initiated [1]. All women reported a large number of lifetime sexual partners and, not surprisingly, 32 (29.1%) of them had circulating IgG antibodies to sperm. Women with antisperm antibodies were significantly more likely ($P = 0.002$) to be HIV antibody-positive than were women without antisperm antibodies. This association was unrelated to the number of lifetime sexual contacts. The data suggested that women who were sensitized to sperm might be at increased risk for acquiring a productive HIV infection following coitus with an HIV-infected man.

HIV infects and proliferates in T-helper/inducer (CD4) lymphocytes only if the lymphocytes are in an activated state. Both sperm

Heterosexual Transmission of AIDS, pages 205–211

TABLE 1. Immunosuppressive Effect of Human Sperm on Autologous and Allogeneic Lymphocyte Proliferation[a]

	Percentage control proliferation	
Sperm ($\times 10^5$)	Autologous	Allogeneic
20	5.9	1.4
10	3.0	5.9
5	5.4	39.5
2	71.1	45.8
1	54.0	44.8

[a]Peripheral blood mononuclear cells were incubated in antigenic fetal bovine serum in the presence or absence of autologous or allogeneic sperm. Lymphocyte proliferation was measured after 7 days by ^{3}H-thymidine incorporation. Isotope incorporation in the absence of sperm was 13,648 cpm.

and seminal plasma are immunosuppressive and, under normal circumstances, inhibit lymphocyte activation. Thus target cells in the female genital tract that are susceptible to infection by HIV are probably in short supply following coitus. Similarly, the ability of HIV-infected male genital tract-derived cells to proliferate and release infectious virus in the female would be severely restricted. Replication of HIV in mononuclear cells is actively inhibited by T-suppressor cells [2].

EFFECT OF ANTISPERM ANTIBODIES ON THE CELLULAR IMMUNE RESPONSE TO SPERM

Human sperm lack major histocompatibility antigens [3] and do not activate autologous lymphocytes in vitro [4]. As has been shown with mouse [5,6] and rabbit [7] sperm, human sperm are highly immunosuppressive for allogeneic and autologous lymphocyte proliferation (Table 1). Although the exact mechanism of sperm-induced immunosuppression is unclear, the increased inhibition of sperm-induced lymphocyte proliferation in direct proportion to the sperm concentration strongly suggests the activation of suppressor cells by sperm. The absence of antibodies to sperm surface antigens in most sexually active women attests to the effectiveness of this suppression. Circulating antisperm antibodies in a woman may, therefore, indicate altered or defective immunosuppression in her genital tract. This could be due to a concurrent infection, a genetic predisposition, or an inability of semen from the specific male partner to activate the female's suppressor cells to inhibit CD4 lymphocyte stimulation. Antisperm antibodies may also be a marker for ineffective immunosup-

TABLE 2. Inhibition of Allogeneic Lymphocyte Proliferation by Sperm With and Without Bound Antibodies[a]

	Percentage control proliferation	
Sperm ($\times 10^5$)	Antibody-bound	Antibody-free
20	16.7	2.1
10	47.2	7.2
5	241.2	56.4
2	248.5	76.2
1	274.9	86.9

[a]Peripheral blood mononuclear cells were incubated with autologous antibody-bound or antibody-free sperm, and lymphocyte proliferation was determined as described for Table 1.

pression in pregnant women, resulting in a high incidence of recurrent spontaneous abortions [8].

Antibodies bind to the sperm surface in men and women sensitized to sperm. This binding drastically alters the sperm's immunosuppressive properties. Sperm with bound antibodies are potent interferon-gamma (IFNγ) inducers [9] and are much less effective in inhibiting lymphocyte proliferative responses (Table 2). These aberrant responses are demonstrable in vitro using lymphocytes from individuals not previously sensitized to sperm. In sensitized women positive for IgG antisperm antibodies, incubation of their lymphocytes with sperm induces the production of IFNγ (Table 3). Thus coitus in situations in which either partner is sensitized to sperm could lead to CD4 lymphocyte activation in the female genital tract. If HIV or HIV-infected cells were also present in the semen, the increased number of target cells in the female would increase the probability of viral infection. IFNγ would also be expected to block immunosuppression and promote proliferation of both semen-derived and female-derived CD4 lymphocytes.

HIV TARGET CELLS IN SEMEN

The typical human ejaculate contains about 10^3–10^4 mononuclear lymphoid cells [9,10]. In semen from most men, T-suppressor/cytotoxic (CD8) lymphocytes predominate over CD4 cells [10,11]. A similar situation occurs in the rete testis, epididymis, and vas deferens [12], suggesting that a state of immunosuppression usually exists in the male genital tract. This state, undoubtedly, inhibits the immune response to autoantigenic sperm surface components.

Antisperm antibodies in men probably arise as a consequence of

TABLE 3. Effect of Prior Sensitization to Sperm on Sperm-Induced IFNγ Production[a]

Lymphocyte donor	Antisperm antibodies	IFNγ (V/ml)
LI	IgG, IgA, IgM	5.0
GR	IgG, IgA	2.0
BI	IgG, IgM	2.0
BU	IgG, IgA	1.5
IM	IgA	0
KA	IgA	0
DI	IgA	0
JA	—	0

[a]Peripheral blood mononuclear cells from women with or without circulating antisperm antibodies were incubated with purified motile sperm for 24 hr at 37°C. Culture supernatants were collected and assayed for IFNγ using a commercial ELISA kit.

increased permeability of the genital tract. This leakage can be due to infection, inflammation, or trauma. The presence in the ejaculate of sperm with bound antibodies is, thus, a marker for male genital tract damage. Genital tract damage also appears to alter the regulatory mechanism that favors CD8 lymphocyte predominance in the tract. In men with antibodies on their sperm, a selective loss of CD8 cells from the semen results in a predominance of CD4 lymphocytes in the ejaculate [11]. Since HIV appears to be sexually transmitted primarily via virus-infected CD4 cells [13], and CD8 lymphocytes suppress HIV production [2], men with antisperm antibodies would transmit more potentially infected CD4 cells to the female partner than would men without antisperm antibodies.

In addition, some men with antibodies on their sperm, but not men with antibody-free sperm, have detectable levels of IFNγ in their semen (Table 4). As described above, this can further promote CD4 lymphocyte activation in the woman exposed to such semen.

SENSITIZATION TO SPERM IN GROUPS AT HIGH RISK FOR AIDS VIA SEXUAL TRANSMISSION

Groups at high risk for contracting AIDS by sexual contact also have a high incidence of antisperm antibodies. A high percentage of homosexual men have antisperm antibodies [14]. These antibodies are readily induced in rabbits by the atraumatic and nonabrasive deposition of semen into their rectums [8]. Antisperm antibodies are also common in female prostitutes [1], possibly due to anal intercourse and to the high incidence of sexually transmitted diseases

TABLE 4. Relation Between IFNγ in Seminal Fluid and Antibodies on Ejaculated Sperm[a]

Patient	Sperm-bound antibodies	IFNγ (V/ml)
649	IgG	12.2
547	IgA	8.5
543	IgG, IgA	7.3
573	IgG, IgA	7.3
605	IgA	3.5
4 Men	IgG, IgA	0
7 Men	—	0

[a]Cell-free seminal fluids from men with and without antibodies on the surface of their ejaculated sperm were assayed for IFNγ as described for Table 3.

(STDs) in this group. The incidence of STDs in male homosexuals also is very high. The presence of an STD has been shown to be a cofactor in the heterosexual transmission of HIV in Africa [15]. To our knowledge, the incidence of antisperm antibodies in this African population has not been evaluated, but it would be expected to be elevated. The lesions in the genital tract induced by STDs can increase genital proliferation and shedding of HIV particles and increase susceptibility to HIV infection.

Thus antisperm antibodies may be a marker for factors increasing the efficiency of HIV sexual transmission. These antibodies may themselves be a factor enhancing the transmission of HIV via coitus. Both infectivity by the male donor and susceptibility of the semen recipient would be increased when the man is sensitized to sperm. Antisperm antibodies in the semen recipient similarly would increase the probability for infection following contact with HIV-infected semen.

The possibility exists that antisperm antibody formation is a consequence of AIDS and not a predisposing factor. HIV is a polyclonal B lymphocyte activator [16] and may induce the production of antibodies that are cross reactive with sperm. Similarly, the disordered immune regulation that is an early consequence of HIV infection may overwhelm sperm-associated immunosuppression and evoke a productive immune response to sperm-specific antigens. Even if sensitization to sperm occurs only after HIV infections, a highly implausible occurrence, each subsequent exposure to semen would still further activate CD4 lymphocytes in the female genital tract and foster further proliferation of the virus.

A proposed mechanism of antisperm antibody-mediated male-to-

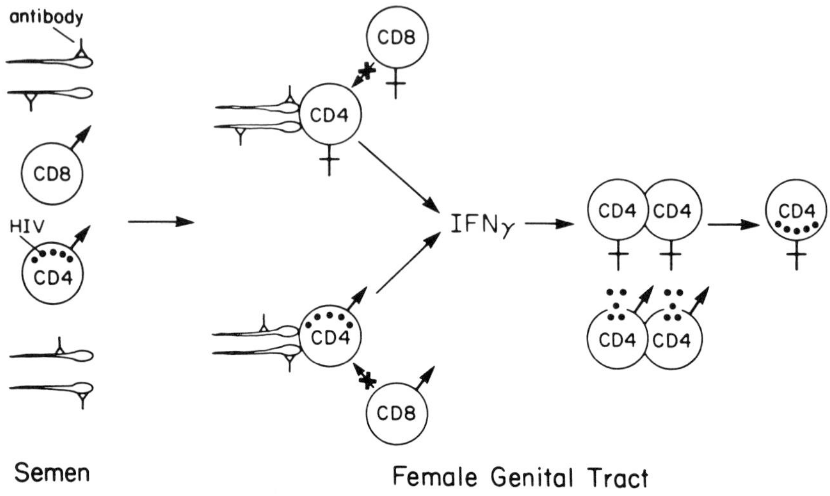

Fig. 1. Effect of sperm with bound antibodies on the male-to-female sexual transmission of HIV.

female sexual transmission of HIV is shown in Figure 1. Semen from an HIV-infected man contains CD4 lymphocytes with internalized HIV as well as CD8 lymphocytes and sperm with antibodies bound to its surface. After being ejaculated into the vagina, antibody-bound sperm activate both male-derived and female-derived CD4 cells to produce IFNγ and to proliferate. In contrast, sperm without bound antibodies react only with CD8 cells and inhibit CD4 proliferation. HIV replicates in the proliferating male CD4 lymphocytes, and infectious virus is released from the cell. Ia antigens, expressed on the surface of replicating female CD4 cells, react with the released HIV, and these cells become infected with the virus. A similar mechanism would occur if the woman was sensitized to sperm and antibodies attached to the sperm after ejaculation or if free IFN was present in the semen.

ACKNOWLEDGMENTS

Studies from the author's laboratory were supported by National Institutes of Health (NIH) grant HD-21909. The outstanding technical assistance of Jan Jeremias is gratefully acknowledged.

REFERENCES

1. **Wallace JI, Beatrice S, Bekes JG, et al.:** The risk of HIV infection in former intravenous drug-abusing women. In Schinazi RF, Mahmias AJ (eds): AIDS in Children, Adolescents, and Heterosexual Adults. New York: Elsevier, 1988, pp 202–206.

2. **Walker CM, Moody DJ, Stites DP, Levy JA:** CD8$^+$ lymphocytes can control HIV infection in vitro by suppressing virus replication. Science 234:1563–1566, 1986.

3. **Anderson DJ, Bach DL, Yunis EJ, Dewolf WC:** Major histocompatibility antigens are not expressed on human epididymal sperm. J Immunol 129:452–454, 1982.

4. **Witkin SS:** Production of interferon gamma by lymphocytes exposed to antibody-coated sperm: A mechanism for sperm antibody production in females. Fertil Steril 50: 498–502, 1988.

5. **Hurtenbach U, Morgenstern, Bennett D:** Induction of tolerance in vitro by autologous murine testicular cells. J Exp Med 151:827–838, 1980.

6. **Hurtenbach U, Shearer GM:** Germ cell-induced immune suppression in mice. Effect of inoculation of syngeneic spermatozoa on cell-mediated immune responses. J Exp Med 155:1719–1729, 1982.

7. **Richards JM, Bedford JM, Witkin SS:** Rectal insemination modifies immune responses in rabbits. Science 224:390–392, 1984.

8. **Haas GG Jr, Kuboto K, Quebbeman JF, Jijon A, Menge AC, Beer AE:** Circulating antisperm antibodies in recurrently aborting women. Fertil Steril 45:209–215, 1986.

9. **Wolff H, Anderson DJ:** Immunohistologic characterization and quantitation of leukocyte subpopulations in human semen. Fertil Steril 49:497–504, 1988.

10. **Witkin SS:** Mechanisms of active suppression of the immune response to spermatozoa. Am J Reprod Immunol Microbiol 17:61–64, 1988.

11. **Witkin SS, Goldstein M:** Reduced levels of T suppressor/cytotoxic lymphocytes in semen from vasovasostomized men: Relationship to sperm autoantibodies. J Reprod Immunol 14:283–290, 1988.

12. **El-Demiry M, James K:** Lymphocyte subsets and macrophages in the male genital tract in health and disease. A monoclonal antibody-based study. Eur J Urol 14:226–235, 1988.

13. **Levy JA:** The transmission of AIDS: The case of the infected cell. JAMA 259:3037–3038, 1988.

14. **Witkin SS, Sonnabend J:** Immune responses to sperm in homosexual men. Fertil Steril 39:337–342, 1983.

15. **Padian NS:** Heterosexual transmission of acquired immunodeficiency syndrome: International perspectives and national projections. Rev Infect Dis 9:947–960, 1987

16. **Pahwa S, Pahwa R, Good RA, Gallo RC, Saxinger C:** Stimulatory and inhibitory influences of human immunodeficiency virus on normal B lymphocytes. Proc Natl Acad Sci USA 83:9124–9128, 1986.

18

Presence of HIV in Cervical and Vaginal Secretions

Gerald S. Bernstein

Individuals infected with the human immunodeficiency virus (HIV) can demonstrate virus in various body fluids, including blood, genital secretions, saliva, tears, cerebral spinal fluid, and milk. Since HIV can be acquired through sexual transmission, the presence of virus in the male and female genital tracts and the factors that influence virus shedding are important in understanding and preventing this mode of transmission.

RESULTS OF STUDIES

The passage of HIV through intercourse between an infected woman and a noninfected man depends, at least in part, on the presence of virus in the vagina and cervix. This chapter summarizes research findings on the presence of HIV in the lower female genital tract.

In 1986, two groups of investigators reported the results of their studies of HIV in the genital tracts of seropositive women [1,2]. Vogt and coauthors [1] studied 14 women, 11 of whom were intravenous drug users and three of whom were partners of high-risk men. Three subjects were healthy; the remaining subjects had acquired immune deficiency syndrome (AIDS)-related complex (ARC) or persistent generalized lymphadenopathy. The investigators obtained cervical mucus by inserting a cotton swab or a glass rod into the endocervical canal. Collection was made between days 7 and 21 of the menstrual cycle to avoid contamination with blood. On microscopic examination, the mucus did not contain any spermatozoa or blood. In all but one case, blood also was collected at the time the cervix was sam-

Heterosexual Transmission of AIDS, pages 213–224

TABLE 1. Prevalance of HIV in Seropositive Women

Study	Genital (%)	Blood (%)
Vogt et al. [1]	4/14 (28.6)	7/13 (53.8)
Wofsy et al. [2]	4/8 (50.0)	7/8 (87.5)

pled. The cervical material was tested for HIV in lymphocyte culture, and the supernatant was analyzed for reverse transcriptase (RT) activity. Positive cultures were confirmed by HIV antigen expression on immunofluorescence.

HIV was detected in four of 14 (28.6%) cervical samplings and in seven of 13 (53.8%) blood specimens (Table 1). All women with positive cervical mucus had positive blood cultures, but some subjects had positive blood and negative cervical mucus (Table 2).

Four of the women were pregnant, and two of them had HIV in their cervical mucus and peripheral leukocytes. One pregnant woman was negative for virus at both sites; the fourth had negative cervical mucus but did not have her blood tested. Vogt et al. [1] suggested that the virus was cell-associated because, when mucus from one patient was passed through a 0.45 μm filter prior to culture, the filtrate was negative, whereas the retained fraction contained HIV.

Wofsy and coworkers [2] evaluated eight seropositive women who were intravenous drug users or sexual contacts of men at high risk of being infected with HIV or both. Six of the subjects had lymphadenopathy and two had other symptoms of infection. Material was collected by swabbing the vagina with cotton and by scraping the exocervix and lower cervical canal with a wooden spatula ordinarily used to collect cells for cervical cytology. Collections were made at random times during the menstrual cycle.

The samples were clarified by centrifugation, and in some cases both the supernatant and cellular fractions were evaluated for HIV by means of lymphocyte culture and determination of RT activity. Positive tests were confirmed by an immunofluorescence assay. Peripheral mononuclear cells from each subject were also cultured for HIV.

Virus was isolated from peripheral leukocytes of seven of the eight women, and HIV was recovered from the vaginal or cervical fluids of four (Table 1). The vaginal and cervical collections could not be compared directly because not all subjects were sampled at both sites. As in the Vogt et al. study, women with positive genital samples also had HIV present in peripheral leukocytes (Table 2).

Virus was not positively identified in the first genital sample of one

TABLE 2. Pattern of HIV Detection in Female Genital Secretions and Blood From Seropositive Women

Study	No. of women	Results (cervix/blood)[a]			
		+/−	+/+	−/+	−/−
Vogt et al. [1]	13	0	4	3	6
Wofsy et al. [2]	8	0	4	3	1

[a]Results for cervix and vagina combined for the Wofsy et al. data.

woman, but was in the second collection, which was made by placing gauze in the vagina and having the woman stimulate herself to orgasm. The authors speculated that sexual stimulation may enhance viral recovery. Low amounts of replicating HIV were detected in the vaginal and cervical samples, suggesting that inflammation, by causing an influx of leukocytes into the lower genital tract, may increase the number of lymphocytes in that area. Virus also could be detected in the supernatant as well as cellular fractions of some vaginal samples.

LATER STUDIES

In a later investigation, Vogt and coauthors [3] studied seven seropositive women at weekly intervals throughout their menstrual cycle to determine whether detection of HIV in specimens obtained from the endocervical canal showed a cyclic pattern. The collection technique was similar to that used in this group's earlier work, except that two samples were usually taken from the endocervix with cotton swabs. Material from one swab was placed into lymphocyte culture, and the second swab specimen was filtered through a 0.45 μm filter before being cultured. The cultures were tested by RT assay, and positive samples were confirmed by immunofluorescence studies and a capture radioimmunoassay for p24 core protein. Peripheral blood also was obtained, sometimes simultaneously with the cervical samples. Four of the study subjects were healthy, two had ARC, and one had persistent generalized lymphadenopathy.

Four of the seven women had at least one positive cervical specimen, and four had HIV in at least one blood sample (Fig. 1). As is shown in Table 3, the pattern of viral detection differed from the earlier studies [1,2] in that three women had HIV in cervical specimens but not in the blood. Table 3 also shows the results for the 18 instances in which blood and cervical samples were obtained simultaneously. Cervical mucus was often positive when the blood was negative; in no case were both specimens positive at the same time

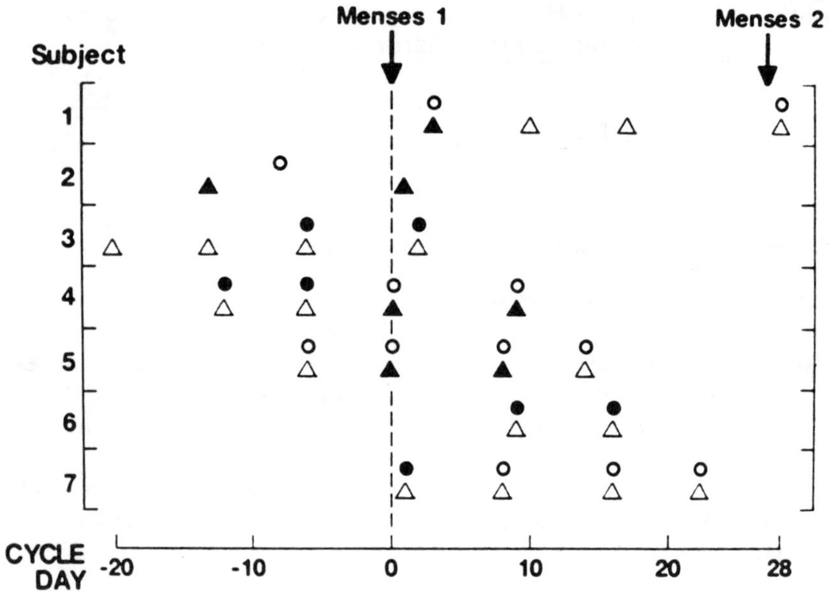

Fig. 1. Pattern of isolation of HIV from blood and cervical mucus of seven seropositive women at different times during the menstrual cycle. ○, HIV-vegative blood; ●, HIV-positive blood; △, HIV-negative cervical mucus; ▲, HIV-positive cervical mucus. (Reproduced from Vogt et al. [3] with permission of the publisher.)

TABLE 3. Pattern of HIV Detection in Cervical Specimens and Blood From Seropositive Women[a]

		Results (cervix/blood)			
Data	N	+/−	+/+	−/+	−/−
All subjects	7	3	1	3	0
Simultaneous Samples[b]	18	5	0	7	6

[a]Reproduced from Vogt et al. [3] with permission of the publisher.
[b]Blood and cervical samples collected at same time.

The investigators concluded that seropositive women have HIV in genital secretions at various times during the menstrual cycle, that viral shedding may be intermittent, and that viral detection shows no cyclic pattern. The investigators recognized, however, the limitations of their small sample and of the detection methods available.

If the phases of the menstrual cycle are estimated from Figure 1, no positive cervical cultures are obtained in the luteal phase (positive

TABLE 4. OKT4 and HIV p17 on Lymphocytes From Cervicovaginal Fluid of 34 Women[a]

Sero status	OKT4-positive	Mean percent positive (SD)	No. HIV p17 positive women	Percent positive cells
Positive	17/17	22 (11)	9/14	0.02–0.5
Negative	17/17	36 (12)	0/13	0

[a]Reproduced from Van de Perre et al. [4] with permission of the publisher.

cervical samples/total number of samples: during menses, 4/7; follicular phase, 2/6; midcycle, 1/3; and luteal phase, 0/8). The pattern is similar if only women with at least one positive cervical culture are included in the tally.

Although three of the four women in whom HIV was detected in the cervix were healthy, only one of the four women with positive blood was healthy. In this subject, HIV was detected at both sites. None of the 18 tested filtered samples were positive for HIV, whereas four of the 18 cell-containing specimens collected at the same time were positive. This finding suggests that the virus was associated with the cellular fraction. Finally, based on the time required for RT to appear in the culture supernatants, the estimate of titers of virus was higher in the peripheral blood than in the cervical secretions.

CYTOIMMUNOLOGICAL AND HISTOIMMUNOLOGICAL STUDIES

In 1988, Van de Perre and coinvestigators [4] reported a study of 17 seropositive women and a similar number of seronegative controls in Rwanda. During a gynecological examination, a clinician obtained vaginal and cervical secretion by means of cotton swabs and wooden spatulas. The secretions were combined in a liquid medium. Cells were obtained by centrifugation and the mononuclear cells were separated in ficoll-hypaque. The investigators studied the lymphocytes and vaginal and exocervical cells using indirect immunofluorescence with monoclonal antibodies and identified and counted T-helper cells and cells containing HIV p17 core antigen.

All women had T4 cells (OKT4-positive) in their cervicovaginal samples (Table 4). The seronegative women had a significantly greater proportion of T4 cells among their lymphocytes than the seropositive women ($P = 0.01$ by t test). Specimens from 27 women had enough lymphocytes (600 or more) for evaluation for HIV p17. Nine of 14 seropositive women had lymphocytes positive for this antigen, but the antigen was not identified in seronegative women (Table 4). The proportion of positive cells ranged from 0.02% to 0.5%. Epithelial cells were negative for HIV p17 in all subjects.

This report did not specify when during the menstrual cycle specimens were collected, except that the menstrual period was avoided. Six women (five of them seropositive) bled from the collection procedures because of cervicitis. The investigators concluded that, within the limits of the detection assay, epithelial cells were not reservoirs or targets for HIV. They also emphasized that genital infections increase the local lymphocyte population and possibly enhance the heterosexual transmission of HIV.

In 1988, Pomerantz and coauthors [5] described studies of cervical tissue obtained from seropositive and seronegative women. The study subjects were four female intravenous drug users, who had antibodies to HIV, and two seronegative drug users. These women had cervical biopsies from the squamocolumnar junction taken at the time of colposcopy. Cervical tissue was also obtained from the extirpated uteri of two women who had no risk factors for HIV. Specimens were collected during the postmenstrual phase of each subject's cycle.

The tissues were divided into three parts. One was frozen for later immunohistological staining; one was fixed in formalin for conventional histological studies; and the third part was homogenized and cultured for HIV with normal peripheral blood lymphocytes. Supernatants from the cultures were tested for HIV p24 antigen, and positive tests were confirmed by assaying cells from the cultures for HIV antigens by means of indirect immunofluorescence. The immunohistological studies involved staining frozen sections with monoclonal antibodies to distinguish and classify leukocytes and to detect HIV proteins gp120 and p24.

HIV was present in the cervical cultures of the four seropositive women but not in the controls. Table 5 summarizes the histological features of the cervical tissue. All seropositive women except one subject had a significant inflammatory infiltrate of mononuclear cells in the mucosa and submucosa, and all had some changes in the vascular endothelial cells in the submucosa.

In the sections studied by immunological methods, one seropositive subject had no epithelium (Table 6). The cellular infiltrates present in the epithelium of two other subjects consisted of leukocytes. Nearly all lymphocytes in all three subjects were T lymphocytes, and, in each case, CD8 cells predominated over CD4 cells. The findings in the submucosa were similar to those in the cervical mucosa.

TABLE 5. Histological Features of Cervix in HIV Seropositive (Subjects 1–4) and Seronegative (Subjects 5–8) Women[a]

Finding	Subject
Nonspecific chronic cervicitis; mononuclear cell inflammation mild to moderate in mucosa and moderate to marked in superficial submucosa	1–3
Submucosal lymphoid aggregates	1,2
Prominent vascular submucosal endothelial cells	1–4[b]
Normal tissue	5–8[c]

[a]Adapted from Pomerantz et al. [5] with permission of the publisher.
[b]Subject 4 was otherwise normal.
[c]Subjects 5–8 were controls.

TABLE 6. Immunohistological Features of the Cervix in HIV Seropositive Women[a]

Epithelial finding	Subject
Leukocytes	
No epithelium	1
Dense infiltrates of leukocytes	2,3
Almost all infiltrating cells are T lymphocytes	2–4
CD8 cells predominate over CD4 cells	2–4
Detection of HIV gp120, p24	
Specific staining of endothelial cells and mononuclear cells in mucosa and submucosa	1–3

[a]Adapted from Pomerantz et al. [5] with permission of the publisher.

Cells positive for HIV antigens were identified in tissue from three of the four seropositive women (Table 6). Viral antigens were found in endothelial cells in the submucosa and in mononuclear cells in the submucosa and mucosal layer. The investigators were unable to double label the tissue sections; as a result, the infected cells could not be characterized definitely. However, the submucosal cells containing HIV antigens were consistent with macrophages, monocytes, and endothelial cells. In the epithelial layer, most of the cells that stained with HIV antibody were round cells that resembled lymphocytes. They did not appear to be T6 or Langerhans cells. Langerhans cells of the skin may contain HIV antigen in some infected patients [6], and similar cells can be found in the cervix [7]. No squamous epithelial cells were positive for HIV antigens.

The authors' findings support the concept that HIV enters the fluids of the lower genital tract by the sloughing of infected cervical cells. Also, inflammation of the cervix, accompanied by infiltrates of mononuclear cells, may enhance heterosexual transmission of HIV by increasing the infectiousness of seropositive women or the susceptibility to infection of seronegative women.

BIOLOGY OF FLUID FROM THE FEMALE GENITAL TRACT

The vagina and cervix contribute most of the secretions found in the lower female genital tract. Although Bartholin's and Skene's glands are present at the entrance to the vagina, the vaginal epithelium contains no glands. The liquid component of vaginal fluid consists of a serum transudate across the vaginal wall, the amount of which varies with sexual stimulation [8]. In addition, epithelial cells produce a hydrophilic layer of glycoprotein, which covers the epithelial surface [9]. Vaginal fluid also contains exfoliated epithelial cells, bacteria, and leukocytes, which are present in small numbers in a healthy vagina [10].

The cervix contributes cervical mucus, which is produced in secretory cells in the endocervical crypts. The quality and quantity of cervical mucus are regulated by estrogens and progesterone. Mucus is made up of a mucin gel, a fluid phase, and a varying number of cells [11,12]. Estrogen causes the mucin to form thread-like macromolecules that form long parallel bundles with fluid-filled channels. This is most marked at midcycle when the mucus is watery, has low viscosity, and is most hospitable to sperm penetration. In the early follicular phase, when estrogen levels are low and influenced by progesterone in the secretory phase, there is no micelle formation. The macromolecules form an irregular, dense network that does not allow sperm penetration. The mucus contains few cells during the estrogenic phase of the menstrual cycle but contains many epithelial cells and leukocytes at other phases.

The vaginal tissue contains lymphocytes and macrophages as does the cervix [5,7,13,14], and the tract is an immunocompetent organ [15]. The genital secretions also contain various antibodies, including those directed against HIV [16].

When cervical mucus extrudes into the vagina, it becomes part of the vaginal fluid. Other genital fluids are derived from the endometrium (menstrual blood as well as other endometrial fluids), the oviduct, and ovarian follicular fluid. These fluids and cells from these areas of the female tract can enter the vagina. Abnormal cells from other parts of the genital tract and from the peritoneal cavity can appear in specimens obtained for cervical cytology. However, apart from menstrual fluids, the other sources do not appear to contribute substantively to the environment of the lower female genital tract.

HIV IN THE LOWER FEMALE GENITAL TRACT

The studies reviewed indicate that HIV can be cultured from cervical and vaginal fluid [1–4] and that HIV antigens can be identified in cells taken from the cervix [4] and in round cells in the mucosal and submucosal layers of tissue from cervical biopsies [5]. Viral antigens were not found in, nor was virus cultured from, epithelial cells [4,5]. These studies suggest that HIV is cell-associated, that viral shedding is not related to stage of disease, and that the detection of HIV in blood and in genital secretion has no consistent relationship. This conclusion suggests that regional infected cells can be a source of virus apart from blood lymphocytes.

FACTORS THAT MAY INFLUENCE VIRAL SHEDDING IN THE VAGINA AND CERVIX

More information is needed to determine the factors that affect viral shedding into the lower female tract. Some possible influences are the stage of disease, phase of the menstrual cycle, other endocrine factors, and inflammation. The stage of disease has been discussed. Although Vogt and coauthors [3] have suggested that viral detection in cervical samples is not related to the menstrual cycle, these data are incomplete. Better assessment of the hormonal status of the study subject is needed. Sex steroids influence the cells of the immune system and their function in the tract of female animals [17] and women [14] and the structure and cellularity of the cervical mucus. In addition, the suppression of T-cell proliferation by vaginal fluid may vary with the menstrual cycle [10]. Oral contraceptives also can affect hormonal environment; the effect of these products should be assessed.

The investigators in most of the studies reviewed above commented on the potential role of inflammation in enhancing the shedding of HIV from the vagina and cervix. Vaginitis and cervicitis can increase the numbers of leukocytes in the vagina and in cervical mucus. Whether this will increase the number of HIV infected cells in the vagina is unknown. Inflammation also can occur secondary to frank trauma or microtrauma caused by the use of mechanical barrier contraceptives [18,19], tampons, and sexual intercourse [20]; the effect of these common practices should be assessed. Additional information is needed to clarify these issues and improve our understanding of how the vagina and cervix relate to viral shedding and the transmission of HIV.

REFERENCES

1. **Vogt MW, Witt DJ, Craven DE, et al.:** Isolation of HTLV-III/LAV from cervical secretions of women at risk for AIDS. Lancet 2:525–527, 1986.

2. **Wofsy CB, Cohen JB, Hauer LB, et al.:** Isolation of AIDS-associated retrovirus from genital secretions of women with antibodies to the virus. Lancet 2:527–529, 1986.

3. **Vogt MW, Witt DJ, Craven DE, et al.:** Isolation patterns of the human immunodeficiency virus from cervical secretions during the menstrual cycle of women at risk for the acquired immunodeficiency syndrome. Ann Intern Med 106:380–382, 1987.

4. **Van de Perre P, De Clercq A, Cogniaux-Leclerc J, et al.:** Detection of HIV p17 antigen in lymphocytes but not epithelial cells from cervicovaginal secretions of women seropositive for HIV: Implications for heterosexual transmission of the virus. Genitourinary Med 64:30–33, 1988.

5. **Pomerantz RJ, De La Monte SM, Donegan SP, et al.:** Human immunodeficiency virus (HIV) infection of the uterine cervix. Ann Intern Med 108:321–327, 1988.

6. **Tschachler E, Groh V, Popovk M, et al.:** Epidermal Langerhans' cells–A target for HTLV-III/LAV infection. J Invest Dermatol 88:233–237, 1987.

7. **Edwards JN, Morris HB:** Langerhans' cell and lymphocyte subsets in the female genital tract. Br J Obstet Gynaecol 92:974–992, 1985.

8. **Wagner G.** Vaginal transduction. In Beller FK, Schumacher GFB (eds): The Biology of the Fluids of the Female Genital Tract. New York: Elsevier, 1979, pp 25–34.

9. **Cohen MS, Black JR, Proctor RA, Sparling PF:** Host defences and the vaginal mucosa. In Mardh PA, Taylor-Robinson D (eds): Bacterial Vaginosis. Stockholm: Almqvist and Wiksell International, 1984, pp 13–22.

10. **Hill JA, Anderson DJ:** Quantitation of human vaginal leukocytes and effects of vaginal leukocytes and effects of vaginal secretions or mechanism of HIV transmission. Abstract 2551: IV International Conference on AIDS, Stockholm, June, 1988.

11. **Odeblad E:** The biophysical aspects of cervical mucus. In Jordan JA, Singer A (eds): The Cervix. Philadelphia: W.B. Saunders, 1976, pp 155–163.

12. **Chantler E, Elstein M:** Structure and function of cervical mucus. Semin Reprod Endocrinol 4:333–342, 1986.

13. **Burgos MH, De Vargas-Linares CER:** Ultrastructure of the vaginal mucosa. In Hafez ESE, Evans TN (eds): The Human Vagina. Amsterdam: North-Holland Publishing Company, 1978, pp 63–93.

14. **Murdoch AJM, Buckley CH, Fox H:** Hormonal control of the secretory immune system of the human uterine cervix. J Reprod Immunol 4:23–30, 1982.

15. **Haas GH Jr.:** The uterine cervix as an immune organ. Semin Reprod Endocrinol 4:357–370, 1986.

16. **Archibald DW, Witt DJ, Craveo DE, Vogt MW, Hirsch MS, Essex M:** Antibodies to

human immunodeficiency virus in cervical secretion from women at risk for AIDS. J Infect Dis 156:1240–1241, 1988.

17. **Wira CR, Savdoe CP:** Endocrine regulation of the mucosal immune system in the female reproductive tract. Specific antibody responses to antigen presentation. In Strober W, Lamm NTC, Mcghee JR, James SP (eds): Mucosal Immunity and Infection at Muscosal Surfaces. Oxford: Oxford University Press, 1988, pp 457–465.

18. **Bernstein GS, Kilzer L, Coulson AH, et al.:** Studies of cervical caps: I. Vaginal lesions associated with use of the Vimule cap. Contraception 26:443–456, 1982.

19. **Bernstein GS, Clark V, Coulson AH, et al.:** Comparative study of the cervical cap and diaphragm: Differences in occurrence of genital trauma and changes in cervical cytology. Abstract 3109: 116th Annual Meeting of the American Public Health Association, Boston, 1988.

20. **Norvell MK, Benrubi GI, Thompson RJ:** Investigation of microtrauma after sexual intercourse. J Reprod Med 29:269–271, 1984.

DISCUSSION

DR. HILL: I have a comment about the potential HIV host cells in the vagina, especially in regard to the African study. We are currently in the process of looking at similar things, and we have thus far processed 190 vaginal secretions from 123 women. Eighteen of these women were in various stages of HIV positivity. We have studied five women in low-risk groups who are HIV negative from whom we obtained samples once per week for three straight months. We found no potential HIV host cells in the vaginal secretions of two normal women who were on oral contraceptives, except during menses. Even then they were very few, less than 10,000 cells/ml; however, in the first part of the cycle we do see increased numbers of granulocytes and macrophages, but of no other cell. However, in 18 HIV-positive women, the CD4 lymphocytes and monocyte-macrophages may be as high as 600,000/ml. In those women who are CDC class 4, the cell number may be as high as 800,000–1,000,000 cells/ml; however, in women with fulminant AIDS, these numbers drop off dramatically to about 12,000, the same as the normal women during menses. But, if you correct for the time and the cycle, there is no difference between menses and any other part of the cycle, unlike in the HIV-negative women of low-risk groups.

DR. BERNSTEIN: Are there differences in B cells at different times of the cycle?

DR. HILL: We have never found a B cell.

DR. BERNSTEIN: Really? These are based on biopsy results. Did any of these women have any type of inflammatory disease?

DR. HILL: We looked at several normal women who had either yeast vaginitis or trichovaginitis, and these cells increased in response to infection. If there is no evidence of infection, these cells are not present.

DR. BERNSTEIN: There is a tremendous increase in WBCs, including different types of lymphocytes, in those infections.

DR. BURNHILL: I just want to support the previous speaker. In studying perhaps several thousand women's vaginal cytology both with and without vaginitis, you could say reasonably clearly that the nonmenstrual discharge in essentially healthy women has practically no white cells per high-powered field and essentially no monocytic components. If, however, they have some staining pre- or postmenstruation, during the menstruation itself, you see the appearance of what may be macrophages, histiocytes, and other mononuclear cells. Do you have any data on the transmission either to or from hysterectomized women?

DR. HILL: We have looked at three with THs, BS, and Os. They showed HIV-positive cells. I believe that two of these women were on estrogen.

DR. BERNSTEIN: Right. Well, certainly, you can have lymphoid collections in the vagina as well as in the cervix, particularly if there is an inflammatory response.

19

Relationship Between Contraceptive Technology and HIV Transmission: An Overview

M.F. Fathalla

A number of mechanisms that account for the interaction between contraceptive technology and infection caused by the human immunodeficiency virus (HIV) are possible, but most are still theoretical. Contraceptive technology may have an impact on HIV transmission, influencing infectivity, susceptibility, or both. This technology may also influence the course of the disease or interfere with diagnostic tests or therapeutic regimens. HIV infection, on the other hand, may change contraceptive effectiveness, contraceptive safety, or both; it may also affect contraceptive prevalence, contraceptive choice, and the field of contraceptive research and development. This paper addresses one aspect of these potential interactions: the relationship of contraceptive technology to HIV transmission.

HIV TRANSMISSION

The modes rather than the mechanisms of HIV transmission are now well established: sexual, perinatal, and parenteral. The relationship between contraceptive technology and HIV transmission should be discussed with respect to each of these modes, as described in Chapter 1 (this volume). The three modes of transmission differ in importance from one region of the world to another. Three patterns of HIV infection have been described [1]. In pattern I—prevalent in western Europe, North America, some areas of South

Heterosexual Transmission of AIDS, pages 225–237

America, Australia, and New Zealand—sexual and parenteral transmission predominate. Sexual transmission is mostly homosexual; heterosexual transmission is limited but is expected to increase. Parenteral transmission occurs predominantly through intravenous drug abuse. In pattern II—prevalent in Africa, the Caribbean, and some areas of South America—all three modes of transmission are prevalent. Sexual transmission is predominantly heterosexual. Parenteral transmission occurs mostly through transfusion of HIV-infected blood and the use of nonsterile needles and syringes. Perinatal transmission is a significant problem since relatively large numbers of women are HIV-positive. In pattern III—prevalent in Asia, the Pacific region (except for Australia and New Zealand, which are pattern I), the Middle East, eastern Europe, and some rural areas of South America—infection has been introduced only recently and is still of low prevalence. Both homosexual and heterosexual transmission have been documented, and parenteral and perinatal transmission are not in general a problem. Although most persons with acquired immune deficiency syndrome (AIDS) in the United States and Europe have been male homosexuals and intravenous drug abusers, on a global scale heterosexual transmission of HIV is probably the most common way that HIV is spread [2].

CONDOMS, SPERMICIDES AND THE TRANSMISSION OF HIV

A number of in vitro and in vivo studies have investigated the protective effect of condoms and spermicides in preventing HIV infection. A recent review of the literature by Feldblum and Fortney [3] questioned the assumed protective effect and outlined gaps in knowledge. To be protective against HIV infection, condoms must be used for all acts of intercourse when pregnancy is not at risk, for example, when one or both partners are sterile, or during anal intercourse, oral intercourse, or vaginal intercourse during menstruation.

Pregnancy rates under actual conditions of condom and spermicide use reflect variable degrees of inconsistent or incorrect use. Although the motivation for disease prophylaxis in condom users may be greater than the motivation for contraception and may lead to better compliance and effectiveness, condom use is no substitute for mutually faithful monogamous sexual behavior. It is, however, the only method that reduces the risk of sexual transmission if one partner is seropositive. Vigorous research is needed on how to improve the effectiveness and acceptability of the condom for both contraception and protection against sexually transmitted disease (STD).

The use of spermicide-lubricated condoms is likely to offer additional protection in the case of condom rupture [4]. The use of spermicides alone has a definite in vitro inhibiting effect on HIV, but studies are needed to demonstrate effectiveness in vivo. Recent evidence [5] that the HIV-infected cell rather than the free virus is the important mechanism for heterosexual transmission challenges the validity of extrapolating from in vitro studies on spermicides. A toxic concentration of the spermicide may be needed to kill the HIV-infected cell. The need to resolve this issue through research is pressing, since there are opportunities to exploit this property of spermicides in developing effective methods of contraception, for example, in sustained-release systems in combination with steroids (such as the vaginal ring) or with vaginally administered hormonal contraceptive tablets.

With the present state of contraceptive technology, a woman at risk of both pregnancy and HIV infection (to herself or to her partner) should be advised to use a reliable contraceptive method and to have her partner use a condom. The female condom is still too new to draw conclusions about its effectiveness and acceptability.

Condoms and spermicides used for protection against HIV infection have the additional benefit of preventing other STDs. Evidence is growing that at least some STDs enhance the efficiency of sexual transmission of HIV. In a cohort study of seronegative female prostitutes, the presence of genital ulcers or *Chlamydia trachomatis* infection increased the risk of acquiring HIV infection [6,7]. Genital ulcers may permit easier penetration of HIV by disrupting the integrity of the mucosal epithelium. Chlamydial and possibly other STDs that elicit an inflammatory reaction in the female genital tract may increase the risk of HIV transmission by increasing the population of infected cells in an HIV-infected person or the pool of potential target cells in seronegative women. Another prospective study in Nairobi [8], of men who acquired an STD from prostitutes known to have a high rate of HIV infection, found that men who acquired genital ulcers had five times the rate of HIV infection of men who acquired urethritis.

OTHER CONTRACEPTIVE METHODS AND HETEROSEXUAL TRANSMISSION OF HIV

HIV has been isolated from semen and from cervical secretions of infected individuals [9]. However, the mechanisms involved in the heterosexual transmission of HIV are not well understood. Moreover, few studies have examined the relation of contraceptive methods, other than the condom and spermicides, to HIV transmission. Given our present knowledge, we can only speculate on a number of mechanisms whereby contraceptive methods may alter HIV transmission, and review the few studies of these mechanisms.

These other methods of contraception will modify the level of risk only for individuals who have unprotected sexual intercourse with an infected partner. Whether the method increases or decreases the risk of transmission should not influence advice about using a condom or the decision to use a condom when risk for HIV transmission is possible. The role of modern contraceptive methods is unlikely to be more than marginal in heterosexual HIV transmission. In fact, heterosexual transmission is most common in areas with low prevalence of contraceptive use and least common in areas with high prevalence.

A World Health Organization (WHO) group [10] studying contraceptive methods and HIV, after considering both adverse and beneficial theoretical interactions, found conclusions difficult to draw because of the paucity of basic and epidemiologic data. In the light of current information, no changes in existing recommendations concerning contraceptive use were warranted. The choice of a contraceptive method for an individual or couple should continue to be made considering the risks and benefits of each method and the circumstances and lifestyles of the individuals concerned. In particular, because of the risk of pelvic inflammatory disease, the intrauterine device was recognized not to be a method of choice for women who are at high risk for STDs, including HIV infection.

POSSIBLE MECHANISMS FOR MODIFICATION OF HIV TRANSMISSION

Cell-free virus in body fluids is unlikely to be a meaningful source of sexual transmission of HIV [5]. In HIV-positive women, no HIV could be recovered from any of 18 cell-free vaginal or cervical fluid samples [9]. It follows that conditions that increase the amount of leucocytes in the vaginal and cervical fluid would increase both infectivity and susceptibility. This explanation could be the basis for a theoretical increased susceptibility to HIV transmission among couples who practice periodic sexual abstinence and in women who use an intrauterine device or an oral contraceptive (because of increased incidence of chlamydial infection).

The effect of vasectomy on the infectivity of the semen is worth studying in light of the growing realization that the infected cell is important in transmission. The site of entry of the virus to the semen also requires clarification.

Uterine Bleeding

Information on the importance of menstrual blood on infectivity is incomplete. Several small studies [7,11] have not found a correlation between the risk of infection and sexual intercourse during menstruation. Methods of contraception affecting the menstrual cycle, increasing or decreasing the amount of bleeding, or causing irregular spotting, could influence HIV transmission.

Break in Continuity of the Epithelial Surface

Certain contraceptive methods may be associated with the possibility of breaks or microabrasions in the continuity of the epithelial surface of the vagina, cervix, and endometrium. Vaginal barrier mechanical methods may traumatize the vaginal epithelium. Cervical erosions in relation to oral contraceptive use are more easily traumatized than the surrounding stratified squamous epithelium. Endometrial trauma may occur with the intrauterine device. Endometrial disruption and bleeding occur with hormonal methods of contraception. The significance of these changes is difficult to determine, especially since the site of entry of the virus in heterosexual transmission is unknown.

Immunologic Changes

Apart from the local mechanisms discussed above, contraceptive methods may also influence HIV heterosexual transmission through a systemic effect on the immune system. This could influence both infectivity and susceptibility. Some studies have correlated immunologic parameters with infectivity.

Evidence suggests that synthetic sex steroids used for contraception modify the immune response. This effect was shown in laboratory animals [12], in vitro [13], and in women [14]. Although estrogen-progestagen contraceptives are expected to suppress some points in the immune reaction, the significance of this suppression for HIV transmission is not clear for two reasons. First, the suppressive effects on one part of the immune reaction may be compensated for by stimulated effects elsewhere. Second, since lymphocyte activation may be involved in replication of the virus, a chronic down-regulation, such as that induced by hormonal contraceptives, might not be favorable for the establishment of the infection.

Recent evidence [15] that pregnancy does not alter the course of AIDS suggests that steroid-mediated changes in the immune reaction are not significant in HIV infection. The development of vaccines for fertility regulation raises questions about possible interactions with HIV infection that cannot be answered given our present knowledge. Information gained from experience with childhood vaccination in areas with high prevalence of HIV infection could be relevant to these questions.

Direct Effect on the Virus

Whether the copper released by intrauterine devices has any effect on the virus is still not known. Steroid hormones may be involved in the replication of the virus, as has been suggested for retroviruses of mice [16]. One study has shown that the expression of HIV is enhanced by hydrocortisone and other hormones, although not by progesterone or testosterone in the model investigated.

STUDIES REPORTING ON CONTRACEPTIVE METHODS AND HIV TRANSMISSION

Few studies have examined contraceptive practice as a risk factor for HIV transmission. The studies that have been done were not designed to answer questions about contraceptive use; therefore, the findings are not conclusive. One study [18] reported on HIV seroprevalence and risk factors in 640 prostitutes in the United States who had no evidence of intravenous drug abuse. Thirty women were HIV-positive, and there was no relationship between susceptibility and oral contraceptive use. Another study [11] of risk factors in heterosexual HIV transmission in the steady female sexual partners of 124 HIV-positive adult hemophiliacs found no association with contraceptive practices. A study in Nairobi [7] found seroconversion in 87 (71%) of 123 seronegative prostitutes during a 54 month period. Seroconversion was reported to be independent of genital ulcers, chlamydial infection, and use of oral contraceptives (see, respectively, Chapters 20, 23, and 21, this volume). More definite answers may be available from a number of ongoing studies designed to investigate the relationship between contraceptive practice and HIV infection.

CONTRACEPTIVE TECHNOLOGY AND PERINATAL TRANSMISSION OF HIV

Vertical transmission of HIV from mother to child is a major health problem where large numbers of women are infected. The risk of HIV transmission from mother to fetus has not been accurately determined. Preliminary reports cite risks of 22% to 51% [19,20]. Factors governing the risk of vertical transmission are not yet clear. Only effective contraception to prevent pregnancy, or pregnancy termination, will decrease the prevalence of this mode of transmission. A sexually active, HIV-positive woman needs both effective contraception to prevent pregnancy and to have her partner use a condom for protection against transmitting HIV.

BREAST FEEDING

Breast feeding is a method of contraception. When associated with lactational amenorrhea during the first 6 months postpartum, its effectiveness is about 98% in women who are exclusively or almost exclusively breast feeding. Breast feeding probably prevents more births, worldwide, than any other method of contraception.

Some evidence suggests that HIV is transmitted from mother to infant through breast milk. The virus has been isolated from cell-free breast milk of healthy virus carriers [21]. In a number of documented cases in which the infant had HIV infection, the infection could only have been transmitted through breast milk since the mother was infected only after delivery [10,22]. Although this criterion is important for documenting this mode of transmission, these cases are not typical of breast feeding. They relate to a phase of high infectivity. Breast feeding during the phase of seroconversion may carry more risk than an antibody-positive pregnancy, whereas breast feeding after an antibody-positive pregnancy may not involve additional risk [23]. A recent study in Haiti [24] followed infants born either to the seropositive spouses of AIDS patients or to AIDS mothers. Thirty-five infants who were seronegative at the time of initial evaluation and breast fed for a mean of 7 months remained seronegative. In addition, 16 of 47 infants who were seropositive and were breast fed for a mean of 5 months became seronegative. Four of eight infants who were born seropositive to mothers with HIV seropositivity documented during pregnancy and who were breast fed for periods up to 1 year became seronegative.

Available evidence indicates that breast feeding represents only a small incremental risk of mother-to-infant transmission compared to in utero transmission [25]. The WHO [26] recommended that, when the safe and effective use of alternatives is not possible, breast feeding by the biological mother should continue to be the feeding method of choice irrespective of her HIV infection status. The U.K. Department of Health and Social Services [27] has advocated that all women known to be HIV antibody-positive, or those at high risk who have not been serologically tested, should be discouraged from breast feeding. The U.S. Centers for Disease Control also recommended that HIV-positive women should be advised against breast feeding.

CONTRACEPTIVE TECHNOLOGY AND PARENTERAL TRANSMISSION OF HIV

HIV can be transmitted from one person to another through the use of unsterile needles, syringes, and other skin-piercing and invasive instruments. Certain methods of contraception involve skin piercing, such as injectables, implants, and vaccines currently under development. The insertion of an intrauterine device involves the use of instrumentation with possible injury to mucosal surfaces. Vas and tubal occlusion are surgical procedures. In areas where infection is prevalent and where sound clinical practices for disinfection and sterilization are not observed, patient-to-patient transmission may be a risk. Any risk to health care personnel involved in delivering contraceptive services should be rare and completely avoidable if sound clinical practices are observed.

HIV is sensitive to standard methods of sterilization and high-level disinfection, and methods that inactivate other viruses (e.g., hepatitis B virus) also inactivate HIV. The WHO has recently issued guidelines on sterilization and high-level disinfection methods effective against HIV [28].

CONCLUSION

Contraceptive technology can influence HIV transmission through a number of possible mechanisms. However, gaps in our knowledge about factors involved in the transmission of the virus and the paucity of studies on contraceptive use allow only tentative conclusions or, in some cases, mere speculation.

Barrier methods, particularly the condom, remain the only effective way to prevent heterosexual transmission for individuals exposed to the risk of infection. The role of other methods of contraception in modifying the risk of infectivity or susceptibility to heterosexual transmission remains unclear, and they are probably of marginal significance to the problem of spread of the disease. The use of effective contraception to prevent pregnancy in a sexually active, HIV-positive woman is the only sure way to deal with the problem of perinatal transmission. The relationship of breast feeding (a widely prevalent birth-spacing method) and HIV transmission is still to be resolved.

In areas with high prevalence of infection, the use of unsterile needles, syringes, and instruments could be a potential risk for patient-to-patient parenteral transmission with certain contraceptive methods. This potential risk should be completely avoidable by observing sound clinical practices for disinfection and sterilization.

REFERENCES

1. **Piot P, Plummer FA, Mhalu FS, Lamboray J-L, Chin J, Mann JM:** AIDS: An international perspective. Science 239:573–579, 1988.

2. **Johnson AM:** Heterosexual transmission of human immunodeficiency virus. Br Med J 196:1017–1020, 1988.

3. **Feldblum PJ, Fortney JA:** Condoms, spermicides, and the transmission of human immunodeficiency virus: A review of the literature. Am J Public Health 78:52–54, 1988.

4. **Reitmeijer CAM, Krebs JW, Foerino PM, Judson FN:** Condoms as physical and chemical barriers against human immunodeficiency virus. JAMA 259:3037–3038, 1988.

5. **Levy JA:** The transmission of AIDS: The case of the infected cell. JAMA 259:3037–3038, 1988.

6. **Plummer FA, Simonsen JN, Ngugi EN, Cameron DW, Piot P, Ndinya-Achola JO:** Incidence of human immunodeficiency virus (HIV) infection and related disease in a cohort of Nairobi prostitutes. Abstract M.8.4 : III International Conference on AIDS, Washington, DC, June, 1987.

7. **Plummer F, Cameron W, Simonsen N, et al.:** Cofactors of male-female transmission of HIV. Abstract 4554: IV International Conference on AIDS, Stockholm, June, 1988.

8. **Piot P, Kreiss JK, Ndinya-Achola JO, et al.:** Heterosexual transmission of HIV. J AIDS 1:199, 1987.

9. **Vogt MW, Witt DJ, Craven DE, et al.:** Isolation patterns of the human immunodeficiency virus from cervical secretions during the menstrual cycle of women at risk for the acquired immunodeficiency syndrome. Ann Intern Med 106:380–382, 1987.

10. **World Health Organization Global Program on AIDS and Special Program of Research, Development and Research Training in Human Reproduction. Joint Statement:** Contraceptive Methods and HIV Infection. SPA/INF/87 9. Geneva: WHO, 1987.

11. **Goedert JJ, Eyster ME, Ragni MV, Biggar RJ, Gail MH:** Rate of heterosexual transmission and associated risk with HIV antigen. Abstract 4019: IV International Conference on AIDS, Stockholm, June, 1988.

12. Hulka JF, Mohr K, Lieberman WM: Effect of synthetic progestational agents on allograft rejection and circulating antibody production. Endocrinology 77:897–901, 1965.

13. Kontula K, Paavonen T, Luukainen T, Andersson LC: Binding of progestins to the glycocorticoid receptor. Biochem Pharmacol 32:1511–1518, 1983.

14. Baker DA, Hameed C, Tejani N, et al.: Lymphocyte subsets in women on low dose oral contraceptives. Contraception 32:377–381, 1985.

15. MacCallum LR, France AJ, Jones ME, et al.: The effects of pregnancy on the progression of HIV infection. Abstract 4032: IV International Conference on AIDS, Stockholm, June, 1988.

16. Hirschman SZ, Funke V: Effects of steroid hormones on replication of murine sarcoma virus in mouse embryo cultures. Proc Soc Exp Biol Med 149:790–795, 1975.

17. Markham PD, Salahuddin S, Verren K, et al.: Hydrocortisone and some hormones enhance the expression of HTLV-III. Int J Cancer 37:67–72, 1986.

18. Darrow WW, Bigler B, Deppe D, French J, Gill P, Potterat J, et al.: HIV antibody in 640 US prostitutes with no evidence of intravenous drug abuse. Abstract 4054: IV International Conference on AIDS, Stockholm, June, 1988.

19. Editorial: HIV infection: Obstetrics and perinatal issues. Lancet 1:806–807, 1988.

20. Mok JQ, Giaquinto C, de Rossi A, Grosch-Worner I, Ades AE, Peckham CS: Infants born to mothers seropositive for human immunodeficiency virus: Preliminary findings from a multicentre European study. Lancet 1:1164–1168, 1988.

21. Thiry L, Spencer-Goldberger S, Jonckheer T, et al.: Isolation of AIDS virus from cell-free breast milk of three healthy virus carriers. Lancet 2:891–892, 1985.

22. Munyakho D: Breast-feeding and HIV infection. Lancet 1:1394, 1987.

23. Ziegler JB, Stewart GJ, Penny R, Stuckey M, Good S: Breast-feeding and transmission of HIV from mother to infant. Abstract 5100: IV International Conference on AIDS, Stockholm, June, 1988.

24. Stanback M, Paper JW, Verier R, Jean S, Johnson WD Jr.: Breast-feeding and HIV transmission in Haitian children. Abstract 5101: IV International Conference on AIDS, Stockholm, June, 1988.

25. Editorial: HIV infection, breast-feeding and human milk banking. Lancet 2:143, 1988.

26. World Health Organization: Breast-Feeding/Breast Milk and HIV. WHO document SPA/INF/87.8 Geneva: WHO, 1987.

27. Department of Health and Social Security: Present Day Practice in Infant Feeding: Third report. Report on Health and Social Subjects 32. London: Her Majesty's Stationery Office, 1988.

28. World Health Organization: Guidelines on Sterilization and High-Level Disinfection Methods Effective Against Human Immunodeficiency Virus (HIV). WHO AIDS series 2. Geneva: WHO, 1988.

DISCUSSION

DR. ALEXANDER: I noticed that you did not mention the possibility that IUDs might increase the risk that a male partner could be exposed to cells carrying the disease. Would you like to comment on that possibility?

DR. FATHALLA: One can speculate on a number of possibilities with the IUD. One that I have already mentioned is that the mechanism of action of the IUD is through mobilization of macrophages in the uterine cavity, so, presumably, that is going to increase the number of cells that can become infected or that can become targets for infection. One can also speculate about the increased bleeding with some IUDs and whether that may increase HIV transmission, but one should keep in mind an important consideration, and that is, for an HIV positive woman or for a woman in the high-risk category, in the majority of cases the IUD is not a method of choice because of the liability for other sexually transmitted diseases. The IUD is not the method of choice for the great majority of women who are exposed, or who have been exposed, to the risk of heterosexual transmission of HIV.

DR. ROSENFIELD: Just a comment on the breast feeding issue. We have noticed in New York City, where there is a high prevalance of the disease, that the prevalence still is very low, in the range of perhaps 2%, among our prenatal populations. As a result of the fear of transmitting HIV through breast milk, attempts to educate women about breast feeding in some of the inner-city hospitals in New York City has been stopped because they consider all patients at high risk. In terms of cost or risk-benefit, the benefits of breast feeding in this population more than offset the very small risk of transmission due to breast feeding over in utero transmission.

DR. WILLIAMSON: I want to comment on the double method issue: that we should be recommending the use of both an effective contraceptive method and condoms to prevent STDs. I think there are several problems with this. One is that virtually no one in the world is doing this, especially in the developing world. Telling people in countries where the contraceptive use prevalence is around 5% that they are supposed to be using two methods instead of one method is ridiculous. That is one problem.

The second problem is that there are not enough supplies available for the world's population to use two methods.

The third problem relates to condom use. It really undercuts the perceived effectiveness of condoms to say, "You cannot possibly count on condoms for protection against pregnancy" and that "You really have to use another method." Why are we providing condoms in family planning programs if they are so poor? I just do not see how we can make recommendations about using two methods, although I am not sure what we should be recommending.

DR. FATHALLA: I do not disagree with that. I am offering that recommendation as a demonstration of one that is neither very practical nor satisfactory. We need data to show whether this recommendation is really valid or that it should be changed. If it is valid, then we have to admit that it is unsatisfactory, and we have to try to develop methods that could have an equally protective effect against pregnancy and HIV, by either improving existing methods, developing new methods, or combining methods that will utilize spermicides together with other effective modalities.

DR. CATES: I would like to follow up on both Dr. Rosenfield's and Dr. Williamson's questions. The statement was that women at risk for both unplanned pregnancy and STDs should be advised to use two methods. But if we could, in fact, define "at risk" more appropriately, perhaps we could target messages more specifically and, therefore, get better acceptability for either or both methods.

Could you give us your definition of women at risk for both unwanted pregnancy and HIV? The term "at risk" was used in the WHO slide you showed advising both methods, and I am just asking for clarification of the term. How would you define the term "at risk"?

DR. FATHALLA: That is difficult. We have to consider two types of patients. First, we have to consider the HIV-positive woman who is sexually active, so she would be a high risk for infecting her partner, and she would be a high risk for infecting her infant. With this type of high risk, you would advise that her partner should be using a condom, and she should be using an effective method to prevent the unwanted pregnancy and subsequent infection of the infant.

The other category would be the woman who is HIV-negative but her partner is HIV-positive. Now, in that case, she would like to protect herself from the HIV infection, and that would involve the partner using a condom. But if, for one reason or another, she also does not want a pregnancy, depending on how strong her desire is for preventing that pregnancy, she would probably need a reliable contraceptive method unless she would like to resort to pregnancy termination in the event the condom fails.

DR. VOELLER: I was interested and a little troubled yesterday that the discussion of mechanisms of transmission among heterosexuals really focused entirely on semen and vaginal events. Interestingly, the seminal route is almost entirely the concern of the women and the vaginal route of the men. The point is that this discussion excluded mechanisms related to rectal absorption. There have been two or three hypotheses published, mainly in Alaska and elsewhere, of active incorporation of the virus through the rectum by a number of different routes. None of that was discussed yesterday, and I suspect that part of the reason is the focus of this workshop on heterosexual transmission. However, we must not fall into the intellectual trap of making quite such a clean distinction between heterosexual and homosexual sex. Nancy Padian underscored the role of anal intercourse in heterosexual transmission. It certainly has been underscored by others as well. I think the extent of heterosexual anal intercourse in our culture is grossly underestimated. Most physicians are embarrassed to raise the issue with their patients, and this is certainly the case in surveys. For most of us to judge what is going on in the rest of the world is presumptuous and a big error. I bring this up to make the point in itself, but also to say that we must look at those other mechanisms as well as contraceptive methods in the spread of HIV.

DR. FATHALLA: I think that is a very interesting and relevant comment.

DR. BURNHILL: I want to support the statement about double methods. We have talked about this in great length both at the National Medical Committee of Planned Parenthood and the Association of Reproductive Health Professionals. Although it is true that there might be supply problems in the Third World, and perhaps in other regions, one must remember that two-thirds of U.S. contraception users are using methods that afford them no protection against STDs. We have to remember that we have moved beyond family planning. We have to give the unambiguous message that if you indulge in any sex that might increase the risk of HIV or any other STD, you need to use barrier contraception, which means that whether you have a tubal ligation, a hysterectomy, whatever, as far as we know, you must employ the second method. I do not think we should lose sight of this; it is a valuable single piece of advice that must be spread.

20

Identification of Biological Cofactors in Heterosexual Transmission of HIV Infection: Epidemiologic Observation and Intervention in Nairobi, Kenya

Bill Cameron

Pandemic dissemination of human immunodeficiency virus (HIV) infection has occurred primarily through sexual transmission in many parts of the world. In the developing countries, particularly in Africa, acquired immune deficiency syndrome (AIDS) has emerged as a sexually transmitted disease (STD) of heterosexual men and women. Sexually transmitted HIV infection has created a reservoir that fuels secondary transmission from mothers to infants and artificial, indirect parenteral contact. Intervention against the dissemination of HIV infection must focus on this reservoir of sexually acquired infection and the disseminating vectors of transmission. In Nairobi, Kenya, as in other urban centers worldwide, these vectors are prostitutes and their clients. The studies discussed here demonstrate likely biological facilitating cofactors of HIV transmission, including interactions among STDs. These studies highlight the importance of strategic focus on "high-frequency transmitters" in the development of tactics for intervention against pandemic HIV infection, through illustration of the mode of dissemination.

Heterosexual Transmission of AIDS, pages 239–246

The seroepidemiologic observational studies reported here were conducted in Nairobi, in the Collaborative Project on Sexually Transmitted Disease Research and Training from 1985 to 1988. Participating institutions were the Nairobi City Commission; the University of Nairobi; the Kenya Medical Research Institute in Nairobi; the Institute for Tropical Medicine in Antwerp, Belgium; the University of Washington in Seattle; and the University of Manitoba in Winnipeg, Canada. The project was the product of longstanding international collaboration, and many persons worked on these studies under the supervision of Dr. Frank Plummer.

Three studies are presented here to discuss possible biological cofactors of heterosexual transmission of HIV and to evaluate an intervention [1–3]. The setting of these studies is unique and important to the interpretation of results. In the Pumwani residential estate of Nairobi, approximately 1,000 women who practice prostitution have been provided health care and have been enrolled in cohort studies of STDs, including AIDS, since 1985. These women are a major reservoir of conventional STDs and HIV; they report a mean of four to five client sexual partners per day. In repeated cross-sectional surveys, *Neisseria gonorrhoeae, Chlamydia trachomatis,* and *Hemophilus ducreyi* infections were present in 50%, 30%, and 33% of these women, respectively, and reinfection with *N. gonorrhoeae* occurred within days of treatment. An explosive epidemic of HIV infection occurred among these women, with seroprevalence increasing from less than 5% in 1981 to 85% in February, 1986. These women have been reevaluated repeatedly for STD management, treatment, and counseling, and have increasingly adopted use of condoms since their introduction, provision, and promotion. Study visits and clinical care were conducted at community-based maternal and child health clinics.

Another study site has been a centralized dispensing referral dermatovenerology clinic serving all of Nairobi, a city of more than 1,000,000 people. At this clinic, 400–600 clients are seen each day. The most frequent STD syndromes are gonorrhea and genital ulcer disease, which in Nairobi is generally chancroid due to *H. ducreyi* infection. We questioned men presenting to this clinic about their source sexual contact to identify those whose contact was a women in the above group. Reporting prostitute source sexual contact in Pumwani residential estate, diurnal sale of sexual services, ethnicity of the woman (Tanzanian), and the lowest standard fee ($00.30 U.S.) reliably identified the group of women. We established a cohort of men who had recent high-risk sexual exposure to HIV and who had acquired chancroid, gonorrhea, or another STD. We evaluated these men for HIV seroprevalence and seroincidence and provided counselling about HIV and STDs. Subsequent HIV seroconversion was thus a measure of incidence in this prostitute clientele, and seroconversion in men reporting a single source sexual contact was a closer estimate of the transmission risk per sexual contact in the presence of another STD.

These men had initial HIV seroprevalence of 12%, which increased to 30% after 1 year. Simonsen et al. [2] have demonstrated that seropositivity correlates significantly with lack of male circumcision, reported past genital ulcer disease (earlier reported by Greenblatt et al. [1]), frequent prostitute contact, and central African travel or origin. HIV seroincidence confirmed a significant association of increased transmission rate in the presence of multiple, high-risk sexual contacts, and more strongly with the acquisition of genital ulcer disease and lack of male circumcision. These correlates were associated with an apparent increased susceptibility of uncircumcised men to chancroid; multivariate analysis confirmed the independent association of each cofactor.

Analysis of a subgroup of singly exposed men revealed the same associations, identifying no transmission in the absence of genital ulcer disease, but an increased risk in the presence of cofactors. Thus this study identified one behavioral and two potential biological cofactors of HIV transmission, with a likely complex interaction between chancroid and HIV. Presuming a biologically causal influence of lack of male circumcision on increased male susceptibility to HIV and of genital ulcer disease on the infectiousness of the female sexual partner, the interactive attributable risk of HIV transmission to these cofactors was 98%.

Behavioral risk factors are amenable to intervention, but chancroid, which is associated with prostitution worldwide, offers an immediate opportunity to identify high-frequency transmitters, or disseminators, of HIV. Screening and treating prostitutes and their clients have in the past controlled outbreaks of chancroid. We chose to evaluate the impact of prophylaxis on the prevalence of genital ulcer disease in sample groups of female prostitutes.

The intervention was evaluated in two cross-sectional surveys of prostitutes in Pumwani. In 1986 and 1987, more than 400 women were called into the clinic for standardized interview and clinical, microbiologic, and serologic evaluation. Since the introduction of condoms, reported condom use has increased significantly and become generalized and sustained for commercial sexual relations. However, the prevalence of clinically diagnosed chancroid was stable at 33% in 1986 and 1987, despite the concurrent increase in condom use. However, more consistent reported use of condoms was protective against chancroid. We identified that HIV infection and more advanced HIV-associated clinical disease were significantly associated with chancroid. Thus simultaneous protection from chancroid by using condoms and predisposition due to HIV infection and disease would explain the observed stable prevalence of genital ulcer disease in these women.

Analyzing data from repeated evaluations more than 6 months apart, we identified that inconsistent use of condoms protected initially HIV-seronegative women from newly acquired HIV infection or seroconversion indirectly through prevention of genital ulcer disease. As well, initially HIV-seropositive women were more likely to have newly acquired chancroid, independent of the consistency of their use of condoms. Complex biological interaction of HIV and *H. ducreyi,* of both infectiousness and susceptibility, may accelerate dissemination of HIV to or from these high-frequency transmitters—prostitutes and their clients. In corroboration of this presumed interaction, antibiotic treatment of *H. ducreyi* infection in men has failed more frequently in the presence of HIV infection and attributable clinical disease than in the absence of HIV infection.

The simple intervention of promoting and providing condoms to prostitutes may have significantly affected the rate of dissemination of STDs and HIV, however difficult the direct measurement of the impact remains. Mass screening and treatment programs for STDs (specifically, targeting genital ulcer diseases) in prostitutes and their clients would considerably reinforce the impact of STD prophylaxis on HIV control through STD control. This tactic would complement simultaneous mass education to encourage modification of high-risk sexual behavior in the overall strategy to control HIV.

A study by Plummer et al. [3] was designed to measure and identify correlates of HIV seroincidence in Pumwani prostitutes during earlier stages of the local subepidemic. Women recruited to a prospectively followed-up cohort were regularly reevaluated with standardized interviews, examinations, and microbiological and serological tests. Analysis revealed an annualized HIV seroincidence well over 50%, which was associated with genital ulcer disease (chancroid), *C. trachomatis* cervicitis, and the use of oral contraceptives for family planning. The use of condoms as barrier STD prophylaxis was independent of the practice of alternate contraception, and the use of condoms was protective against HIV infection by reducing the incidence of genital ulcer disease. The independence of oral contraceptive use, chancroid, and chlamydial cervicitis as risk factors for HIV seroconversion is suggested by multivariate analysis using stepwise logistic regression, and the evidence of a dose-response affects the former two statistical correlates. Potential sources of bias through selection or confounding were not apparent in analysis of suspect parameters measured in this study, and survivorship analysis demonstrated the influence of oral contraceptive use on cumulative HIV seroincidence.

Thus we have identified several influences on the epidemic of sexually transmitted HIV infection in a select subpopulation of Nairobi. Many of these cofactors are potential tactical intervention points about control strategies through education and behavior modification or mass control of STDs as a group. These cofactors reinforce two central points about the pandemic dissemination of HIV. First, HIV is linked to classic (or conventional) STDs as a group due to sociological, behavioral, and biological influences. Second, high-frequency transmitters, as identifiable reservoirs or vectors of HIV infection, are the group upon whom our intervention efforts must focus.

REFERENCES

1. **Greenblatt RM, Dukehart SA, Plummer PA, et al.:** Genital ulcerations as a risk factor for human immunodeficiency virus infection. AIDS 2:47–50, 1988.

2. **Simonson JN, Cameron DW, Gakinya MN, et al.:** Human immunodeficiency virus infection in men with sexually transmitted diseases. N Engl J Med 319:274–278, 1988.

3. **Plummer FA, Simonsen JN, Cameron DW, et al.:** Cofactors in male-female sexual transmission of HIV. Abstract 4554: IV International Conference on AIDS, Stockholm, June, 1988.

DISCUSSION

DR. ALEXANDER: I have several questions. The first is, do you have evidence from Kenya that AIDS is being spread to the villages from the major cities?

DR. CAMERON: I do not have any data to answer that question. Intuitively, one would think that might be happening.

DR. ALEXANDER: The second question is, has the frequency of genital ulcers risen markedly in the last 10 years? Is it possible that women who are HIV-seropositive are less responsive to treatment for genital ulcer disease?

DR. CAMERON: To answer the first part of that question, one has to look at the past experience of clinicians in the urology clinic. One who has worked there since the mid-1950s reported that chancroid, as a frequent STD diagnosis, appeared in Nairobi in the early 1960s following more contact with people from central Africa. That is anecdotal reporting.

I would like to rephrase the second part of your question. Is there an interaction in prevalence between HIV infection and chancroid, which is the predominant genital ulcer? I have data that show that there is a powerful interaction. The two lines of evidence are: 1) to look in the prostitute cohort, which shows that women with chancroid are more likely HIV-positive in a cross-sectional study, and 2) to look at men treated for chancroid, in whom microbiologic treatment failure is associated with HIV infection.

DR. ALEXANDER: One last question. Did you test for *Chlamydia* using antibodies or culture?

DR. CAMERON: Culture.

DR. FOURCROY: I only want to express a word of caution about circumcision in men. When one looks at the role of circumcision, or risks associated with not being circumcised, you have to consider the other cofactors. Cleanliness in developing countries is the most important cofactor.

DR. CAMERON: I would suggest that the most important cofactor is sexual exposure to HIV, and that circumcision is not going to present itself as a major intervention point. I would also suggest that the control of genital ulcer disease is likely the more operative intervention point.

DR. CONE: The data you presented for transmission from women to men was really clear. If genital ulcers were present, the men would get infected; if not, there was no infection.

DR. CAMERON: The statistical association was very strong.

DR. CONE: Does the same apply when the disease is transmitted from men to women? How likely is a woman to get the infection from a male who has genital ulcer disease? What I am trying to find is the source to source mode of transmission.

DR. CAMERON: If I could rephrase the question, I think you are asking, is the genital ulcer acting as a portal of exit, increasing the infectiousness of a female sexual partner, or does a genital ulcer in a man act as a portal of entry for the virus? The latter is a minor mode, but I would suggest that ulcers in either partner may act as entry or exit portals for the virus.

DR. CONE: Both ways?

DR. CAMERON: Yes. We see this with increased risk to women with ongoing exposure to HIV: Having genital ulcers apparently increases their susceptibility to HIV infection, and, for a man, sexual exposure to a woman with both HIV infection and an ulcer increases that man's likelihood of seroconverting.

DR. POTTS: I would like to ask if you think it would be possible and responsible to treat chancroid on the streets in the sense of asking the woman whether she has the disease, and, if she does, saying, here, take these tablets? Or, do you think you must have clinical back-up to treat genital ulcer disease?

DR. CAMERON: Chancroid is painful, and most people who have it, men more so than women, are aware that they have it. I think what you propose would be an easy starting point for mass control programs.

More important than treatment, although that has to be part of a control program, is prevention. We have data that show that the introduction and acceptance of condom use, which have been quite thorough and sustained in this cohort of women in Nairobi, have had impact on lowering the rate at which they acquire genital ulcer disease. On the other hand, HIV infection in these women is increasing. I think that we need a two-pronged attack, and we should focus on identifiable, high-frequency transmitters. Chancroid, wherever it occurs in the world, is a highly prostitute-associated disease. If we can focus disease control measures on the clientele of male and female prostitutes, and the prostitutes themselves, I think we have a good opportunity to make an impact on sexually transmitted HIV.

DR. PETERSON: You presented a lot of good, hard work. I am really concerned, though, about your interpretation of the oral contraceptive use findings. How have you been able to convince yourself that the increased risk of transmission is due to oral contraceptive use and not the lack of condom use? I am not sure that the information you presented on the model resolves that concern.

I would also like to know how you can sort out the effects of oral contraceptive use from characteristics of the oral contraceptive user? One question that comes quickly to mind is the loss to follow-up. About one-third of the people were lost to follow-up. Are oral contraceptive users not more likely to be followed?

DR. CAMERON: I cannot answer the last question. The introduction of condoms to this group of women was done for the purpose of STD prophylaxis. Oral contraceptive use is an ongoing choice women make for themselves for the purpose of family planning. The oral contraceptives are independently used, and in fact, in the sample, condom use did not correlate with whether a woman has chosen to use oral contraceptives or not.

DR. PETERSON: When one looks at oral contraceptive use for family planning, and one looks at the risk of cancer associated with oral contraceptive use, methodological problems arise. Cervical cancer studies are extraordinarily difficult to carry out and to interpret, in part because women in several studies who chose to use oral contraceptives had certain characteristics that put them inherently at increased risk for STDs, which may increase the risk of cervical cancer. This same issue is very much of concern to me in your study and the analysis of the results.

DR. CAMERON: In measuring the incidence of any STD in the presence of oral contraceptive use, there is always concern about confounded association due to epidemiological interaction, behavioral interaction, or biologic interaction. I share your concerns. What I presented here are the hard, statistical associations to show that oral contraceptive use and the risk of HIV transmission are associated. Whether this represents confounding, bias, or causality is going to come out in corroborative studies designed specifically to answer those questions.

21

Oral Contraceptives and HIV Transmission

Olav Meirik and Timothy M.M. Farley

Concern has been raised that oral contraceptives (OCs) may increase the susceptibility of women to sexually transmitted infection with the human immunodeficiency virus (HIV) [1]. Theoretically, OCs could induce subtle changes in the vaginal and cervical epithelium and sometimes of the vaginal bacterial environment. Changes such as cervical ectropion, which is often found in women using OCs, could theoretically enhance adhesion or penetration of virus or of infected cells. These concerns have prompted studies that are underway to examine a possible increase in susceptibility due to the use of OCs.

Some reported results regarding this theoretical association have received attention in the mass media. A cross-sectional study in Nairobi, Kenya, uncovered an increased prevalence of HIV antibodies in women using OCs, and a follow-up study of the same population disclosed a higher incidence of HIV seroconversion for OC users compared to non-OC users [2]. The association between OC use and antibodies to HIV has so far been observed only in this single population. To our knowledge, no other study has uncovered a similar association.

An increased susceptibility to HIV infection of women using OCs would have serious public health implications in areas where both OC use is prevalent and HIV infection is present. Furthermore, if OCs increase HIV susceptibility, this effect should be widely publicized. Such publication would reduce the acceptability and use of OCs, even among women who are not at risk for HIV infection. Since OCs are a popular and effective method of contraception, their reduced use would lead to unplanned pregnancies and concomitant

Heterosexual Transmission of AIDS, pages 247–254

health consequences. A scrutiny of the association reported in Nairobi and additional studies to confirm or refute the finding are urgently needed.

THE FINDINGS

The positive correlation between OC use and antibodies to HIV found in the Nairobi study [3] was communicated orally at the III International Conference on AIDS and in an abstract in the proceedings of the IV International Conferences on AIDS [2]. For the purpose of this review, the authors were made available two manuscripts [3,4] describing the findings of the cross-sectional study and of the follow-up study. In this chapter, the methodology and main findings of the two Nairobi studies are briefly summarized.

The Cross-Sectional Study [3]

In 1985, women in Nairobi who admitted prostitution were enrolled in a project to study the general epidemiology of sexually transmitted diseases (STDs). The report concerned 429 women who were living in a low socioeconomic status residential area of Nairobi. The women were recruited at a maternal and child health (MCH) clinic after a public community meeting for prostitutes. The researchers arranged the meeting with the assistance of area, city, and national agencies. Participants received free health care as an incentive for participation. The women were interviewed and examined at the MCH clinic, and laboratory specimens were taken. Data analyses disclosed a high prevalence of STDs, and 61% of the women were HIV-seropositive. Current OC use was reported by 27% of the women and no contraception by 69%. Of the HIV-seropositive women, 33% were current OC users; of the HIV-seronegative women, 21% used OCs [crude odds ratio (OR) = 1.9, with 95% confidence limits of 1.2–3.1]. Adjustment for nationality, parity, and duration of prostitution did not substantially alter the OR. Other factors independently associated with HIV seropositivity were Tanzanian origin, younger age, low parity, short duration of prostitution, and genital ulcer disease.

The Follow-Up Study [4]

The follow-up study was a continuation of the cross-sectional study referred to above. A total of 196 HIV-seronegative women from a low socioeconomic status area of Nairobi enrolled for semiannual clinic revisits. Incentive for compliance was free health care at the study center, which was located in an MCH clinic in the area. Serum samples were taken at monthly intervals; a history was taken and genital examinations and gonococcal culture were performed at semiannual visits. In addition, examinations and laboratory investigations were performed at unscheduled visits for medical problems. All women with proved HIV seroconversion and those who did not seroconvert during at least 12 months of follow-up were included.

In analyses, observations on the women were censored at time of seroconversion. Consequently, the duration of follow-up of seroconverters was shorter than for those who did not seroconvert. HIV seroconversion occurred in 83 women (42%), 41 (21%) remained seronegative, and 72 (37%) were lost to follow-up. HIV seroconverters had, on average, nine visits during 16 months, whereas those remaining seronegative had on average eight visits during 21 months of follow-up. Factors associated with seroconversion were OC use [OR = 3.1 (1.1–8.6)], condom use [OR = 0.1 (0.05–0.3)], frequency of genital ulcers ($P < 0.02$), and *Chlamydia trachomatis* infection [OR = 3.6 (1.3–11.1)]. In multivariate logistic regression analyses, including the above-mentioned variables and the number of sex partners per day, the variables OC use and genital ulcer were independently associated with HIV seroconversion, whereas condom use was protective (borderline statistical significance).

CAUSALITY IN EPIDEMIOLOGICAL RESEARCH

Since experimental research on direct transmission of HIV to human beings is unethical, the study of HIV transmission in humans must be observational. Although natural experimental situations often answer important questions and enable us to draw important inferences, they occur rarely and unpredictably. Therefore, answers we seek must come from observational clinical and epidemiological research.

As a consequence of relying on clinical epidemiology to study transmission of HIV, several factors from various studies will be statistically significant but not necessarily causally associated with transmission of the virus. Although some significant associations will appear because of biases or undetected confounding in a study, others will occur haphazardly because multiple comparisons are made. Some of these statistically significant factors will be important to public health, and the need to evaluate the question of causality will be urgent. As indicated, the reported association between heterosexual transmission of HIV and use of OC is one that, if substantiated, will have considerable public health importance. It is, therefore, imperative to scrutinize the evidence about this reported association and, if necessary, pursue research to determine whether the association is causal.

An epidemiologist [5] wrote the following about causality in medical research: "The final strategy to the epidemiologist for making inferences about cause depends on his subjective judgement. Such judgements are reached by weighing the available evidence; there are no absolute rules, and different workers often come to conflicting conclusions." Although rules are not absolute in this context, other epidemiologists [6] have suggested how to assess a single epidemiological study's scientific soundness and how to proceed from an "observed association to a verdict of causation" [7].

SCIENTIFIC CRITERIA

Feinstein [6] identified five basic scientific standards for epidemiological studies: a stipulated research hypothesis, a well-specified cohort, high-quality data, analysis of attributable actions, and avoidance of detection bias. Three of the five standards are not fulfilled in the two studies under review here.

The objective of the research project that led to the cross-sectional study and to recruitment of the cohort was stated to be the epidemiology of STDs in general. The question of heterosexual HIV transmission was considered after the cohort had been assembled. The hypothesis of an association between OC use and HIV seropositivity and HIV transmission was generated by the data and not postulated a priori. Distinguishing between an a priori and a post hoc hypothesis may be difficult in this case; others [1] have raised theoretical concerns about OC influence on heterosexual transmission of HIV. The lack of an a priori hypothesis in this project has, in addition, influenced data collection. In particular, data to evaluate possible mechanisms by which the OCs facilitate HIV transmission have not been ascertained, for example, by noting the presence or absence of cervical ectropion. Furthermore, indicators of possible selection and detection biases were not collected.

The subjects for the cross-sectional study, on which the follow-up study was based, were obtained through a call for voluntary participation supported by the provision of free health care during the study period. Subjects were not recruited by active sampling from a well-defined population. Admittedly, the task of obtaining a representative sample of a population such as the one studied here is formidable. Nevertheless, an estimate of the total number of prostitutes in the study area and information about their basic characteristics would have been useful. The applied sampling procedure may have generated a group in which certain subcategories of persons were overrepresented (e.g., individuals with previous health care contact or in need of health care) while individuals with high-risk behavior may have been underrepresented. In the cross-sectional study, the population of current OC users was probably well represented because of their recent contact with health care facilities. In particular, OC-using women with high-risk behavior (including risk for HIV infection) would be more likely to participate than non-OC users with high-risk behavior.

The provision of free health care to participating subjects may have led to considerable detection bias in the follow-up study. Subjects who had unscheduled visits to the research facility for symptoms and complaints, or for contraceptive advice and prescription, would be more likely to have HIV seropositivity demonstrated. The reported higher number of visits during a shorter follow-up period for HIV-seroconverting women compared to the nonseroconverting women suggests that important detection bias may have occurred in this study. In the analysis, the varying observation periods for seroconverting and nonseroconverting women have not been adjusted for in all instances, which has led to a bias towards zero in some of the reported ORs. Another disturbing factor in the follow-up study is the very high proportion of women (37%) lost to follow-up.

Regarding the requirements of high-quality data and analysis of attributable actions suggested by Feinstein [6], the data collected were relatively straightforward, and their validity is not controversial. However, the data that were not collected are more important. The lack of indicators of selection and detection bias and of mechanisms of action for important variables such as OCs has hampered the analysis of attributable actions.

CONCLUSIONS

The scrutiny of the two papers discloses important sources of bias, which, in our opinion, may explain the finding of a positive correlation between OC use and HIV seropositivity in the cross-sectional study and the increased risk of HIV seroconversion associated with OC use in the follow-up study. Further examination in a broader context of the causality of the associations of OC use and risk of HIV infection reported from Nairobi leads us to a similar conclusion. Not all nine criteria suggested by Hill [7] apply to the association under examination because of the paucity of knowledge and the lack of data from independent sources. Of the nine criteria—the strength of the association and its consistency, specificity, temporality, biological gradient, plausibility, coherence, analogy, and experimental evidence—only the important sine qua non criterion of temporality is fulfilled in the follow-up study. The strength of the association as demonstrated by the increased OR and its biological gradient as claimed by the authors can be explained by systematic sampling errors and detection bias, as indicated above. To our knowledge, no other study in Africa or from other continents as reported recently [8,9] has confirmed the association between OC use and increased susceptibility of HIV infection. However, that OCs modify the risks of transmission of HIV is plausible. On the other hand, because little is known about the mechanisms of HIV transmission, many hypotheses are biologically plausible on the basis of current knowledge.

In conclusion, we find no scientifically valid evidence that OCs increase women's susceptibility to HIV infection. In view of the public health importance of such an effect of OCs, additional studies should be undertaken to confirm or refute this hypothesized side effect of OCs.

ACKNOWLEDGMENTS

Funding was provided by the World Health Organization. The views expressed by the authors do not necessarily represent those of the WHO.

REFERENCES

1. **World Health Organization:** HIV and contraception; Report from a WHO consultation 1987. Geneva, 1987 (unpublished document).

2. **Plummer FA, Cameron W, Simonsen N, et al.:** Cofactors of male-female transmission of HIV. Poster session: IV International Conference on AIDS, Stockholm, June, 1988.

3. **Simonsen JN, Plummer FA, Ngugi EN, et al.:** Human immunodeficiency virus infection among lower socioeconomic strata prostitutes in Nairobi. Submitted for publication, 1988.

4. **Plummer FA, Simonsen JN, Cameron DW, et al.:** Co-factors in male-female transmission of HIV. Submitted for publication, 1988.

5. **Susser M:** Causal Thinking in the Health Sciences. New York: New York University Press, 1973.

6. **Feinstein AR:** Scientific standards in epidemiological studies of the menace of daily life. Science 242:1257–1263, 1988.

7. **Hill AB:** The environment and disease: Association or causation. Proc Med 58:295–300, 1965.

8. **World Health Organization:** WHO consultation on prevention and control of sexually transmitted disease in population groups at risk. Geneva, 1988 (unpublished document).

9. **World Health Organization:** WHO meeting on STD as cofactors for HIV transmission. Geneva, 1988 (unpublished document).

DISCUSSION

DR. ROSENFIELD: My question is addressed to both Dr. Meirik and Dr. Cameron. As the data on the potentially increased risk of HIV in women who use oral contraceptives becomes publicized, what should be the rational decision on the part of public health officials in high-prevalence countries vis-á-vis their family planning programs and oral contraceptive use? In both scientific and practical terms, what would be the outcome of publication of this type of data on such programs? What advice would you give them?

DR MEIRIK: I cannot find any reason to change recommendations with regard to OC use based on any findings so far.

DR. CAMERON: I would like to direct my comment to Dr. Meirik. That was an excellent presentation and I would like to congratulate you on your analysis of this study. I share your concerns, and we agree that an association between OC use and HIV has been found. We do not think it is due to chance, but whether there is causality will have to be answered in a study specifically designed to address that question. I would suggest to Dr. Rosenfield that such a study is the next step to proceed with, rather than making recommendations based on an interpretation of existing data.

DR. CATES: Some of you heard me speak on this issue before. I always begin by saying I feel like Billy Martin in the beer commercial, "Does it taste great or is it less filling?" In this case, it depends on whether you are really talking to an audience dealing with contraceptives or infectious diseases (ID). A lot of times, the ID audience picks up a finding such as this and then extrapolates to the beliefs that oral contraceptives have no value, that they increase the risk of transmission, and that they should be taken off the market. And then you speak to the family planning community and they say, "This study is hogwash, scientifically invalid." Depending on which audience I am addressing, I am always on the other side.

As Dr. Cameron explained in beautifully objective terms, this [the Nairobi study] was a well done cohort study. I am wondering whether many of our family planning colleagues would have been as strong in their dissection of the scientific validity of that particular study had the data shown that OCs protected against AIDS transmission. I caution, also, the ID researchers to consider the risks of advocating OC removal, or even cautioning against their use, in terms of major public health issues of this sort in the developing world. My position is one of temperance, and I think the presentations by Drs. Cameron and Meirik at this conference certainly support that.

22

Barrier Contraceptives and the Interaction Between HIV and Other Sexually Transmitted Diseases

Peter Lamptey

Acquired immune deficiency syndrome (AIDS) and infection with the human immunodeficiency virus (HIV) constitute a worldwide public health problem. AIDS epidemics in Europe, most of North and South America, and Asia predominantly have been in homosexual men and intravenous drug abusers. In Africa, the pattern of transmission is primarily heterosexual, with perinatal transmission an increasingly important mode of spread. The groups at greatest risk of HIV infection are urban prostitutes, their male clients, and other men and women with multiple sexual partners. Studies in Nairobi [1–4] have shown that sexually transmitted diseases (STDs) and other risk factors play an important role in HIV infection in both men and women. These findings have been corroborated by studies [5] in the United States. The interaction between STDs and HIV infection is one reason accounting for the high prevalence of infection in prostitutes and other persons who exhibit high-risk sexual behavior. In the absence of a vaccine for HIV infection and of a cure for AIDS, behavior change—reducing the number of sexual partners and using effective contraception, including condoms—is seen as the most feasible way to reduce sexual transmission of HIV infection. Promoting the use of condoms already is the mainstay of AIDS intervention programs.

Several issues about the association between contraception and HIV infection have arisen. Although it makes intuitive sense that

Heterosexual Transmission of AIDS, pages 255–265

condoms would protect against HIV just as they protect against other STDs, the epidemiological evidence for protection against HIV is inadequate, and even less evidence supports the effectiveness of spermicides in preventing HIV transmission.

Of equal importance is whether any method of contraception increases a person's risk of acquiring HIV infection. One study [4] indicated that oral contraceptive use by prostitutes may enhance the risk of acquired HIV infection. Until additional data are available on the interaction between hormonal contraceptives and HIV infection, conclusions cannot be drawn.

This chapter examines evidence about the interaction between HIV and other STDs and about the effectiveness of condoms and spermicides in preventing STDs and HIV infection. Recommendations also are made about the research needed to fill our knowledge gaps.

INTERACTION BETWEEN HIV AND OTHER STDs

Evidence shows that the presence of some STDs, especially genital ulcer disease caused by chancroid, syphilis, and herpes, increases the risk of acquiring HIV infection [6–8]. Earlier studies had not determined whether this association is causal or merely that genital ulcers correlate with a large number of sexual partners. A prospective study [4] of seronegative prostitutes from Nairobi that controlled for number of sexual partners, duration of prostitution, and use of condoms found that the presence of genital ulcer disease greatly increases the risk of HIV acquisition. This study also showed that chlamydial infection increases the risk of HIV infection, whereas gonococcal infection has no effect on HIV infection. In a second prospective study [9], men with STDs, recent prostitute exposure, and genital ulcers were more likely to seroconvert during a 2–6 month period than were men with urethritis. Men who had sex with a prostitute in Nairobi had a 7% chance of acquiring HIV infection after a single exposure, and this risk increased fourfold if the men had genital ulcers [9]. These studies suggest that STDs that produce genital ulcerations greatly increase the vulnerability of seronegative persons.

Recent studies of homosexual men support this hypothesis. After controlling for number of sexual partners, Handsfield and coauthors [5] showed that HIV seropositivity is associated with a history of genital, anorectal, or oral herpes; a history of syphilis; or a positive serological test for herpes simplex virus (HSV) type 2 or *Treponema pallidum.* The study also showed that HIV seroconversion is associated with anogenital lesions. These findings suggest that STDs are not covariates of sexual activity but are independent risk factors for HIV infection.

Two theories have been postulated to explain the interaction between STDs and HIV infection. First, conditions that increase the number of lymphocytes in the genital tract, such as STDs, may potentiate the risk of HIV transmission by increasing the pool of target cells in a seropositive or seronegative person. Second, the disruption of the genital epithelium by STDs permits penetration by HIV [10].

Some data suggest that the presence of HIV infection also may adversely affect coexisting STDs, such as syphilis and chancroid. One study showed that standard penicillin therapy fails to cure secondary syphilis in HIV-seropositive persons [11]. A similar finding was reported in HIV-seropositive persons with chancroid [10].

CONDOMS AND STDs

In vitro studies have shown that an intact condom provides an effective barrier against HSV, HIV, cytomegalovirus, *Neisseria gonorrhoeae, Chlamydia trachomatis,* and mycoplasma [12–14]. Other laboratory studies have demonstrated that HIV cannot pass through plain latex condoms despite the use of virus concentrations higher than those found in semen [15]. A condom lubricated with nonoxynol-9 (N-9) may be effective against HIV even when the condom ruptures. Three studies found that intact condoms lubricated with N-9 did not leak HIV; when these condoms were deliberately ruptured, the HIV was still inactivated [15]. Several clinical studies demonstrated that condoms protect men and women against bacterial and viral infections [13,14]. The correct use of a condom provides an effective mechanical barrier: for a man, a condom reduces the risk of infection acquired through penile exposure to cervical, vaginal, vulvar, or rectal secretions or lesions; for a woman, a condom prevents exposure of the female genital mucosa to urethral discharge, semen, and lesions of the penis.

When condoms are used with other barrier methods, the condom's protective effects appear to be enhanced. In one case-control study, condoms used alone reduced the risk of gonorrhea in women by 13%. In women using both condoms and spermicides, the risk of gonorrhea was reduced by 59% [16].

A few studies have shown that condoms offer some protection against HIV. In a study of Danish prostitutes, condoms were used in 68% of episodes of vaginal intercourse, 54% of episodes of fellatio, and 3% of anal sex episodes. None of the prostitutes was seropositive for HIV [17]. In another study of 448 German prostitutes who used condoms extensively, 97.5% with vaginal intercourse and 55% with anal intercourse, none of the 399 tested for HIV was seropositive [18]. An ongoing multicenter study of U.S. prostitutes by the Centers for Disease Control found that 11% of prostitutes who reported unprotected vaginal intercourse were seropositive for HIV. None of the prostitutes who used condoms for every episode of vaginal intercourse was seropositive [19]. However, the absence of control groups in these studies greatly reduces the validity of the findings.

SPERMICIDES AND STDs

Several studies have shown that N-9, the active ingredient of most spermicidal products, is effective in vitro against a variety of STD pathogens, including *Neisseria gonorrhoeae, Treponema pallidum,* HSV-1 and HSV-2, chlamydia, *Candida albicans,* and *Trichomonas vaginalis* [12–22]. The mechanism of action of N-9 is based primarily on its surfactant properties; it immobilizes sperm, bacteria, and viruses by disrupting cell membranes and viral envelopes [23]. A few studies also have shown that N-9 and active ingredients in other spermicidal preparations inactivate HIV in vitro. In one study [24], HIV inactivation occurred within 60 sec of exposure to an N-9 concentration of 0.05% or greater; this concentration was also toxic to the lymphocytes infected by the virus. Other studies have confirmed that a concentration of 0.05% N-9 disrupts free HIV.

In vivo studies support the in vitro findings that spermicides offer protection against STDs. For women, this protection is enhanced when spermicide use is combined with another barrier method, such as a diaphragm or condom. In one case-control study [16], the use of spermicide with a diaphragm reduced the risk of gonorrhea by 55%. The use of spermicide alone reduced the risk of gonorrhea by only 10%. In a study by Family Health International (FHI) in Bangkok, the use of the N-9 contraceptive sponge reduced the women's risk of acquiring gonorrhea by 69% and of acquiring chlamydia by 33% [25].

Few studies have evaluated the effectiveness of spermicides in preventing HIV transmission. A study of the protective effects of the contraceptive vaginal sponge (Today®; containing 1 gm of N-9) against the transmission of HIV is ongoing in Kenya, but results are not yet available [26]. In another study, FHI is evaluating the acceptability of a new female condom.

DISCUSSION

The AIDS epidemic has drawn attention to other STDs, which, until recently, have received little notice from policy makers and health providers. Sexual transmission of HIV is the most important mode of spread of the AIDS epidemic in developing countries. STD control is an important component of AIDS prevention activities for several reasons:

1 AIDS is spread predominantly by sexual intercourse. Public health measures used to control other STDs are applicable in AIDS prevention.
2 Epidemiological evidence strongly suggests that individuals who practice high-risk sexual behavior are at risk of acquiring a range of STDs, including HIV infection. The highest rates of HIV infection usually are found in prostitutes and other persons who have multiple sexual partners and high rates of STDs.
3 Evidence is increasing that the presence of STDs increases the risk of HIV infection.
4 Prevention of STDs, whether through reducing the number of sexual partners or through use of barrier methods, will reduce HIV transmission.

The effects of condoms in preventing most STDs, including HIV, are assumed to be protective enough to justify their widespread use in AIDS intervention programs. Condoms are safe, relatively cheap, devoid of side effects, and effective when used correctly and consistently for birth control. The major drawback of condom use in family planning programs has been the relatively high failure rates. Failure of condoms to protect against pregnancy is explained by user failure more often than by product failure. The factors that influence use effectiveness are important in preventing both pregnancy and STDs, including HIV. Most research about condoms has focused on their use as a contraceptive to prevent pregnancy. Whereas the risk of pregnancy usually occurs during a narrow time span (2–3 days) during a woman's menstrual cycle, STD and HIV transmission can occur each time a couple has sex. To be effective in preventing HIV and other STDs, condoms must be used correctly with every sexual act, especially by persons for whom the risk of HIV infection is high. This caveat is important for high-risk groups, such as prostitutes, who have a large number of sexual partners and other cofactors, such as genital ulcer disease.

Some evidence shows that the correct and regular use of condoms protects against several STDs, including HIV, but further research is required. However, the protective effect of condoms against STDs and HIV may be synergistic because STDs, such as chancroid, syphilis, chlamydia, and herpes, appear to increase the risk of HIV infection. On the other hand, condoms may not protect against infections acquired from an open genital ulcer disease that is not located on the penis. The acceptability and extent of use of condoms, and other factors that affect condom failure, also should be studied. Ultimately, we may have an acceptable and effective method that protects against pregnancy and HIV and other STDs.

Spermicides appear to offer some protection for both men and women against STDs, particularly when used with other barrier methods [16,25]. The protection may be only slight when a spermicide is used alone [16]. Insufficient information is available to determine the effectiveness of spermicides in preventing HIV transmission. However, use of a spermicide with a condom or diaphragm may reduce the risk of HIV indirectly by reducing the risk of STDs. Despite the need for a female-driven barrier method to prevent HIV infection in high-risk groups such as prostitutes, promoting the use of spermicides alone does not appear to be justified by the available evidence [27,28]. FHI is supporting a study to assess the efficacy of N-9 spermicides in preventing HIV infection in Zambia, and another study is planned for the Cameroon.

THE NEED FOR FURTHER RESEARCH

In the past few years, our knowledge of the epidemiology and prevention of AIDS has lagged behind our increasing knowledge of HIV. Studies are urgently needed to help us understand the interaction between STDs and HIV more thoroughly and to evaluate the protective effects of condoms and spermicides or virucides against STDs and HIV transmission. Answers to the following questions are needed:

1 Interaction between HIV and STDs:

   a. What is the pathophysiology of the interaction between STD and HIV infection?
   b. What is the relative risk of STDs, especially genital ulcer disease, in different subpopulations, including groups at relatively low risk of HIV infection?
   c. Do STDs accelerate the progression from HIV infection to AIDS?

d. Does a preexisting HIV infection adversely affect the response to treatment of an existing or newly acquired STD?
e. Do the treatment and control of STDs lower the risk of HIV infection in a high-risk population?

2 Barrier contraception and STDs/HIV:

a. Does the regular and correct use of condoms alone prevent STDs? What level of protection is afforded for each STD? Does the regular and correct use of condoms alone prevent HIV infection?
b. Does the regular and correct use of spermicides alone prevent STDs? What level of protection is offered for each STD? Does the regular and correct use of spermicides prevent HIV infection?
c. What effect does each of these combinations of barrier contraceptives have on preventing STDs or HIV infection: condom with spermicide, diaphragm with spermicide, spermicidal sponge, female condom with spermicide?
d. Do spermicides other than N-9, or virucides, prevent the sexual transmission of HIV infection?

Even if we demonstrate unequivocally that barrier methods prevent STDs, including HIV, these contraceptives must be used regularly and correctly to be effective. Further research is required on ways to increase the acceptability and use of these methods to reduce failure rates.

Barrier contraceptives do not constitute the primary solution to the AIDS epidemic. Reduction or elimination of sexual activity with persons who exhibit high-risk behavior, reduction in the number of sexual partners, and mutual monogamy are the most effective preventive measures. Although barrier contraceptives may only reduce the risk of STDs and HIV infection rather than eliminate the risk entirely, they should be recommended for persons at risk.

REFERENCES

1. **Piot P, Plummer FA, Rey MA, Ngugi EN, Rouzioux C:** Retrospective seroepidemiology of AIDS virus infection in Nairobi populations. J Infect Dis 155:1108–1112, 1987.

2. **Kreiss JK, Koech F, Plummer FA, Holmes KK, Lighfoote M:** AIDS virus infection in Nairobi prostitutes: Spread of the epidemic to East Africa. N Engl J Med 314:414–418, 1986.

3. **Plummer FA, D'Costa LJ, Nsanze H, Dylewski J, Karasira P, Ronald AR:** Epidemiology of chancroid and H ducreys in Nairobi Kenya. Lancet 2:1293–1295, 1983.

4. **Plummer FA, Simonsen JN, Ngugi EN, Cameron DW, Piot P, Ndinya-Achola JO:** Incidence of human immunodeficiency virus (HIV) infection and related disease in a cohort of Nairobi prostitutes. Abstract M84: III International Conference on AIDS, Washington, DC, 1987.

5. **Handsfield HH, Ashley RL, Rompalo AM, Stamm WE, Wood RW, Corey L:** Association of anogenital ulcer disease with HIV infection in homosexual men. Abstract F16: III International Conference on AIDS, Washington, DC, 1987.

6. **Greenblatt RM, Lukehart SA, Plummer FA, et al.:** Genital ulceration as a risk factor for HIV infection. J AIDS 2:47–50, 1988.

7. **Kreiss J, Caral M, Meheus A:** Role of sexually transmitted diseases in transmitting HIV. Genitonim Med 64:1–2, 1988.

8. **Simonsen JN, Cameron DW, Gakinya MN, et al.:** Human immunodeficiency virus infection among men with sexually transmitted diseases. N Engl J Med 319:274–278, 1988.

9. **Cameron DW, Plummer FA, Simonsen JN, Ndinya-Achola JO, D'Costa LJ, Piot P:** Female to male heterosexual transmission of HIV infection in Nairobi. Abstract MP91: III International Conference on AIDS, Washington, DC, 1987.

10. **Piot P, Plummer FA, Mhalu FS, Lamboray JL, Chin J, Mann JM:** AIDS: An international perspective. Science 239:573–579, 1988.

11. **Lukehart SA, Hook EW, Baker-Zander SA, Collier AC:** Invasion of the central nervous system by treponema pallidum. Ann Intern Med 109:855–862, 1988.

12. **Feldblum PJ, Fortney JA:** Condoms, spermicides, and the transmission of HIV: A review of literature. Am J Public Health 78:52–54, 1988.

13. **Stone KM, Grimes DA, Magder LS:** Primary prevention of STDs. JAMA 255:1763–1766, 1986.

14. **Conant MA, Spicer D, Smith C:** Herpes simplex virus transmission: Condom studies. Sex Transmitted Dis 11:94–95, 1984.

15. **Judson FM, Bodin GF, Levin MJ, Ehret JM, Rietmeijer CA:** In vitro evaluations of condoms with and without nonoxynol-9 as physical and chemical barriers against chlamydia trachomatis, HSV type 2 and HIV. Sex Transm Dis 16:51–56, 1989.

16. **Austin H, Louv W, Alexander J:** A case control study of spermicides and gonorrhea. JAMA 251:2822–2824, 1984.

17. **Krogsgaard K, Gluud C, Pdersen C, et al.:** Widespread use of condoms and low prevalence of STDs in Danish non-drug addict prostitutes. Br Med J 293:1473–1474, 1986.

18. **Smith GL, Smith KF:** Lack of HIV infection and condom use in licensed prostitutes [letter]. Lancet 2:1392, 1986.

19. **Centers for Disease Control:** Antibody to HIV in female prostitutes. MMWR 36:157–161, 1987.

20. **North B:** Vaginal contraceptives: Effective protection from STDs for women? J Reprod Med 33:307–311, 1988.

21. **Kappus E, Quinn T:** The spermicide nonoxynol-9 does not inhibit chlamydia trachomatis in vitro. Sex Transmitted Dis 13:134–137, 1986.

22. **Berger KL, Remington K:** The prophylactic properties of the Today® sponge and other spermicides containing contraceptives. Adv Contraception 3:125–131, 1987.

23. **Centers for Disease Control:** VD Fact Sheet, 1975, 32 ed. Atlanta; CDC, 1976.

24. **Hicks DR, Martin LS, Getchell JP:** Inactivation of HTLV/LAV-infected cultures of normal human lymphocytes by nonoxynol-9 in vitro [letter]. Lancet 2:1422–1423, 1985.

25. **Rosenburg MJ, Rojanapithayakorn W, Feldblum PJ, Higgins SJ:** Effect of the contraceptive sponge on chlamydia, gonorrhea and candidiasis: A comparative clinical trial. JAMA 257:2308–2312, 1987.

26. **Kreiss J:** Nonoxynol-9 and Prevention of Sexual Transmission of HIV [report]. Seattle: University of Washington, 1988.

27. **Kreiss J, Cameron DW, Ngugi E, et al.:** Efficacy of the spermicide nonoxynol-9 (N-9) in preventing heterosexual transmission of HIV. Abstract 6525: IV International Conference on AIDS, Stockholm, June, 1988.

28. **World Health Organization:** Consultation on Prevention and Control of Sexually Transmitted Diseases in Population Groups at Risk. Consensus Statement, Chemical Prophylaxis. Geneva; WHO, 1988.

DISCUSSION

DR. MARX: Can you indicate the prevalence of HIV-1 and HIV-2 cases between western Africa and central Africa?

DR. LAMPTEY: I am sorry, I do not have the data, but most of the HIV-2 cases diagnosed so far have been in western Africa. There have been isolated cases in Angola and Mozambique. Probably the countries with the highest prevalence of HIV-2 are Guinea Bissau and then Burkina Faso. Some studies showed that 30% of the cases of HIV infection were with HIV-2.

DR. MARX: So HIV-2 is in the minority?

DR. LAMPTEY: Yes.

DR. MATA: Do you have any suggestions regarding changing policies towards the use of contraceptives?

DR. LAMPTEY: The data from Africa may not be relevant to Latin America, where we are just beginning to learn things that we did not suspect. For instance, in Cali, Colombia, a recent study showed that 60% of heterosexual couples regularly have anal sex. In Costa Rica, one in every five men who come to our clinic seeking HIV testing regards himself as homosexual. The word gay is not much used in Central America. Some homosexual men, even married men, have regular sex with women. We have to urge couples to use condoms.

For people who are not very well educated, we have to promote the idea that it protects against infection too.

DR. GUINAN: I would just like to endorse what Dr. Lamptey said about looking at different subpopulations and their risk for STD and HIV transmission. In the United States, one of the things that would bear considerably on the heterosexual transmission of HIV is the crack epidemic. This epidemic, which was not mentioned except by Dr. Potts earlier, is now pervasive in the United States, and not only in the inner cities but also in smaller towns. The epidemic of STDs that Dr. Ward Cates' group has been detecting recently, including much of the increase in syphilis, is associated with crack and crack houses, where sex is exchanged for drugs. This affects women very much. In the United States, women are less likely to be IV drug users, but crack apparently affects men and women equally. There seems to be a great desire to have sex while on crack.

In this particular situation, where there is no rational behavior, talk of condoms or contraceptives is not something that is very relevant. The increasing problem that we are seeing in this country is the fact that these women, especially those who are exchanging sex for drugs, are highly susceptible to HIV. This is because the men who come to the crack houses are likely to be IV drug users, such as IV cocaine users, and are likely to be HIV-positive and to infect the women. This population must be studied.

In the United States, when we are thinking about prevention, we have to realize, as Ward Cates' group has shown, that the risk of STDs is directly related to these crack houses. That is an observation that we as public health workers have to recognize and put into our strategy for preventing the heterosexual transmission of HIV.

DR. CAIN: I agree with your statement about the data on sexual behavior being woefully inadequate throughout the world, so I was very interested in your comments about Brazil and the increase in the heterosexual spread of HIV. Could you comment on your source of data, particularly the sexual behavior data on the use of transvestite prostitutes by married men?

DR. LAMPTEY: I am sorry but those data are anecdotal. A physician I talked to who has been seeing men with gonorrhea provided this information. He says that he cannot publish his data.

DR. MATA: In Brazil, a psychiatrist published a book in which he described tranvestite prostitutes. In Costa Rica, about two hundred male transvestites who were basically transsexual and used a lot of hormones were studied. Some of them were indistinguishable from a beautiful lady. We have wrong ideas about these people. When we go deeply into their behavior we find that most of them will serve as passive partners, but they have very complex practices. The men who seek them seek beautiful women, but they engage in anal intercourse. They penetrate these men. But some of the men, maybe 15%, also have relations with women. They are certainly a source of STDs, but not HIV in Costa Rica so far.

DR. CONE: We all talk about vaginal intercourse and anal intercourse as if that is the mechanism of transmission. When I talk with students, they are all surprised to discover that the problem is that semen contains the pathogens and white blood cells, and that it is the source of HIV. I think if we could come up with sort of a jingle so that people would understand this better, it would help. One jingle could be, "semen and sores." I guess men do not want to think that their semen can be the vector, but somehow we have to get across the point that it is not intercourse per se, but rather that the ejaculate contains the virus.

General Discussion: Mechanics of Heterosexual Transmission

Murray B. Gardner, Moderator

DR. SCOFIELD: I have some questions for Dr. Anderson. You presented beautiful data demonstrating the presence of leukocytes in the semen of HIV-infected men as compared to controls, but we did not see any infectivity data. How do you determine without doubt that sperm from HIV-infected men were utterly without HIV antigens? In our determinations, they are there in very small amounts. How do you conduct your infectivity studies, by co-culture? In our hands, co-culture always works with blood leukocytes, but, with seminal leukocytes, it only works in a portion of the men. Every HIV-infected man is not going to have infectious semen components. Can you comment, please?

DR. ANDERSON: People have been frustrated by semen culture, because seminal plasma is toxic to target cell systems. It contains what immunologists call immunosuppressive factors, but actually they are antiproliferative factors that in high concentrations are toxic to peripheral blood leukocytes (PBLs) and tumor target cells that are commonly used in HIV culture systems. We bypassed that problem by using human serum instead of fetal calf serum in the culture medium, because it is the polyamine oxidase in fetal calf serum that induces much of the toxic activity in semen. We have also titered both seminal plasma and semen components in our target cell systems to determine the toxic range, and we add nontoxic amounts to the cultures. With spermatozoa, you may also have antiproliferative or toxicity effects. We standardize our cultures to a maximum ratio of sperm per lymphocyte or other target cell type.

We use a 24 well microtiter plate system to compare three types of target cells: sup-T lymphoma cells, U937 monocytic cells, and phytohemagglutinin (PHA)-activated peripheral blood leukocytes. We find we get the best results with PBL cultures. We culture cell-free seminal fluid that is millipore filtered. We also culture the enriched

Heterosexual Transmission of AIDS, pages 267–272

white blood cell fraction and the motile sperm pellet following percoll gradient centrifugation.

DR. SCOFIELD: So are you saying that you have actually cocultured all three different target cell types with all these different components?

DR. ANDERSON: Yes, in our early studies on approximately 12 individuals, we found that PBL target cells provide the highest incidence of successful culture results, so now we are only using the PBL culture system.

DR. SCOFIELD: What do you mean by successful results?

DR. ANDERSON: Conversion of the culture supernatants to p24 antigen-positive; we sampled them every 3 days for 28 days and tested them by DuPont ELISA. We achieved conversion in the U937 and the sup-T models, but the incidence was higher in the PBLs, and we never had a positive conversion with the other models when we did not have a positive result with PBLs.

DR. SCOFIELD: You are saying that the effects of semen components for cocultures were always the cell-free seminal fluid?

DR. ANDERSON: That gave us the best results because it was sterile and we could get results essentially on every individual. With the cell fractions, some of the samples did not have 1,000,000 white blood cells or 1,000,000 sperm, and we often had a contamination problem with long-term cultures. However, we have successfully cultured all three components for 28 days with 12 individuals, and, of those 12, I think six were white blood cell-positive, and the white blood cell positivity correlated with seminal plasma positivity. In none of these cases, including one patient who had extremely high levels of free virus in his seminal plasma, did we observe conversion with the purified sperm fraction. We think that transmission of infectious HIV-1 by sperm is a very rare phenomenon; in our limited number of samples, we have not seen it.

DR. MILLER: With the culture techniques that we use, we have not found any toxicity with sperm. We conducted experiments with tritium uptake by the cells and incubated the sperm at a ratio of ten sperm to one cell. We have, in fact, sometimes found increased tritium uptake under those circumstances, so I do not think that toxicity is a problem. We basically culture all the motile sperm we can get from one patient, so I think we may be maximizing the system to a greater extent than you.

DR. JOHNS: I have a speculative response to Dr. Anderson's comments and then a question. In your specific gradient L separation, there was one fraction containing nonmotile sperm, and, if it so happens that the virus-bearing sperm are actually nonmotile, you would have missed your virus, so I speculate that this is one possible explanation for the difference.

My question to Dr. Martin Dym is in relation to the monkey model that was described earlier. If 1 ml of carrier fluid is inoculated into the monkey's urethra, how far retrograde will it travel? In looking at pathogenesis, one must understand which cell type is first infected; that is, the primary cell of multiplication. I am trying to speculate what that might be in the monkey urethra, and how far back the fluid would have traveled?

DR. DYM: I cannot answer the question, but I suppose the speakers are here. Perhaps they can say something.

DR. ALEXANDER: We never checked that, but we could take some methylene blue fluid and do an evaluation.

DR. WITKIN: One of the outstanding differences now seems to be whether or not there is CD4 on sperm. In our laboratory experiment, as in Dr. Anderson's, we cannot find it. I would like Drs. Miller and Anderson to comment on that.

DR. MILLER: When we talk about the role of sperm in the transmission of HIV, I think whether the CD4 is present on sperm or not is not really such a crucial question. If it is present, then you can envision the virus fusing and actually becoming internalized, and then, of course, you can start thinking in more interesting directions if that is the case.

We have tried antibodies to CD4, including OKT and OKT4A, and have been able to confine the positive finding to a small cell population of sperm. This is not the case every time with every donor, but all the literature that I have read on sperm antigens report an incredible amount of polymorphism, depending on what kind of fixatives were used. There is a lot of donor-to-donor variation as well as day-to-day variation with the same donors, so it does not surprise me that people are reporting differences. I want to stress again that, in terms of our model of HIV transmission, HIV-infected sperm may not necessarily be important.

DR. ANDERSON: To address in more detail the concept that HIV binds to the sperm, we have looked at sperm from more than 20 HIV-seropositive patients by transmission electron microscopy and have never seen HIV attachment to sperm. We have also examined sperm following in vitro coculture with HIV. We have simulated reproductive events in vitro by adding HIV to semen before coagulation, and HIV to semen mixed with fresh vaginal secretions. We also incubated washed sperm with HIV at both 37°C and 4°C, reasoning that 4°C coculture might retard fusion events that could occur between virus and sperm.

In none of our electron microscope studies have we observed HIV attachment to the surface of sperm. We have also taken sperm from these coincubation experiments, passed them through percoll gradients, and added them to culture systems. We have never seen HIV infection with the purified sperm fraction from these samples. Perhaps we are not seeing low-incidence phenomena, but our evidence argues against sperm serving as principal vectors in HIV transmission.

DR. MILLER: Using EM, we have been able to find 120 antigens on the surface of sperm. We have not looked for actual virus particles for exactly the same reasons that were mentioned, because it is going to be very difficult to establish by EM that these are indeed HIV particles. We have found not only that there appear to be increased numbers of immature germ cells but also that the sperm membranes are not quite as healthy-looking as those of normal sperm; therefore, I think it is going to be even more difficult to detect virus by EM.

DR. PADIAN: I have a question for Drs. Miller and Scofield. What is your hypothesis concerning transmission? Let us not discuss whether a virus or sperm is a laboratory phenomenon or an in vitro phenomenon, or even if it occurs in vivo. I will be sending specimens to both laboratories in the hope that this will help resolve some of this controversy. If viral incorporation into sperm is a true phenomenon and it occurs in only a few people, and if those people also have HIV-infected lymphocytes or free virus in seminal fluid, then what is the hypothesis for transmission? You are describing this phenomenon in AIDS patients only but not seropositive patients; we know that asymptomatic patients can transmit the disease. Does it really matter if, in addition to finding HIV in sperm, you find it in much larger quantities in seminal fluid as well?

DR. SCOFIELD: The hypothesis has two parts, the sperm can carry virus into cells through one or both novel receptor-like end pathways described here for the first time: 1) the DR target pathway for normal sperm assuming that a virus-coated sperm is going to have its CD4-like ligand available for fusigenic interactions with DR and 2) the CD4 target pathway that involves HIV-bearing sperm. There is an abundance of 120 antigen on sperm from AIDS patients. It is possible that the spermatozoa in the semen of an AIDS patient would have acquired 120 from another source but that they do not have virus nucleocapsid on the surface; we believe that our infectivity data are quite convincing.

We admit that we do not always get a positive result. Our approach requires sperm penetration of target cells through fusigenic interactions that can drag viral particles into cells, making them available to the cytoplasm.

Sperm may also assist in HIV infection by activating target cells through either or both of the receptor-like end pathways. Independent of that, our preliminary data support our morphological observations of this event. Calcium mobilization occurs, and this event should be physiologically relevant either to virus attached to the sperm or to free virus particles in the seminal fluid.

DR. BURNHILL: Being a humble clinician, I find myself somewhat confused by contradictory statements about the location of virus in genital tract secretions. Is there any consensus on the next two statements? I think they both may offer some clinical help. It seems most likely that the virus, if present, is associated with lymphocytes in the semen; therefore, clinically, if you use a gram stain and if there are no white cells, you might a priori say that virus shedding may not be present. That is a low-tech test that one can perform out in the field.

Similarly, in women, if shedding occurs around the time of menses, one could advise women that they are taking a higher risk if they are bleeding. This would give us another rather simple clinical intervention.

DR. WITKIN: Tell your patients to have safe sex. There is no other way out.

DR. ALEXANDER: Dr. Anderson pointed out that normal men have many white blood cells in their semen, and so you cannot directly correlate the presence of white blood cells with the potential transmission of HIV. Second, Dr. Padian noted that, in epidemiologic studies, there is no association between transmission of HIV and menstrual blood.

DR. BURNHILL: Normal men may have white blood cells, but when a large number of white cells are present in semen, one should consider whether chlamydia or something else may be present. Dr. Anderson simply evaluated the semen of people who did not have HIV. The presence of white cells in any quantity should be looked into.

DR. ANDERSON: We have followed our laboratory donors over time, and several have demonstrated transient spikes in semen white blood cell counts. This suggests that you would want to monitor the HIV patients very frequently, and I do not think it would be practical. I should also mention that semen white cells are difficult to quantify by gram stain because they can resemble immature germ cells, so that poses a second problem. Also, you consider a threshold of 1,000,000 white cells per milliter significant; when you have a hundred-to-one ratio of sperm to white cells, they are not so apparent unless you use monoclonal antibodies.

DR. PAULSEN: For 7 years, King Holmes and I tried to determine some relationship between white cells and infection, and there is absolutely none. You can have as many as 2,000,000 white cells per milliliter of seminal fluid with absolutely no evidence of chlamydia, cytomegalovirus, or anything else.

23

Effectiveness of Vaginal Contraceptives in Prevention of Sexually Transmitted Diseases

Barbara B. North

The alarming rise in the incidence of most sexually transmitted diseases (STDs) in the past several decades has been attributed not only to the ease with which STD microorganisms are transmitted but to an increased frequency of many sexual contacts between individuals. Sexual transmission generally occurs by direct contact with infectious lesions or body fluids. For men, condoms have a significant protective effect in vitro and in vivo against STD transmission [1–3]. For women, vaginal spermicides may offer considerable protection against STDs.

Spermicidal methods available to women include foam, jelly, cream, suppositories, the vaginal sponge, the diaphragm, and the cervical cap [4]. Spermicides function by placing a chemical barrier between infected fluids and vulnerable mucous membranes. The surfactant properties of the most widely used spermicide, nonoxynol-9 (N-9), immobilize not only sperm but also bacterial and viral pathogens by disrupting cell membranes and viral envelopes. In the case of chlamydia, N-9 may function as an antimicrobial agent via action on the chlamydia receptors or on the inclusion membranes present on host cells rather than by disrupting the chlamydia cell membrane itself [5,6].

Since specific STD pathogens may infect different sites, the method by which spermicide is delivered to vaginal tissues may be one determinant of the effectiveness of spermicides in STD prophy-

Heterosexual Transmission of AIDS, pages 273–290

laxis. Gonorrhea and chlamydia organisms infect mainly cervical and endometrial tissue. Thus a contraceptive that covers the cervix may be most effective in prophylaxis of these diseases. Conversely, vaginitis pathogens responsible for bacterial vaginosis or trichomoniasis may be more susceptible to spermicide dispersed throughout the vaginal vault. Similarly, prophylaxis against viral pathogens such as the herpes simplex virus (HSV) and the human immunodeficiency virus (HIV) may depend on adequate spermicide dispersal on all genital surfaces as well as protection of cervical tissues and of the upper genital tract.

IN VITRO STUDIES

Many laboratory studies [7,8] have demonstrated the ability of N-9 and other spermicides in vaginal contraceptives to inhibit growth of *Treponema pallidum, Neisseria gonorrhoea, Candida albicans,* and *Trichomonas vaginalis.* At concentrations as low as 1%, many contraceptives effectively immobilize pathogenic microorganisms in as little as 90 sec. Similar studies have confirmed the in vitro effectiveness of N-9 contraceptive products in inactivating *Chlamydia* and HSV-1 and -2 [9–12]. HIV is also very sensitive to N-9 in vitro. The virus is fully immobilized after less than a 60 sec exposure to concentrations of N-9 likely to be found in the vagina [13,14]. A summary of in vitro studies using various N-9 formulations is shown in Table 1.

Extensive in vitro antimicrobial testing has also been conducted using the vaginal contraceptive sponge (Today® sponge; Whitehall Laboratories). In contrast to other N-9 preparations, the sponge combines a polyurethane sponge (which acts as a barrier and absorbs seminal fluids) with a large reservoir of N-9, which is released over an extended wear time of up to 30 hr. The sponge contains 1 gm of N-9 plus several weak organic acids that act as buffers and preservatives.

Singh [15] reported antibacterial and antiviral activity in the sponge and in foam obtained from a sponge to which water had been added to facilitate spermicidal foam release. Both the intact sponge and the resulting foam were highly active against *N. gonorrhoea* and HSV-2. The foam eluted from the sponge also showed activity against *T. vaginalis, Gardneralla vaginalis,* and *Chlamydia trachomatis.* Another study [16] confirmed in vitro inhibitory activity of the sponge against *N. gonorrhoea, Mycoplasma hominis, Ureaplasma urealyticum, G. vaginalis, C. trachomatis,* and HSV-1 and -2, and a recent laboratory evaluation of sponge eluate confirmed significant activity against HIV in vitro [17]. Vaginal concentrations of N-9 produced by the contraceptive sponge average 80–125 mg/ml, which far exceed minimum virucidal or bactericidal concentrations. Only one study [18] failed to show an antimicrobial effect of the sponge. This may have been due to poor study design and failure to effect spermicide activation and release from the polyurethane sponge [18]. In vitro antimicrobial studies of the vaginal sponge are summarized in Table 2.

Thus laboratory data strongly suggest that N-9 preparations in general should be effective in reducing STD transmission. Evaluation is ongoing of other spermicidal preparations, including octoxynol, benzalkonium chloride, chlorhexidine, and menfegol [19].

RETROSPECTIVE CLINICAL EVIDENCE

Jick and coauthors [20] contrasted the methods of contraception used by 77 women with a positive *N. gonorrhoea* culture to those used by 164 women with a negative culture. The risk ratio (RR) of contracting gonorrhea for spermicide users was 0.13. Kelaghan and coauthors [21] evaluated the protective effect of barrier-method contraception against pelvic inflammatory disease (PID). Ultimately, 645 women with a discharge diagnosis of PID were compared to 2,509 sexually active women having no history of PID. The risk of hospitalization for PID in women using barrier methods of contraception compared to all other women in the study or those using no contraception was significantly reduced (RR = 0.60 for each comparison). Moreover, the type of barrier contraception was found to influence the probability of developing PID, with those subjects using a diaphragm having a lower risk than condom and spermicide users.

A recent study by Cramer and coauthors [22] concluded that "contraceptive users who use barrier methods that combined both a mechanical and chemical barrier, such as diaphragms, cervical caps, and condoms plus spermicides, have the clearest protection against tubal damage."

Austin and coauthors [23] compared women attending an STD clinic who were diagnosed as having gonorrhea to women who either had an STD other than gonorrhea or had no STD. The RR of gonorrhea for barrier contraception and/or spermicide users relative to nonusers was 0.54. The adjusted RR of contracting gonorrhea for individuals using spermicides alone was 0.90. These authors suggested that the much larger protective effect (RR = 0.13) observed by Jick and colleagues [20] for spermicide users at risk of gonococcal infection may have resulted from the high percentage (50%) of subjects who used diaphragms in addition to spermicidal contraceptives. Finally, a preliminary study [24] of 593 spermicide users and

TABLE 1. Summary of In Vitro Antimicrobial Studies on Spermicidal Contraceptive Preparations

Reference	Investigator(s)	Year	Test method/ preparation	Organism(s) tested	Effect
7	Singh et al.	1972a	20 Different preparations	*T. pallidum* *N. gonorrhoeae*	Treponemes immobilized Bactericidal
8	Singh et al.	1972b	20 Different preparations	*T. vaginalis* *C. albicans*	Trichomonacidal Some antifungal activity
40	Singh and Cutler	1982	5 Different preparations	*T. pallidum*	Spirocheticidal
41	Cowan and Cree	1973	Nonoxynol-9 alone	*N. gonorrhoeae*	Bactericidal
42	Todd et al.	1984	4 Different preparations	*N. gonorrhoeae*	Bactericidal
43	Bolch and Warren	1973	Emko vaginal foam	*N. gonorrhoeae* *T. vaginalis*	Bactericidal Trichomonacidal
10	Benes and McCormack	1985	Conceptrol and nonoxynol-9 alone	*C. trachomatis*	Inhibited growth
11	Kelly et al.	1985	Conceptrol, Koromex, and nonoxynol-9 alone	*C. trachomatis*	Inhibited growth
5	Kappas and Ouinn	1986	Nonoxynol-9 alone	*C. trachomatis*	No direct effect but prevented cell infection

12	Singh et al.	1976	5 Different preparations	HSV-2	Virucidal
9	Asculai et al.	1978	Nonoxynol-9 alone	HSV-1	Virucidal
				HSV-2	Virucidal
44	Rapo and Wrzos-	1985	Nonoxynol-9 and interferon	HSV-2	Synergistic reduction in viral activity
45	Barbi et al.	1987	Nonoxynol-9 alone	HSV-2	Virucidal
				RSV	Virucidal
				Polio type 2	No effect
13	Hicks et al.	1985	Nonoxynol-9 alone	HIV and HIV-infected lymphocytes	Inactivation
3	Rietmeijer et al.	1988	Nonoxynol-9 containing condoms	HIV	Virucidal
14	Malkovsky et al.	1988	4 Different preparations and nonoxynol-9 alone	HIV	Inactivation
46	Eglin	1988	Nonoxynol-9 treated condoms and nonoxynol-9 suppositories	HIV	Virucidal

(continued)

TABLE 1. Continued.

Reference	Investigator(s)	Year	Test method/ preparation	Organism(s) tested	Effect
19	Coulson et al.	1988	Nonoxynol-9 alone	HIV	All lethal
			Chlorhexidine alone	HSV-2	All lethal
			Benzalkonium chloride alone	*C. trachomatis*	All toxic to host cell
				Giardia intestinalis	All lethal
			Menfegol alone	*Entamoeba histolytica*	All lethal
			Octoxynol alone	Genital mycoplasma	No effect
			Nonoxynol-9 and chlorhexidine	Cytomegalovirus	All toxic to host cell except octoxynol and benzalkonium
				Epstein-Barr virus	All toxic to host cell except octoxynol

TABLE 2. Summary of In Vitro Antimicrobial Studies on the Today® Contraceptive Sponge

Reference	Investigator(s)	Year	Test method/ preparation	Organism(s) tested	Effect
15	Singh	1983	Eluates in the presence of sponge	*N. gonorrhoeae*	Bactericidal
				HSV-2	Virucidal
47	Smith et al.	1987	Sponge eluates	*G. vaginalis*	Bactericdal
				T. vaginalis	Trichomonacidal
				N. gonorrhoeae	Bactericidal
				M. hominis	Bactericidal
				U. urealyticum	Bactericidal
				HSV-1	Virucidal
				HSV-2	Virucidal
				C. trachomatis	Infectivity inhibited
					Bactericidal
16	Berger and Remington	1987	Sponge eluates	*G. vaginalis*	Bactericidal
				T. vaginalis	Trichomonacidal
				N. gonorrhoeae	Bactericidal
				HSV-1	Virucidal
				HSV-2	Virucidal
				C. trachomatis	Infectivity inhibited
48	Alden and Spence	1987	Sponge eluates	*T. vaginalis*	Trichomonacidal
17	Polsky et al.	1988	Sponge eluates	HIV	Virucidal, infectivity inhibited
18	Hammill et al.	1986	sponge pieces or in vitro vaginal model	*S. aureus*	None
				E. coli	None
				C. perfringens	None
				B. fragili	None
				N. gonorrhoeae	None
49	Tierno and Hanna	1985	Sponge	*S. aureus*	Growth inhibited
50	Stumpf et al.	1986	Sponge pieces	*S. aureus*	Growth inhibited
51	Remington et al.	1987	Sponge	*S. aureus*	Growth inhibited

TABLE 3. Summary of Clinical Studies on Vaginal Contraceptives and STD Prophylaxis

Reference	Investigator(s) (year)	Preparation(s) tested	Type of study	Study site	Study population	Number of subjects	Results
31	Rosenberg et al. (1987)	Today sponge	Randomized, controlled clinical trial, parallel and crossover phases	Bangkok, Thailand	Prostitutes	149 Users 163 Nonusers	Results of parallel phase suggested that sponge users were less likely to contract chlamydial and gonococcal infections (RR = 0.67 and 0.31, respectively) but more likely to develop candidiasis (RR = 2.76)
27	Cutler et al. (1977)	Conceptrol	Randomized, controlled clinical trial	Allegheny County, Pennsylvania	Women attending health department preventative medicine clinics	37 Users 50 Nonusers	During first 6 months of study, 97% of users remained uninfected compared to 75% of nonusers based on cumulative life-table proportions
30	Rendon et al. (1980)	Phenylmercuric acetate Nonoxynol-9 and placebo–suppositories	Randomized, placebo controlled clinical trial	Nueve Laredo, Mexico	Women attending health department outpatient clinics	24 Phenylmercuric acetate 24 Nonoxynol-9 29 Placebo	Incidence rates for gonorrhea of 0.08 for PMA users, 0.17 for N-9 users, and 0.28 for placebo users

28	Cole et al. (1980)	Lorophyn suppositories	Controlled clinical trial	Tampa and Orlando. Florida	Women attending venereal disease clinics	570 Subjects during pretrial control phase; 312 users and 363 nonusers during trial phase	Cumulative gonococcal reinfection rates of 19% in users and 40% in nonusers
21	Keeghan et al. (1982)	Chemical and mechanical barriers	Retrospective, case-control study	Nationwide multicenter	Women hospitalized for a first episode of PID. Data for controls and cases obtained from records of the Women's Health Study	645 Women with PID; 2,509 Women without PID	Relative risk for hospitalization for PID was 0.6 for users when compared to all others

(continued)

TABLE 3. Continued.

Reference	Investigator(s)	Preparation(s) tested	Type of study	Study site	Study population	Number of subjects	Results
20	Jick et al. (1982)	Any spermicide	Retrospective, case-control study	Seattle, Washington	Women with positive *N. gonorrhoeae* cultures; data obtained from records of the Group Health Cooperative of Puget Sound	77 Cases of gonorrhea; 164 Controls	RR for gonorrhea of 0.23 for spermicide users compared to all others
29	Austin et al. (1984)	Any spermicide	Retrospective, case-control study	Jefferson County, Alabama	Women attending STD clinics for treatment of gonorrhea	733 Cases of gonorrhea; 958 Controls	After correction for IUD, tubal ligation, and oral contraceptive use, RR for gonorrhea in users was 0.47; before correction RR was 0.67
24	Feldblum et al. (1988)	Any spermicide	Retrospective, case-control study	New York City	Women attending gynecologic or STD clinics	593 Spermicide users; 449 Oral contraceptive users	Odds ratios of 0.4 for trichomonal infection, 0.7 for bacterial vaginosis, 0.9 for candidiasis for spermicide users compared to oral contraceptive users
32	Louv et al. (1988)	Koromex gel	Double-blind, placebo-controlled trial	Jefferson County, Alabama	Women attending STD clinic	408 Users; 410 Nonusers	RR of chlamydial infections for users compared to nonusers was 0.79; RR of gonorrhea for users compared to nonuser was 0.75

449 oral contraceptive users who attended a reproductive health clinic indicated that spermicide use protected against trichomoniasis and bacterial vaginosis.

PROSPECTIVE CLINICAL EVIDENCE

Obtaining precise in vivo measurements of the protective effects of vaginal contraceptives presents two major problems. First, the frequency of a subject's exposure to STDs is difficult to gauge: patient records of the frequency of intercourse and the number of sexual partners are rarely accurate. Second, compliance with a contraceptive regimen varies widely and is often poor when the regimen is used for STD prophylaxis. A major clinical trial [25] showed that 90% of participants used a spermicidal preparation only 40% of the time. Even when used for contraception, vaginal methods are not used reliably by most women. In a comparative trial [26] of the vaginal contraceptive sponge and the diaphragm, only about 60% of the women reported using the assigned method during every episode of intercourse. Nonetheless, several controlled clinical investigations support the effectiveness of vaginal spermicides in reducing risk of acquiring gonorrhea in vivo.

Cutler and coauthors [27] conducted a clinical trial and reported a reduced rate of gonorrhea reinfection in women given packets of spermicidal cream compared to a control group. In the first 6 months, only 3% of women in the spermicide group were reinfected vs. 25% in the control group. Similarly, Cole and coauthors [28] reported a 19% gonorrhea reinfection rate in the spermicide treatment group vs. 40% in the control group. Jick and coauthors [20] calculated an estimated RR of 0.23 among spermicide users compared with other sexually active women.

The benefits of combining spermicides with a mechanical barrier to reduce risk of contracting gonorrhea was emphasized by Austin and coauthors [29]. These investigators found that women attending an STD clinic who used spermicides with mechanical barriers, such as condoms or diaphragms, received the greatest degree of gonorrhea protection. Another prospective controlled study, conducted by Rendon and coauthors [30], examined the relationship between chemical prophylaxis and the incidence of gonorrhea. Women attending an outpatient health clinic were randomly assigned to receive vaginal suppositories containing a placebo, phenylmercuric acetate, or N-9. After 6 months, the RR gonorrhea for those who used N-9 spermicide compared to controls was 0.60.

In a recent prospective study, Rosenberg and colleagues [31] evaluated the protective effect of the sponge in reducing incidence of gonorrhea and chlamydia infection in women at high risk for contracting these infections. Women wearing the sponge containing N-9 were much less likely than nonusers to contract chlamydia infection (RR = 0.67) and gonorrhea (RR = 0.31) after 400 women-weeks of use.

In another recent prospective study, reported by Louv and associates [32], 818 women from an STD clinic were randomly assigned to 5% N-9 gel or to a placebo gel. After 6 months, subjects using the N-9 gel had fewer chlamydial infections (RR = 0.79) and a reduced infection rate for *Neisseria* (RR = 0.75). A stronger protective effect was observed among women who used the gel for a majority of coital episodes. Reports of human clinical studies of spermicidal prophylaxis of STDs are summarized in Table 3.

DISCUSSION

In vitro data have clearly established the inherent virucidal and antimicrobial qualities of N-9 vaginal contraceptives. Human clinical evidence confirms a reduction in risk of acquiring chlamydia and gonorrhea under realistic use conditions. The apparent susceptibility of HIV to concentrations of N-9 and other spermicides likely to be found in the vagina is reassuring. However, recent discussions of a possible association between genital ulcers and HIV infection create additional concerns [33]. The likelihood that spermicidal products may damage the protective mucosal tissues of the vagina must be considered. Chvapil and coauthors [34] reported an inflammatory reaction in the vaginal wall of rats and rabbits exposed to N-9. However, human clinical trials [26,32] in the United States revealed no association between use of N-9 and gross mucosal damage, genital ulceration, or changes in cervical cytology under average use conditions (five to eight coital episodes per month) in generally healthy women. Nonetheless, since consensual vaginal intercourse without spermicidal use may itself cause microtrauma [35] frequent or continuous exposure to spermicides may exacerbate vaginal microtrauma under extreme use conditions, particularly in populations at risk for genital ulcer disease. However, among the prostitute population studied by Rosenberg and colleagues [31], frequent sponge use was not associated with development of vaginal trauma or genital ulcer disease. These women averaged ten sexual partners per week during the 6 week study period.

For many women, the risk of acquiring an STD is far greater than the risk of accidental pregnancy. STDs are highly contagious and can be transmitted with every coital episode, whereas pregnancy can occur only during fertile periods. In addition, the sequelae of an STD can present health risks to a women as serious as the consequences of an unwanted pregnancy. As indicated by Grimes [36], sexually transmitted pathogens may be directly or indirectly responsible for as many as 20% of all reproductive deaths.

Even when used conscientiously, vaginal contraceptives do not provide flawless contraception, and they are not likely to offer complete protection against STDs. However, from an epidemiological perspective, even imperfect preventive measures can have a significant impact on the incidence of disease. Stone [37] calculated that a 10% reduction in gonorrhea risk to an individual could reduce prevalence of the disease in the population by over 50%. According to the model developed by Lee [38], a dramatic decrease in STDs could be effected by a topical agent that is only 50% effective and used by only 25% of the at-risk population. Furthermore, the combination of vaginal spermicides with mechanical barrier methods, such as the sponge, condom, diaphragm, or cervical cap, may enhance the prophylactic effects, thus reducing any residual risk of transmission incurred by improper or inconsistent use of one method alone. Besides preventing transmission of the primary pathogen, these contraceptive measures may also reduce the transmission of STD cofactors, particularly other viruses.

A study [39] of 10,000 15–44-year-old U.S. women showed that the use of condoms remained low during the years 1982–1987 despite concern over STDs. The study found that only 16% of sexually active, unmarried women and 15% of married women used condoms. Obviously, the addition of a condom to vaginal spermicide would offer optimal protection. In circumstances when one or both partners refuse condoms, a vaginal spermicide allows the woman to participate actively in STD prevention.

REFERENCES

1. **Condoms prove effective against herpes, *Chlamydia*.** Contraceptive Technol Update 4:129, 1983.

2. **Stone KM, Grimes DA, Mageder LS:** Primary prevention of sexually transmitted diseases. JAMA 255:1763, 1986.

3. **Rietmeijer CAM, Krebs JW, Feorino PM, Judson FN:** Condoms as physical and chemical barriers against HIV. JAMA 259:1851–1853, 1988.

4. **North BB:** Vaginal contraceptives. Effective protection from sexually transmitted diseases for women? J Reprod Med 33:307–311, 1988.

5. **Kappus EW, Quinn TC: The spermicide nonoxynol-9 does not inhibit** *Chlamydia trachomatis* in vitro. Sex Transmitted Dis 13:134, 1986.

6. **Knight ST, Lee S, Davis C, Moorman D, Hodinka R, Wyrick P:** In vitro activity of N-9 on McCoy cells infected with *Chlamydia trachomatis.* Sex Transmitted Dis 14:165–173, 1987.

7. **Singh B, Cutler JC, Utidjian HMD:** Studies on the development of a vaginal preparation providing both prophylaxis against venereal disease and other genital infections and contraception. II. Effect in vitro of vaginal contraceptive and noncontraceptive preparations on *Treponema pallidum* and *Neisseria gonorrhoeae.* Br J Vener Dis 48:57, 1972.

8. **Singh B, Cutler JC, Utidjian HMD:** III. In vitro effect of vaginal contraceptives and selected vaginal preparations on *Candida albicans* and *Trichomonas vaginalis.* Contraception 5:401–411, 1972.

9. **Asculai SS, Weis MT, Rancourt MW, Kupferberg AB:** Inactivation of herpes simplex viruses by nonionic surfactants. Antimicrob Agents Chemother 13:686, 1978.

10. **Benes S, McCormack WM:** Inhibition of growth of *Chlamydia trachomatis* by nonoxynol-9 *in vitro.* Antimicrob Agents Chemother 27:724, 1985.

11. **Kelly JP, Reynolds RB, Stagno S, Louv WC, Alexander WJ:** In vitro activity of the spermicide nonoxynol-9 against *Chlamydia trachomatis.* Antimicrob Agents Chemother 27: 760, 1985.

12. **Singh B, Postic B, Cutler JC:** Virucidal effect of certain chemical contraceptives on Type 2 herpes virus. Am J Obstet Gynecol 26:422, 1976.

13. **Hicks DR, Martin LS, Getchell JP:** Inactivation of HTLV-III/LAV-infected cultures in normal human lymphocytes by nonoxynol-9 in vitro. Lancet 2:1422, 1985.

14. **Malkovsky M, Newell A, Dalgleish AG:** Inactivation of HIV by nonoxynol-9. Lancet 1:645, 1988.

15. **Singh B:** A new contraceptive sponge and its potential in prevention of sexually transmitted diseases. Abstract: 111th Annual Meeting of the American Public Health Association, Dallas, 1983.

16. **Berger KL, Remington K:** The prophylactic properties of the Today Sponge and other spermicides containing contraceptives. Adv Contraception 3:125–131, 1987.

17. **Polsky B, Gold JWM, Baron PA, Smith JL, Jensen RH, Armstrong D:** In vitro inactivation of HIV-I by contraceptive Sponge containing nonoxynol-9. Lancet 1:1456, 1988.

18. **Hammill HA, Ford LC, Suzuki J, Mickus K, Yip D, Finegold S:** In vitro testing of Today® vaginal contraceptive sponge with bacteria. Obstet Gynecol 6:S50–S52, 1986.

19. **Coulson A, Voeller B, Bernstein G, et al.:** Effectiveness of five spermicidal preparations against sexually transmitted disease agents. Abstract: 116th Meeting of American Public Health Association, Boston, November, 1988.

20. **Jick H, Hannan MT, Stergachis A, Heidrich J, Perera DR, Rothman KJ:** Vaginal spermicides and gonorrhea. JAMA 248:1619–1621, 1982.

21. **Kelaghan J, Rubin GL, Ory HW, Layde PM:** Barrier method contraceptives and pelvic inflammatory disease. JAMA 248:184–187, 1982.

22. **Cramer DW, Goldman MB, Sciff I, et al.:** The relationship of tubal infertility to barrier method and oral contraceptive use. JAMA 257:2446–2450, 1987.

23. **Austin H, Louv WC, Alexander WJ:** A case-control study of spermicides and gonorrhea. JAMA 251:2822–2824, 1984.

24. **Feldblum PJ, Bernardik E, Rosenberg MJ:** Spermicide use and sexually transmitted disease. JAMA 259:2851, 1988.

25. **Alexander J:** Prophylaxis of STDs with nonoxynol-9: A review of clinical trials. Abstract: Impact of STDs on Contraceptive Practice, New Orleans, May, 1986.

26. **Edelman DA, McIntyre SL, Harper J:** A comparative trial of the Today® contraceptive sponge and diaphragm. Am J Obstet Gynecol 150:869, 1984.

27. **Cutler JC, Singh B, Carpenter U, et al.:** Vaginal contraceptives as prophylaxis against gonorrhea and other sexually transmissible diseases. Adv Planned Parenthood 12:45, 1977.

28. **Cole CH, Lacher TG, Bailey JC, Fairclough DL:** Vaginal chemoprophylaxis in the reduction of reinfection in women with gonorrhea: A clinical evaluation of the effectiveness of a vaginal contraceptive. Br J Vener Dis 56:314, 1980.

29. **Austin H, Louv WC, Alexander WJ:** A case control study of spermicides and gonorrhea. JAMA 251:2822, 1984.

30. **Rendon AL, Covarrubias J, McCarney KE, Marion-Landais G, Luna del Villar J:** A controlled comparative study of phenylmercuric acetate, nonoxynol-9 and placebo vaginal suppositories as prophylactic agents against gonorrhea. Curr Ther Res 27:780–783, 1980.

31. **Rosenberg MJ, Rojanapithayakorn W, Feldblum PJ, Higgins JE:** Effect of the contraceptive sponge on chlamydial infection, gonorrhea, and candidiasis: A comparative trial. JAMA 257:2308–2312, 1987.

32. **Louv WC, Austin H, Alexander WJ, Stagno A, Cheeks J:** A clinical trial of nonoxynol-9 for preventing gonococcal and chlamydial infections. J Infect Dis 158:518–523, 1988.

33. **Alexander NJ:** Heterosexual transmission of AIDS. Am J Reprod Immunol Microbiol 16:163–164, 1988.

34. **Chvapil M, Droegemueller W, Owen JA, Eskelson C, Betts K:** Studies of nonoxynol-9. I. The effect on the vagina of rats and rabbits. Fertil Steril 33:445–450, 1980.

35. **Norvel MK, Benrubi GI, Thompson RJ:** Investigation of microtrauma after sexual intercourse. J Reprod Med 29:269–271, 1984.

36. **Grimes DA:** Deaths due to sexually transmitted diseases. JAMA 255:1727, 1986.

37. **Stone KM:** Personal protection against sexually transmitted diseases. Am J Obstet Gynecol 155:180, 1986.

38. **Lee TY:** Potential impact of chemical prophylaxis on the incidence of gonorrhea. Br J Vener Dis 48:376, 1972.

39. Forrest JD, Fordyce R: US Women's contraceptive attitudes and practice: How have they changed in the 1980s?. Fam Plann Perspect 20:112–118, 1988.

40. Singh B, Cutler JC: Demonstration of a spirocheticidal effect by chemical contraceptives on *Treponema pallidum*. Pan Am Health Org Bull 16:59–64, 1982.

41. Cowen ME, Cree GE: A note on the susceptibility of *N. gonorrhoea* to contraceptive agent Nonyl-P. Br J Vener Dis 49:65–66, 1973.

42. Todd MJ, Hockin JC, Ashton JE, Collins J: Inhibitory effect in vitro of four vaginal contraceptives on *Neisseria gonorrhoea*. Abstract: International Conjoint STD Meeting, 32nd General Assembly of the International Union Against Venereal Diseases and Treponematoses, Montreal, June, 1984.

43. Bolch OH Jr, Warren JC: In vitro effects of Emko on *Neisseria gonorrhoea* and *Trichomonas vaginalis*. Am J Obstet Gynecol 115:1145–1148, 1973.

44. Rapp F, Wrzos H: Synergistic effect of human leukocyte interferon and nonoxynol-9 against herpes simplex virus type 2. Antimicrob Agents Chemother 28:449–467, 1985.

45. Barbi M, Bertoli GL, Miceli G: Attivita antiverale di un contraccettivo chimico (nonoxynol-9). Bol Inst Sieroter [Milan] 66:158–160, 1987.

46. Eglin RP: Nonoxynol-9 pessaries and condoms prevent transmission of HIV in vitro. Br J Sexual Med, July, pp 237–238, 1988.

47. Smith JL, Allicoti GM, Jensen RH, Berger KL, Saxena SJ: The in vitro activity of nonoxynol-9 in eluates from the Today contraceptive sponge against several sexually transmitted disease pathogens. Abstract: 87th Annual Meeting of the American Society for Microbiology, Atlanta, March, 1987.

48. Alden M, Spence MR: In vitro effect of the contraceptive sponge on *Trichomonas vaginalis*. Abstract: 87th Annual Meeting of the American Society for Microbiology, Atlanta, March, 1987.

49. Tierno PM Jr, Hanna BA: In vitro amplification of toxic shock syndrome toxin-1 by intravaginal devices. Contraception 31:185–194, 1985.

50. Stumpf PG, Byers G, Lloyd T: Effect of vaginal contraceptive sponges on growth of toxic shock syndrome-associated *Staphylococcus aureus* in vitro. Contraception 33:395–399, 1986.

51. Remington KM, Buller RS, Kelly JR: Effect of the Today contraceptive sponge on growth and toxic shock syndrome toxin-1 production by *Staphylococcus aureus*. Obstet Gynecol 69:563–569, 1987.

DISCUSSION

DR. GREENSLADE: Would you be willing to speculate on the pros and cons of using a douche product containing nonoxynol-9 as a protection from STDs, including HIV?

DR. NORTH: Well, I would be a bit concerned about that for

several reasons. One is that intercourse itself, of course, produces some microtrauma, and if the ejaculate is deposited prior to the presence of the N-9, I would be concerned that there may be immediate penetration of whatever infectious agents we are talking about, either infectious cells or viral particles. In addition, the time required for the virucidal effect may be a matter of minutes rather than seconds, and douches are not often retained that long, depending on the technique that is used, but there may be others who have a different opinion about that.

DR. WITKIN: On the douching question first, there was a good study by Lawson from Seattle that commercial aerosol douches increase the risk of PID, because they shoot the organisms up. So I do not think that would be a good thing. Second, HIV is mainly transmitted by infected cells and not the free virus. So, we need to know how these spermicides act on the cells. Finally, if the sponge is in place for 24 hr, does that increase the concentration of cervical lymphocytes, which could be a problem?

DR. NORTH: These are two important questions. First, in terms of infected cells, I believe, Dr. Voeller, in your study, you looked at the lethal effects of N-9 on infected lymphocytes, and the lymphocytes themselves, I think, were inhibited by 1% N-9.

DR. VOELLER: Yes, but it varies from study to study and from person to person.

DR. NORTH: Different people may have different resistance.

DR. VOELLER: The figure we published was the highest. The lymphocytes are more sensitive than sperm.

DR. NORTH: Absolutely. So if we are talking about a good dose of spermicide and getting the vaginal levels up to 5% or even 10%, then we may be in a good range in terms of killing infected lymphocytes, but obviously that needs to be examined. In terms of wearing time of the sponge (24 hr), again, I think one can make the argument that, as with all vaginal barrier methods, the recommendation is to wear it for at least 6 hr after intercourse. Again, given the exquisite sensitivity of the HIV virus itself, presumably there will not be any viable infectious agent after 6 hr, so, even if there is some lymphocytic response in the cervix, it would not matter. Furthermore, I am unaware of any real problem. The sponge, unlike the cap or the diaphragm, does not really collect or enclose cervical secretions.

DR. HARRIS: I have two concerns about your recommendations. First, what data do we have on contraceptive sponges? Joan Kreiss was not allowed to present her data in Stockholm, but they are published in the book of abstracts. Her data showed that the sponge did decrease chlamydial infection and gonorrheal infection, but it did not decrease HIV infection. It does not mean that we throw out contraceptive sponges or N-9, but it does mean that we should be cautious in what we tell people so that they can make an informed choice. If we are telling people that they can substitute spermicides for condom use, then we ought to be careful not to push them into something that is not as efficacious, even though you made it quite clear that you are not suggesting that spermicides be the primary means of prevention.

The second point I would like to make is that there are going to be costs associated with the use of spermicidal condoms. The estimates that the Agency for International Development has gathered to date indicate that we will pay 20% more for spermicidal condoms than we do for nonspermicidal condoms. Again, if there is no demonstrated benefit, I do not think we should accept that increased cost. It is going to be hard to look at that, because, as you know, the major reasons that condoms fail are that people do not use them at all, or they do not use them properly. So it is going to be hard to detect the benefit of spermicidal condoms.

DR. NORTH: That is a good point. I have not talked to Joan Kreiss for several months, so I am not up to date on where she is with her study. My understanding, though, is that there are some complexities with her study involving genital ulcers as a cofactor.

Really, my remarks are primarily concerned with what is going on in the United States, not necessarily with a high-risk prostitute population in Nairobi, although it would be wonderful if N-9 were found to be an effective intervention there.

I am afraid I may not have made my point clear. I am not terribly interested in promoting spermicidal condoms, although I think adding N-9 is probably helpful. I am concerned about giving women an option for a method that they can use independently that is certainly effective in preventing gonorrhea and chlamydia and may have some benefit in preventing HIV under average use conditions.

I am a family planning clinican. I am in the trenches a lot, and I am concerned that we cannot depend on condom use because, at this point in time, we all know there is enormous resistance to it in the United States.

24

Design of Clinical Studies of Spermicides for Prophylaxis Against Sexually Transmitted Diseases

Robin G. Foldesy, M. Gaston Farr, Deborah C. Thompson, and Diane N. Catotti

The current concern with acquired immune deficiency syndrome (AIDS) and other sexually transmitted diseases (STDs) has focused attention on prophylactic measures that individuals can take to reduce their risk of becoming infected. Among these measures is the use of vaginal spermicides. None of these products is approved by the U.S. Food and Drug Administration for prophylaxis, and no such use is suggested in the product labeling. Indeed, laboratory and clinical evidence suggests that spermicides provide some protection, but the evidence is not compelling, and the degree of protection afforded by regular use remains unquantified [1–7].

The need for effective prophylactic agents has forced the clinical community to evaluate potentially effective agents in cultural and social settings that have not been used traditionally for drug evaluations. Specifically, measuring the protective effect that a drug or device may have against STDs requires study in a population among whom STDs are relatively prevalent, for example, prostitutes. Otherwise, an unusually large number of study participants and an unacceptably long time are required to complete each study. Unfortunately, individuals who practice behaviors that put them at risk for STDs often do not lead lifestyles that are conducive to participation

Heterosexual Transmission of AIDS, pages 291–301

in a regimented clinical trial [8]. Too often, problems are encountered with inconsistent product use, irregular and untimely return visits to the clinic, and unreliability of information provided by the study subjects. These obstacles are rarer in studies involving curative treatments for STDs, since such subjects are highly motivated to cooperate with clinic requests. It is the study of prophylactic agents, in which uninfected individuals participate, that these problems characterize.

The present work discusses the experience of Family Health International (FHI) in conducting four clinical trials—one each in Costa Rica and the Dominican Republic and two in Colombia—of spermicides and other compounds for prophylaxis among women at high risk for STDs. Because FHI had limited prior experience with this type of population, initial studies of product acceptability were conducted to gain insight into product preferences and to develop strategies that would maximize the chance for success of a clinical study. The present work focuses on the difficulties encountered in these studies and the problems and possible solutions that can arise with the study design, the subject population, and the clinic and subject follow-up and compliance.

STUDY DESIGN

Great care and attention to detail must be given to research protocol development. As with all good clinical trials, the clinical investigator, and perhaps the staff, should review the protocol before it is finalized to ensure that the requirements, procedures, and data collection forms are logical and clear. Several aspects of the study design, however, require particular attention for studies involving subjects at high risk for STDs.

The two most troublesome aspects of these studies are the lack of compliance with or inconsistency of product use, and the unpredictability of subjects in returning for follow-up evaluations. The first problem largely reflects the convenience and acceptability of the study product. The second, in part, relates to the number and frequency of required return visits to the clinic. Frequent follow-up visits hinder the cooperation of study subjects, but too-infrequent visits make it difficult to estimate the date of infection. Regardless of the follow-up scheme chosen, a balance must be struck that achieves high compliance and follow-up rates while maintaining a follow-up schedule that allows a reasonable estimate of date of infection. Deterioration in the rates of follow-up and compliance is usually more severe in long-term studies. Because of this and other factors in the

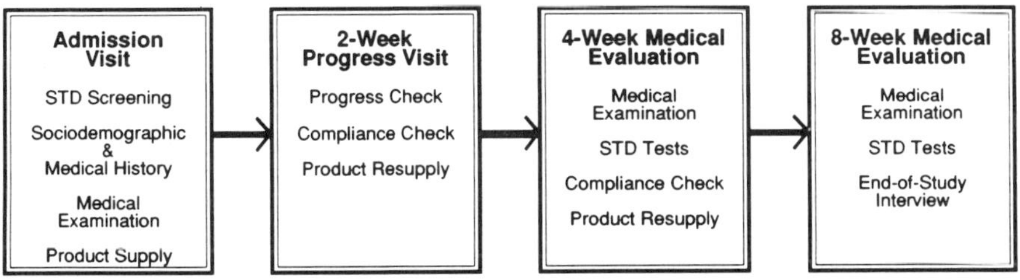

Fig. 1. Suggested scheme for clinical trials involving high-risk subjects at STD clinics.

participant's lifestyle that are discussed below, study participation for each subject should be minimal in length. Although situations differ, FHI has found that 8 weeks of participation are optimal. Figure 1 outlines one scheme for the frequency and activities of follow-up visits.

High-risk subjects frequently fail to return to the clinic for their scheduled follow-up visit. The protocol must include policies to deal with these situations and to define when to discontinue a patient from the study due to loss to follow-up. In our current clinical trials, FHI provides a 4-day grace period within which a subject may return for a follow-up visit and still be retained in the study.

Since many STD clinics are understaffed, the complexity of protocols involving high-risk subjects requires particular attention. In an early clinical trial in Costa Rica, the protocol required that subjects who became infected with an STD be discontinued from the study, cured, and then reentered to complete the full duration of product use. In addition, the protocol stipulated many more laboratory tests than were required to measure product efficacy and ensure the subject's general health. These facets of the study design created administrative and record-keeping difficulties that hindered completion of the study.

POPULATION

Our study definition of an individual at high risk for an STD is one who has had at least one clinically proved and verifiable STD within the past 12 months and also has had two or more sexual partners in the past 30 days. Most individuals recruited at STD clinics, particularly where FHI studies were implemented, exceeded these minimum requirements. Once these criteria have been met, the most critical elements about the study population are lifestyle, attitude, and reliability.

TABLE 1. Interim Data on Selected Sociodemographic Characteristics of 195 High-Risk Women Participating in a 4-Week Trial of Spermicides in Bogota and Ibague, Colombia, 1988

	Mean	Standard Deviation
Age (years)	29.2	5.4
Education (years)	5.3	2.9
Parity	2.1	1.4
Self-reported frequency of intercourse per week in the three months prior to study	14.5	10.6

Table 1 presents sociodemographic characteristics for the women participating in a 4-week trial in Bogota and Ibague, Colombia. These women on average were 29 years of age, had completed about 5 years of schooling, and had borne two children. The women reported frequent sexual activity, averaging over 14 acts of intercourse per week in the 3 months prior to their admission to the study.

When considering the appropriateness of a clinic as a site for any clinical trial, it is obvious that the clinic must have a sufficiently large pool of clients with the disease or diseases to be studied. From this pool, the most cooperative, reliable subjects must be identified. These subjects must also be willing to use the product and return to the clinic once enrolled in the study.

In trials involving individuals at high risk for STDs, the lifestyles and cultural habits of the subjects are of great importance. Many of the women make their livelihood from prostitution and lead a transient lifestyle in which sexual practices are characterized by frequent, sometimes hurried sexual intercourse and a willingness to meet customer demands. These women generally are reluctant to use products that are time-consuming to apply, messy, or otherwise offensive to them or their sexual partners. In addition, reusable applicators, if provided, are not always cleaned between use. In our study in Costa Rica, a cream containing a nonspermicidal, antifungal formulation was applied intravaginally just prior to intercourse by means of a reusable applicator that was filled halfway from a tube of medication. This cumbersome, time-consuming process was believed to have contributed to inconsistent product use. In another example, approximately one in seven women in our study in Bogota reported that their partners generally did not like the spermicidal foam they were using. In the Dominican Republic, a few complaints were made of excessive vaginal wetness by users of liquid-filled gelatin capsules and of dysuria by foam users. Although the extent to which these factors contributed to inconsistent product use is unknown, some women reported these reasons for nonuse.

The cultural and legal setting of the study site also affects the regularity of follow-up visits to the clinic. In Colombia, where prostitution is unofficially allowed, enforced guidelines require women to report monthly to a clinic to ensure the absence of STDs. In both study clinics in Colombia, follow-up visits were missed infrequently. In the Dominican Republic and Costa Rica, on the other hand, the lack of an enforced contact system contributed to greater difficulties in getting women to return to the clinic. In Costa Rica, frequent migration of the women to rural areas to meet farm workers also contributed to many missed clinic appointments and a high loss to follow-up rate. Thus follow-up rates are higher in settings where the subjects are accustomed to returning to the clinic on a regular basis. The rates can be further enhanced by scheduling follow-up visits that coincide with scheduled nonstudy visits.

STUDY CLINIC

A well equipped facility that is run by an organized, dedicated staff optimizes the success of any clinical trial. Unfortunately, many STD clinics have the lowest priority when government funds are allocated. A facility may be outdated, a clinic housed in inadequate quarters, and staff greatly overworked or undertrained or both. These conditions can damage any clinical trial, but they especially affect a trial that involves individuals at high risk for STDs and that must carefully recruit reliable subjects and give them extra attention during their participation.

FHI has encountered two other problems in clinic studies: the overcommitment of the principal investigator to other obligations and the failure of the diagnostic laboratory to complete the required tests in a timely manner. The first problem can be overcome somewhat by delegating duties to responsible support staff. The second is troublesome because it slows both the admission of subjects into the study and processing of study data. In Costa Rica, the FHI experience was hampered by an overburdened diagnostic laboratory. In addition, the laboratory director worked in a department different from that of the principal investigator and was not obligated to the study. In Bogota, most laboratory tests were done on the clinic premises, and the remaining tests were sent to an efficient laboratory that responded to the clinic's needs. It is important, therefore, to

TABLE 2. Interim Data on Nonoxynol-9 Gel and Foam Product Use and Satisfaction Among 150 High-Risk Women Participating in a 4-Week Trial of Spermicides in Bogota and Ibague, Colombia, 1988

	4-Week visit
Median (range) of biweekly frequency of intercourse	19.0 (0–198)
Median (range) of biweekly number of different sexual partners	13.8 (0–98)
Regularity of product use (% women)	
Always	54.3
Frequent	34.4
Occasional	4.6
Not used	6.6
Product acceptability (% women)	
Very favorable	66.7
Favorable	22.0
Unfavorable	6.0
Very unfavorable	3.3
No response	2.0

consider not only the investigator, the staff, and the facilities but also the competence of collaborating centers and their relationship with the investigator.

COMPLIANCE WITH PRODUCT USE AND REGULARITY OF FOLLOW-UP VISITS

The success of trials in high-risk populations using prophylactic agents depends in part on a good relationship between the investigator or other members of the clinic staff and the study participants. A good relationship optimizes subject compliance and the subjects' willingness to return to the clinic for follow-up visits. The FHI studies in Colombia were successful because almost 90% of the eligible subjects reported for follow-up visits and completed the study using either a nonoxynol-9 gel or foam; by the end of the study, almost 90% reported using these assigned products frequently or always (Table 2). These investigators and their staff established an excellent rapport with their clients because of their personalities and the clinics' philosophy and mission, and this rapport contributed to the high compliance and follow-up rates. The clinics not only provided exam-

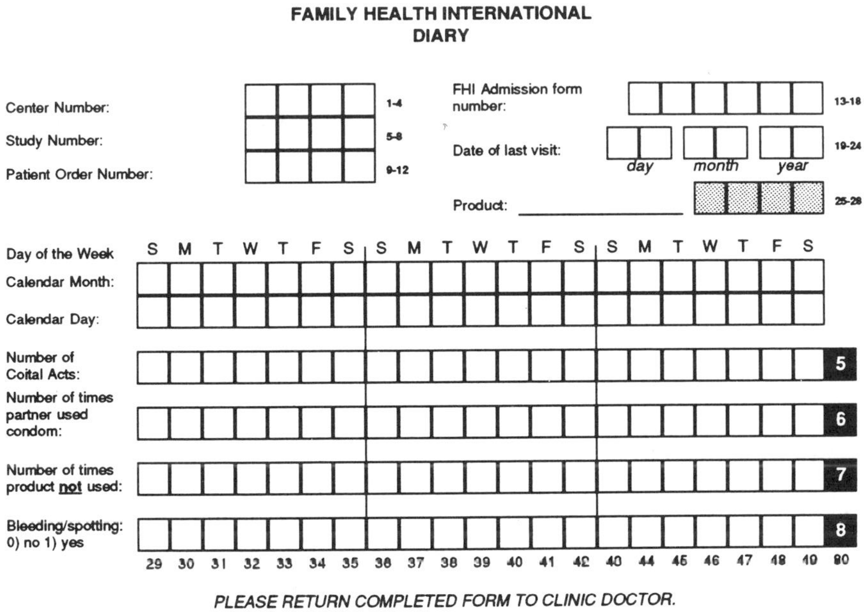

FAMILY HEALTH INTERNATIONAL
DIARY

Center Number: 1-4
Study Number: 5-8
Patient Order Number: 9-12

FHI Admission form number: 13-18
Date of last visit: day month year 19-24
Product: 25-28

Day of the Week: S M T W T F S | S M T W T F S | S M T W T F S
Calendar Month:
Calendar Day:
Number of Coital Acts: 5
Number of times partner used condom: 6
Number of times product **not** used: 7
Bleeding/spotting: 0) no 1) yes 8

29 30 31 32 33 34 35 36 37 38 39 40 41 42 43 44 45 46 47 48 49 50

PLEASE RETURN COMPLETED FORM TO CLINIC DOCTOR.

Fig. 2. Coital log used in clinical trials of spermicides with high-risk subjects at STD clinics.

inations, diagnostic tests, and treatment for STDs but also contraceptives, counseling, and education on reproductive health issues.

The consistency and diligence of spermicide use by study subjects are of paramount importance for estimating the clinical efficacy of these products against STDs. With many medications, failure of subjects to comply with the dosing schedule can be uncovered by periodic analysis of blood or urine samples. With the use of vaginal spermicides or other barrier contraceptives, this detection is not possible. FHI often requests that subjects participating in clinical studies of barrier contraceptives complete coital logs (Fig. 2). Although diaries initially were developed to indicate only sexual activity, they evolved into documents that indicate the consistency of product and condom use. The coital logs are an important means of measuring subject compliance, and the candid completion of these documents helps establish the reliability of the follow-up data. For this reason, FHI instructs the clinic to emphasize to the subjects the importance of accurate, truthful logs rather than absolute compliance to product use. It is unreasonable to expect all women to use their assigned product at every act of sexual intercourse, and badgering the subjects to do so is counterproductive. For these women, the threat of being

TABLE 3. Frequency of Spermicide Use Among High-Risk Women Participating in a 4-Week Trial in Bogota, Colombia, 1988

	Percent of women	
Frequency of use	2-Week visit (n = 87)	4-Week visit (n = 78)
Always	30	45
Frequent	43	45
Occasional	23	5
Not used	5	5

dropped from the study if they do not use the study products consistently is, essentially, an invitation to falsify the coital logs. In our earliest study in Costa Rica, many coital logs were believed to have been completed falsely for this reason. On the other hand, underemphasizing consistent use is dangerous as well. In the Bogota study, the frequency of use improved during the second half of the subjects' participation mainly because the importance of consistent product use was explained more fully during the subjects' return visit (Table 3).

CONCLUSIONS

The issues raised throughout this chapter, summarized in Figure 3, all contribute to the success of a clinical trial with individuals at high risk for STDs. These issues involve five major considerations.

1. The subjects' lifestyle and culture must be conducive to the use of the study product and demands of a clinical trial.
2. The impositions of study participation upon the subjects must be kept to a minimum.
3. The clinic must have a good rapport with its clients.
4. The principal investigator and clinic staff must be dedicated to the project.
5. The clinic must be adequately staffed and equipped and have good access to diagnostic testing.

ACKNOWLEDGMENTS

The authors thank Christine Colven and Diego Berrio for their assistance with this project. This project was funded by support from

Clinic

Well-equipped, modern clinic facilities.

Adequate location and space to meet patient load.

Organized, dedicated, trained clinic staff

Committed investigator having adequate time to devote to study.

Organized, efficient record-keeping system.

Availability of a reliable diagnostic laboratory.

Good rapport between clinic staff and study subjects.

Study Populations

Sufficient pool of subjects at risk of contracting disease or diseases to be studied.

Cooperative, reliable subjects.

Subjects willing to use study product as required by protocol.

Subjects willing to return to clinic for follow-up visits.

Subjects do not see study as interfering with their lifestyles or livelihood.

Subjects without transient lifestyles.

Good Compliance and Follow-Up

Study product acceptable to the subjects.

Subjects enthusiastic about the study.

Subjects accustomed to returning to clinic on a regular basis.

Accurate, truthful completion of subject coital logs.

Balanced emphasis at each follow-up visit on the consistent use of study product .

Clinic conveniently located for ease of access.

Fig. 3. Characteristics of a model STD study clinic and its population and the factors that influence subject compliance and follow-up.

Pfizer International and the Advanced Care Products Division of Ortho Pharmaceutical Corporation and by FHI under a cooperative agreement with the U.S. Agency for International Development. FHI is an international, not-for-profit organization that conducts research and provides technical assistance in health, family planning, STDs, and AIDS. The views expressed are solely those of the authors and are not necessarily those of FHI or the funding organizations.

REFERENCES

1. **Benes S, McCormick WM:** Inhibition of growth of chlamydia trachomatis by nonoxynol-9 in vitro. Antimicrob Agents Chemother 27:724–726, 1985.

2. **Hicks DR, Martin LS, Getchell JP, et al.:** Inactivation of HTLV-III/LAV-infected cultures of normal human lymphocytes in vitro. Lancet 2:1422–1423, 1985.

3. **Kelly JP, Reynolds RB, Stagno S, et al.:** In vitro activity of the spermicide nonoxynol-9 against Chlamydia trachomatis. Antimicrob Agents Chemother 27:760–762, 1985.

4. **Singh B, Cutler JC, Utdjian HMD:** Studies on the development of a vaginal preparation providing both prophylaxis against venereal disease and other genital infections and contraception. Br J Vener Dis 48:57–64, 1972.

5. **Stone KM, Grimes DA, Magder LS:** Personal protection against sexually transmitted diseases. Am J Obstet Gynecol 155:180–188, 1986.

6. **Austin H, Louv WC, Alexander WJ:** A case-control study of spermicides and gonorrhea. JAMA 251:2822–2824, 1984.

7. **Louv WC, Austin H, Alexander WJ, Stagno S, Cheeks J:** A clinical trial of nonoxynol-9 for preventing gonococcal and chlamydial infections. J Infect Dis 158:518–523, 1988.

8. **Mertz GJ, Schmidt O, Jourden JL, et al.:** Frequency of acquisition of first-episode genital infection with herpes simplex virus from symptomatic and asymptomatic source contacts. Sex Transmitted Dis 12:33–39, 1985.

DISCUSSION

DR. JOHNSON: One of the problems we have had in practice using nonoxynol-9 in our partner study (and Dr. Cameron has just said he had a similar experience) is that a lot of the women complained of candidiasis, which in itself caused irritation and inflammation. There is some concern about whether this is a sensible product to be advising for people who are at very high risk of HIV transmission.

DR. FOLDESY: Well, nonoxynol-9 is a surfactant, as Dr. Chantler mentioned earlier, and it can cause irritation. I think that the irritation is going to vary with the individual. From the data that I have seen, it seems that just about as many men as women will experience local irritation. Obviously, if you use it more often, say, 10 times a day rather than once a week, you are more likely to experience irritation. I think that in regular use, i.e., a few times a week, the percentage of people who complain of irritation seems to be rather low, maybe in the area of 2–3%.

DR. JOHNSON: My question was, should we be recommending this for people or not? There could be a potentially deleterious effect, with the product causing irritation and abrasion of the vaginal mucosa that could facilitate HIV transmission.

DR. FOLDESY: I think that is a very important consideration and is related to the earlier discussion today. In my mind, the jury is still out on the question of spermicides. There are data to suggest that there is some protective effect, but they are not compelling data.

DR. HEYMANN: I have seen considerable monilial vulvitis from nonoxynol-9-impregnated sponges, but these cases were in women in Nairobi working as prostitutes who put a sponge in all day, every day. It might be a dose-related phenomenon, and may or may not be related to sponge use in other settings.

I would like to ask about attempting to establish a cohort of women to study for incident STDs. Is there a representative community spokesperson who could act as an intermediary between the clinic and the community of women that you would like to study?

DR. FOLDESY: With regard to the latter question, I think it is entirely possible, and, in some of the other work that is being supported by FHI, they have used exactly that strategy.

In the studies we have conducted in Latin America, we have not found it necessary, because the clients come to the clinic. The clinic is the draw in that situation.

DR. CAMERON: The combination of both has been very successful in Nairobi, and I think that is why in Nairobi that cohort is sustained.

DR. FOLDESY: Thank you very much for that comment. With regard to the monilia, an FHI study was completed a couple of years ago in Bangkok, where prostitutes used the N-9 sponge. It was observed there that an increased incidence of monilia accompanied the use of the sponge.

DR. CATES: Dr. Foldesy, that was a delightful presentation, and, to me, it really reflected on a personal odyssey moving from a family planning field, where clinical trials are conducted with individuals who are there to choose contraceptives and who are generally motivated enough to come back to the clinic on a regular basis to obtain their supplies. Conducting studies with populations who are at an STD clinic because they have a symptom or a particular, one-time need to be treated is something else. How to motivate those individuals to become involved in long-term studies that need to be conducted on AIDS is going to be a continuing challenge as we see this overlap of the two fields. We all have to digest this. This is probably one of the most important points made at this conference.

DR. FOLDESY: You are absolutely right. The real problem is that when people are not well they take their medicine, and as soon as they start to feel better they stop taking it.

DR. CAMERON: You alluded to an interesting sociologic point, and that is that women with STDs are required to report monthly for surveillance, I presume, in some countries. Is there any attention to, or is there any voice directing public policy towards, men with STDs?

DR. FOLDESY: That is a fascinating question. I do not know the answer. I would think, at least from what I have heard in my work in these countries, that the answer is no, but I am really not sure.

25

New and Existing Spermicides With Virucidal Properties

Eric N. Chantler

The concept that some spermicides may restrict the spread of sexually transmitted diseases (STDs) is not new. In 1972, it was reported that *Treponema pallidum, Neisseria gonorrhoea, Trichomonas vaginalis,* and *Candida albicans* were inactivated by exposure in vitro to nonionic surfactant spermicides at levels expected to be present in the vagina during intercourse when a spermicide is used [7]. In vivo, a decrease in the rate of reinfection was seen in a group of women at high risk of reinfection when a surfactant spermicide was used following eradication of the infection [2,3]. The authors noted that the spermicide, although it did not cure a preexisting infection in the female partner, significantly limited the transmission of infection. Although the majority of pathogens in that study were bacterial, nonoxynol-9 (N-9) has been shown to be active against vaginal infections of *Herpesvirus hominis* [4,5] as well. It was proposed that nonionic surfactants that have ether or amide linkages between the hydrophobic and hydrophilic domains of the molecule have a virucidal action because of their ability to dissolve lipid components in the membrane of the viral envelope. This observation is based on destruction of the envelope that is seen after exposure in vitro of herpes to N-9 [6]. Several authors [4,5] have suggested that this compound may play a role in regulating the transmission of herpesvirus during intercourse. Much less is known about the transmission of the human immunodeficiency virus type 1 (HIV-1) during vaginal heterosexual intercourse from either an infected male or female partner. Many aspects of the infectivity of HIV are only now being determined. The following

Heterosexual Transmission of AIDS, pages 303–310

questions are relevant in considering the control of transmission of the virus during intercourse.

1 What is the most significant infective agent, the virus or the transformed lymphocyte?
2 Which of the male genital tract secretions in the ejaculate carry the infection, the vesicular or prostatic secretions? In an infected woman, is the infection present in the serum transudate in the vagina, resident in the mucus, or residual from menstrual blood?
3 Does the risk of transmission of infection vary with the progress of the disease? Similarly, does the major infectious particle change during the progress of the disease?
4 Are the motile spermatozoa a significant factor in the transmission of the infection by infected men?

EXISTING VIRUCIDAL SPERMICIDES

Two spermicides—N-9 and benzalkonium chloride (BZK)—that are used in commercially available preparations have been shown to inactivate HIV-1 in vitro. However, the conditions under which the activity is assessed should be considered, because the vaginal environment could limit the virucidal properties of a spermicide demonstrated to be active in vitro. Two major uncertainties exist. The first is the extent to which the transmission of the virus depends on the use of spermatozoa as a vector. This method of movement of the pathogen from the vagina to the upper genital tract has been demonstrated in the case of *Escherichia coli* [7] and is potentially available to other pathogens. This route is important when considering vaginal spermicides, since they are associated with a significant number of contraceptive failures compared to oral contraceptives or intrauterine devices (IUDs). This obviously indicates that spermatozoa enter the upper genital tract in a number of cases, even though a supposedly spermicidal concentration of the contraceptive exists in the vagina. Such failures may be associated with user procedures rather than method failures [8]; however, if sperm reach the uterus and hence the peritoneum, the risk of infection remains even if they have lost fertilizing ability.

The second consideration, which is linked to the first, is the extent to which the vaginal spermicide is active throughout the female genital tract. We have shown that N-9 does not exhibit spermicidal activity in the cervical mucus even though it is at high concentration and in surface contact with midcycle mucus [9]. Furthermore, a high proportion of the spermicidal activity is lost when mucus and spermicide mix. This effect restricts much of the spermicidal potential of N-9 to the vagina, since N-9 is incompatible with cervical mucus. Indeed, N-9 probably does not enter cervical mucus to any significant extent following vaginal application, thus limiting the extent of both its contraceptive action and its potential activity against sperm that carry HIV-1.

The same conditions apply to BZK, the other virucidal spermicide, with respect to the rate of contraceptive failure inherent in vaginal contraception generally. However, unlike N-9, BZK has some compatibility with cervical mucus and has been reported to enter midcycle mucus while retaining its spermicidal activity [10]. This compatibility probably relates to its charge-bearing structure. Although it shows surfactant properties in common with N-9, BZK differs in that it has a positive charge on the molecule at physiological pH. This positivity facilitates charge-related interaction between BZK and mucin (the latter being a large polyanionic glycoprotein that is present in cervical mucus and responsible for its rheological properties).

The interaction of BZK with mucus results in a modification of the macromolecular structure of the mucus as examined by scanning electron microscopy [11]. Midcycle mucus changes from a fine reticular network to a nonuniform structure in which some areas appear where the reticular structure is replaced by a compact "crushed" structure, comparable to the organization seen in luteal-phase mucus. The heterogeneity of the mucus structure seen in women using BZK as a vaginal spermicide may arise from an uneven distribution of the compound in the mucus.

Our preliminary studies have shown a compatibility between mucus and BZK similar to that previously reported [12,13] for the entry of biguanides into cervical mucus. In this situation, entry of biguanides occurs at low concentrations but is restricted at higher concentrations. This effect is thought to stem from the thickening of mucus that occurs with high concentrations of biguanides; the resulting modified mucus acts as a barrier at the interface between mucus and biguanide, restricting the further entry of the biguanide into the mucus.

In the case of BZK, anomalous entry into mucus begins to occur at concentrations of BZK above 1 mg/ml. This level is considerably lower than the concentration that exists in the vagina when this compound is used as a spermicide, for example, from a Pharmatex sponge containing 60 mg BZK.

The assay of the activity of these two spermicides against HIV-1 infective material has been made in a comparable manner, that is, by measuring the retrovirus-specific enzyme reverse transcriptase. However, in both cases, the activity has been measured in vitro and in the absence of female genital tract secretions, which, as previously discussed, can modify the availability of the spermicide. In the case of BZK, an inhibition of reverse transcriptase activity and the "loss of infectivity of the AIDS virus for human lymphocytes" is reported after 10–15 min exposure of a solution containing HIV-1 to 120 μg/ml [14] or 500 μg/ml [15] BZK followed by addition of normal human peripheral blood lymphocytes. Subsequent virus production is monitored by assay of reverse transcriptase activity in the cell-free supernatant of the culture medium.

Two reports relate to the activity of N-9 against HIV. The first study [16] reported that, following a 1 min exposure to levels of N-9 greater than 0.5 mg/ml, an abolition of reverse transcriptase activity occurred in the culture medium of peripheral blood lymphocytes that had been exposed to HIV-1. Much higher levels of N-9 (on the order of 50 mg/ml) were required to reduce the viability of the lymphocytes, although levels five times lower significantly reduced the counts of live target lymphocytes. The second report [17] confirmed these findings but showed that only a 30 sec exposure to N-9 inactivated HIV-1 isolates (using reverse transcriptase as a criterion). The previously reported [16] differential between the inactivation of HIV-1 and the doses of N-9 required for toxicity towards human lymphoid cell lines was confirmed. The authors concluded that, if vaginal contraceptive preparations of the types tested were not diluted by more than 100-fold, a significant effect on the transmission of HIV-1 during sexual intercourse could be expected.

In summary, the value of existing vaginal spermicides in limiting the spread of HIV during intercourse is as follows.

1. Data exist only about the use of spermicides when applied vaginally. Nothing is known of their action when applied rectally, although this route is recognized as one of high risk for transmission of HIV.
2. Nothing is known of the spread of these spermicides from the vagina to the cervix, a process that would extend their scope in preventing the spread of infection.
3. Little is known about the infectivity of the semen or the route of transmission of the infection from semen to the female partner; similarly, changes in the infectivity of the semen as a function of the stage of HIV infection are not known. Even less is known about the transmission of the infection from the female to the male partner, though this

route is considered less common as HIV-1 is present in the cervical mucus and vaginal secretions of only about 50% of women who are serum antibody positive [18–20].

4 Nothing is known of the persistence, extent, and retention of virucidal spermicides following vaginal application.

NEW DEVELOPMENTS

An extension to the available virucidal spermicides is offered by the use of the bisbiguanide chlorhexidine. This compound is a long-established, broad-spectrum antiseptic with a good safety record. Its spermicidal activity is comparable to that of N-9, although the loss of spermicidal activity upon its dilution is less marked than that occurring with N-9 [9]. In contrast to both N-9 and BZK, chlorhexidine has other properties that make it a more suitable candidate as a vaginal spermicide that can be used to prevent the transmission of HIV. These properties include the following.

1 Chlorhexidine shows activity towards HIV. Treatment of the active virus, in a virus-permissive cell line, with 400 μg/ml chlorhexidine gluconate destroys infectivity when monitored by indirect immunofluorescence of the cells for HIV p24 antigen (ICI Pharmaceuticals, United Kingdom, unpublished communication).

2 Chlorhexidine is compatible with midcycle cervical mucus at concentrations up to 10 mg/ml and shows unimpeded entry into the mucus at this concentration. Chlorhexidine retains undiminished spermicidal activity in the mucus at these concentrations [12].

3 Chlorhexidine has a mucospissic action on midcycle cervical mucus that prevents motile spermatozoa from entering the mucus at levels that are not spermicidal in semen [12].

4 Chlorhexidine has been used in an obstetric cream for many years. It has also been investigated as a potential local method for treating vaginitis (from *Gardinerella vaginalis* and *Bacteroides bivius*) [21], with a good rate of success. It is not absorbed systemically [22] and has no reported long-term effects on the vaginal flora.

These facts combine to make chlorhexidine a preferred candidate for a virucidal spermicide compared to N-9 or BZK. The most important novel properties of chlorhexidine in this respect are its mucospissic action and its compatibility with mucus. The mucospissic action enhances contraceptive protection, preventing sperm from gaining access to midcycle cervical mucus, which is probably a major factor in the failure rate of other vaginal spermicides. N-9, in particular, is not compatible with mucus and, as a result, is probably active only in the vagina [13].

The compatibility of chlorhexidine with mucus produces a thicker mucus that would inhibit the entry of both the infection-bearing spermatozoa and infected lymphocytes into the upper region of the genital tract, and hence into the peritoneal fluid, via the pouch of Douglas. Furthermore, this chlorhexidine-mucus complex, with its increased viscoelasticity, can form a layer on the vaginal and cervical epithelium that contains active chlorhexidine, protecting against the transfer of infection from either the male or female partner. Additionally, the generation of a more viscoelastic mucus may retard its expulsion from the cervix by reducing the efficiency of the ciliary propulsive effect that propels it from the cervix to the vagina [23]. These local actions would form a cervical reservoir of chlorhexidine, prolonging its duration in the genital tract, in contrast to conventional spermicides that drain out after intercourse. Study of the clinical application of the vaginal use of chlorhexidine in controlling the spread of HIV is presently underway.

ACKNOWLEDGMENTS

Much of the work cited here is or has been supported by grants from: the U.S. Agency for International Development in the Contraceptive Research and Development (CONRAD) Program, the British Medical Research Council, London International PLC, and ICI (Pharmaceuticals) PLC.

REFERENCES

1. **Singh B, Cutler JC, Ujidjian HMD:** Studies on development of a vaginal preparation providing both prophylaxis against venereal disease, other genital infections, and contraception. Br J Vener Dis 48:52–62, 1972.

2. **Stone KM, Grimes DA, Magder LS:** Personal protection against sexually transmitted diseases. Am J Obstet Gynecol 155:180–188, 1986.

3. **Singh B, Cutler JC:** Vaginal contraceptives for prophylaxis against sexually transmitted diseases. In Zatuchni GI, Sobrero AJ, Speidel JJ, Sciarra JJ (eds): Vaginal Contraception: New Developments. Hagerstown, MD: Harper and Row, 1979, pp 175–185.

4. **Singh B, Postic B, Cutler JC:** Virucidal effect of certain chemical contraceptives on type 2 herpes virus. Am J Obstet Gynecol 126:422–425, 1976.

5. **Postic B, Singh B, Sequeglia NL, Guevarra LO:** Inactivation of clinical isolates of Herpes hominis, types 1 and 2, by chemical contraceptives. Sex Transmitted Dis 5:22–24, 1978.

6. **Asculai S, Weis M, Rancourt M, Kupferberg A:** Inactivation of Herpes simplex viruses by nonionic surfactants. Antimicrob Agents Chemother 13:686–690, 1978.

7. **Toth A, O'Leary WM, Ledger W:** Evidence for microbial transfer by spermatozoa. Obstet Gynecol 59:556–559, 1982.

8. **Sciarra JJ:** Vaginal contraception: Historical perspective. In Zatuchni GI, Sobrero AJ, Speidel JJ, Sciarra JJ (eds): Vaginal Contraception: New Developments. Hagerstown, MD: Harper and Row, 1979, pp 2–12.

9. **Sharman D, Chantler E, Dukes M, Hutchinson F, Elstein M:** Comparison of the action of nonoxynol-9 and chlorhexidine on sperm. Fertil Steril 45:259–265, 1986.

10. **Chretien FC:** Mise en évidence expérimentale des modifications induites au sein du mucus cervical par un spermicide tensio-actif. Contra Fertil Sex 12:1211–1220, 1984.

11. **Enry R, Siborni C:** The effect of benzalkonium chloride on ovulatory cervical mucus. Acta Eur Fertil 18:109–111.

12. **Sharman DA:** The Interaction of Polymers With Cervical Mucus. PhD Thesis, University of Manchester, 1987.

13. **Chantler E, Sharma R, Sharman D:** Changes in cervical mucus that prevent sperm penetration. In Chantler E, Ratcliffe N (eds): Society for Experimental Biology Symposium Series: Mucus and Related Topics, in press.

14. **Chermann J-C, Barre-Sinoussi F, Henin Y, Marechal V:** HIV inactivation by a spermicide containing benzalkonium chloride. AIDS Forschung 2:85–86, 1987.

15. **Wainberg M, Bleau G:** Effect of benzalkonium chloride on HIV and related infections and on other infectious agents. Arch AIDS Res 1:57–68, 1988.

16. **Hicks DR, Martin LS, Getchell JP, et al.:** Inactivation of HTLV-III/LAV-infected cultures of normal human lymphocytes by nonoxynol-9 in vitro. Lancet 2:1422–1423, 1985.

17. **Malkovsky M, Newell A, Dalgleish AG:** Inactivation of HIV by nonoxynol-9. Lancet 1:645, 1988.

18. **Archibald DW, Witt DJ, Craven DE, Vogt MW, Hirsch MS, Essex M:** Antibodies to immunodeficiency virus in cervical secretions from women at risk from AIDS. J Infect Dis 156:240–241, 1987.

19. **Vogt MW, Witt DJ, Craven DE, Byington R, Crawford DF, Schooley RT, Hirsch MS:** Isolation of HTLV-III/LAV from cervical secretions of women at risk from AIDS. Lancet 1:525–527, 1986.

20. **Wolfsy CB, Cohen JB, Hauer LB, Padian NS, Michaelis BA, Evans LA, Levy JA:** Isolation of AIDS-associated retrovirus from genital tract secretions of women with antibodies to the virus. Lancet 1:527–529, 1986.

21. **Ison CA, Taylor RFH, Link C, Buckett P, Harris JRW, Easmon CS:** Local treatment for bacterial vaginosis. Br Med J 295:886, 1987.

22. **Vorherr H, Vorherr UF, Mehta P, Ulrich JA, Messer RH:** Antimicrobial effect of chlorhexidine and povidone-iodine on vaginal bacteria. J Infect 3:195–199, 1984.

23. **Elstein M:** Cervical mucus: Its physiological role and clinical significance. Adv Exp Med Biol 144:301–318, 1982.

DISCUSSION

DR. POTTS: What is the evidence that chlorhexidine is not absorbed across the vagina? Can you measure it in the blood?

DR. CHANTLER: Yes, it can be measured in the blood. There is an HPLC procedure for measuring it and also a colorimetric method. Buttar et al. (Teratology 35:61) demonstrate transvaginal absorption of chlorhexidine in rats.

DR. POTTS: Very impressive. Thank you.

DR. KANGAS: Does chlorhexidine have any effects on latex?

DR. CHANTLER: Per se, I do not think it would have an effect. The vehicle it is put in, obviously, is more likely to affect the latex than the compound itself. I cannot see, looking at its structure, why it should affect latex. Chlorhexidine is particularly sensitive to the vehicle. If you were going to use it, you would certainly have to use it in something phosphate- or chloridine-free. Something like methyl cellulose would be a good vehicle. It is known to have little effect on latex, so I do not think it will be a problem.

DR. PHANUPHAK: I would suggest that any developer of a spermicide also consider that the drug work orally, because oral sex is one of the main problems, as was previously mentioned. I have been asked by both male and female prostitutes, which mouth gargles might be effective in killing HIV.

DR. CHANTLER: Well, serendipitously, this particular compound is also marketed as a mouthwash.

26

Anti-HIV Screening Technology

Lionel Resnick, Mariano E. Busso, and
Robert C. Duncan

The human immunodeficiency virus (HIV) is the etiologic agent of acquired immune deficiency syndrome (AIDS) and its related disorders [1,2]. Transmission of HIV occurs primarily through intimate sexual contact. Therefore, judicious use of barrier methods of contraception by individuals at risk for infection may reduce the likelihood of sexual transmission of HIV [3]. Although HIV does not penetrate latex condoms, it has not been established that condoms alone, with documented failure rates of 10–15%, represent sufficiently reliable barriers for HIV during sexual intercourse, given the gravity of HIV infection [4–7]. Epidemiologic studies have shown that condoms in combination with spermicides can reduce the incidence of sexually transmitted diseases in a variety of clinical settings [8–10]. Although an additional margin of safety in the prevention of HIV transmission may not be achievable, the need for a back-up virucidal chemical barrier has become apparent. Chemical spermicides have demonstrated efficacy in the inactivation of enveloped viruses, such as herpes simplex virus and HIV in vitro [11–15]. Nonoxynol-9 (N-9), a nonionic surfactant, in concentrations available in commercial contraceptive preparations, has been reported to inactivate HIV in vitro [13–15]. If condoms in combination with spermicidal agents could reduce the transmission of HIV, they could provide an important means of containing the epidemic.

The need to identify spermicidal agents with potent HIV inactivation properties requires the development of in vitro screening systems. These systems should be the initial testing ground for agents prior to consideration for clinical trials. A quantitative determination

Heterosexual Transmission of AIDS, pages 311–325

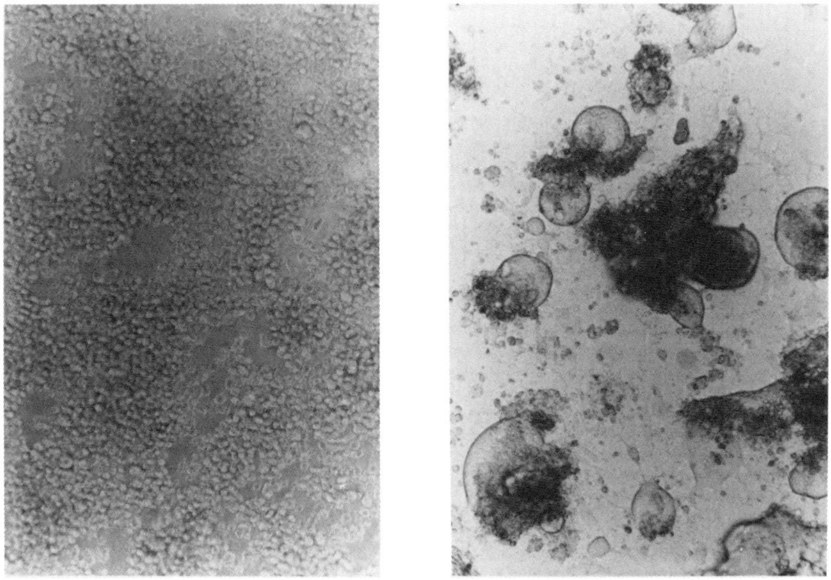

Fig. 1. Uninfected MT-2 cell culture **(left)** and HIV-infected MT-2 cell culture with syncytium-formation **(right)**. ×400.

of the anti-HIV properties of spermicidal agents in vitro will allow for prioritizating and selecting agents. The availability of standardized, reproducible, and validated in vitro assays renders such an approach feasible. With these goals in mind, we report our experience in the development and performance of a rapid, quantitative screening assay that determines the relative potency of HIV (cell-free) inactivation by spermicidal agents. Once an agent with potent HIV-inactivating properties has been identified, a comprehensive evaluation of that agent can be performed.

METHODS AND RESULTS

In establishing the primary screening assay, the goal was to devise a standardized, reproducible, and valid assay that provides a high-capacity, sensitive, rapid, and quantitative method for identifying potent HIV (cell-free) inactivating agents.

Syncytium-Forming (Primary Screening) Assay

The following discussion focuses on the development of the syncytium-forming assay and the experimental design (Table 1). To

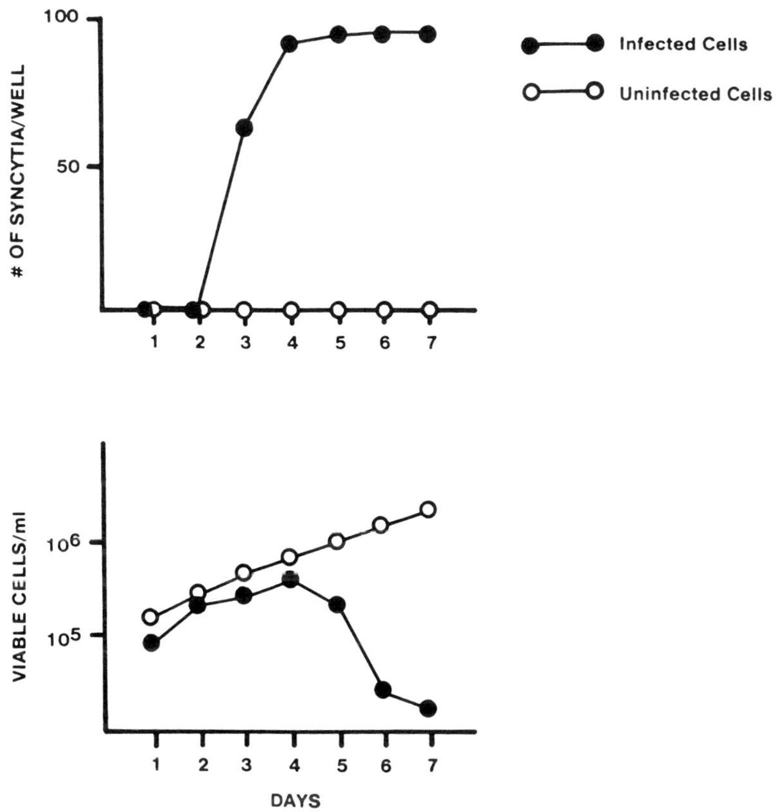

Fig. 2. Number of syncytia per well **(top)** and viable MT-2 cell count **(bottom)** after HIV infection (MOI = 0.01).

quantitate infectivity of a virus preparation, an in vitro biological system susceptible to infection and a method for detecting infection are required. Two commonly used methods for monitoring virus expression in culture are cytoplasmic staining for HIV antigens and the reverse transcriptase assay. These methods are labor-intensive, cumbersome, and expensive, and they do not lend themselves easily to experiments with hundreds of cultures. The HIV p24 antigen capture assay can be used, but it is relatively expensive, and the removal of residual inactive p24 antigen requires manipulations that enhance the capacity for errors and contamination [16]. A sensitive system that allows for the visual detection of HIV expression would be ideal.

After HIV inoculation of MT-2 cells [human T-lymphotropic virus I (HTLV-I)-infected CD4 lymphocyte cell line], giant syncytia (multi-

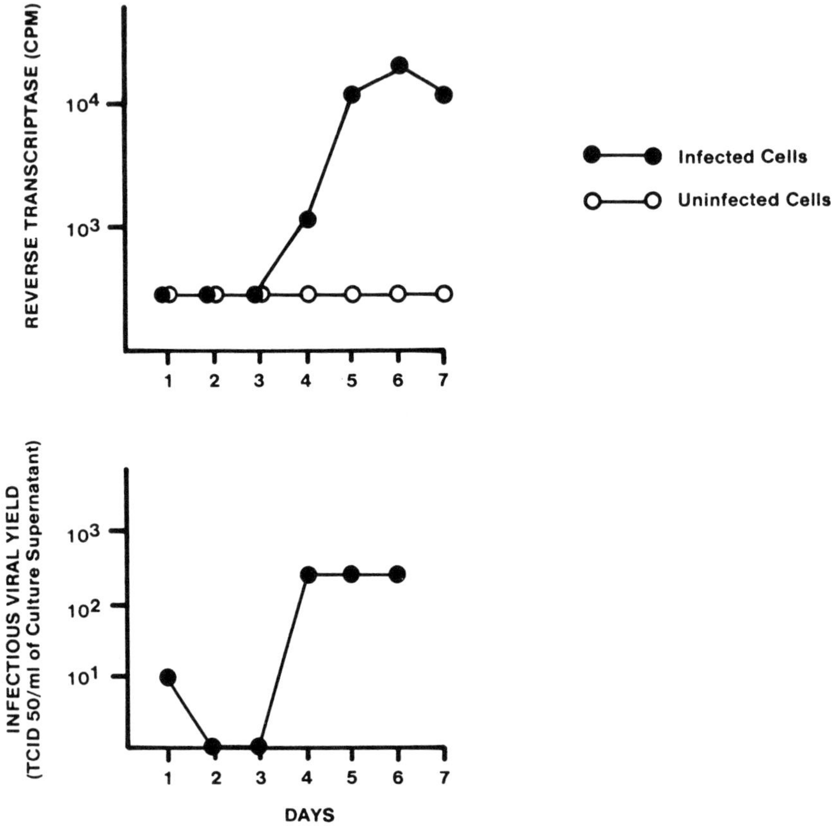

Fig. 3. Reverse transcriptase activity **(top)** and infectious viral yield **(bottom)** after HIV infection of MT-2 cells (MOI = 0.01).

TABLE 1. Primary Screen Experimental Design

Target cells: MT-2 cell line
Target cell concentration: 3×10^5 cells/ml
Virus strain: HIV-1 (IIIB)
Virus stock concentration: $10^{8.23}$ $TCID_{50}$/ml[a]
Spermicide concentration: 1% or 0.1%
Contact time: 1 min
Temperature: 30–33°C
pH: 7.0–7.5

[a]$TCID_{50}$, tissue culture infectious dose 50%.

TABLE 2. Calculation of Virus Titer (stock)

Log virus dilution	Syncytium[a] +	Syncytium[a] −	Cumulated HIV-positives (%)
1	4	0	100
2	4	0	100
3	4	0	100
4	4	0	100
5	4	0	100
6	4	0	100
7	2	2	60
8	1	3	16
9	0	4	0
10	0	4	0

[a] + Denotes the presence and − the absence of syncytia (quadruplicate samples per dilution). Virus titer = 8.23 log $TCID_{50}$/ml (Reed-Muench method) (Virus titer Is ten times calculation due to volume adjustments: 1:1 dilution with PBS and total volume of 0.2 ml).

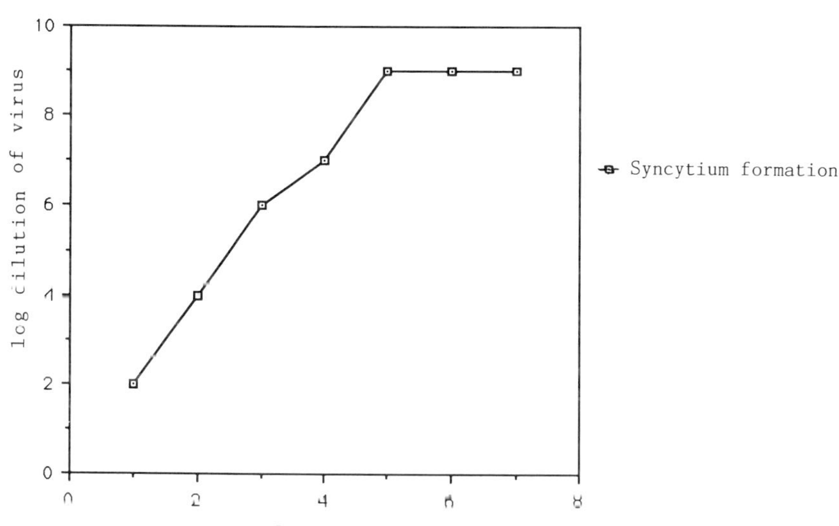

Fig. 4. Effect of virus input on syncytium formation over time.

TABLE 3. Experimental Controls

Virus/no spermicide (phosphate-buffered saline) ($TCID_{50}$ control)
Virus/1% nonoxynol-9 (inactivation control)
No virus/spermicide (toxicity control)
No virus/no spermicide (cell control)

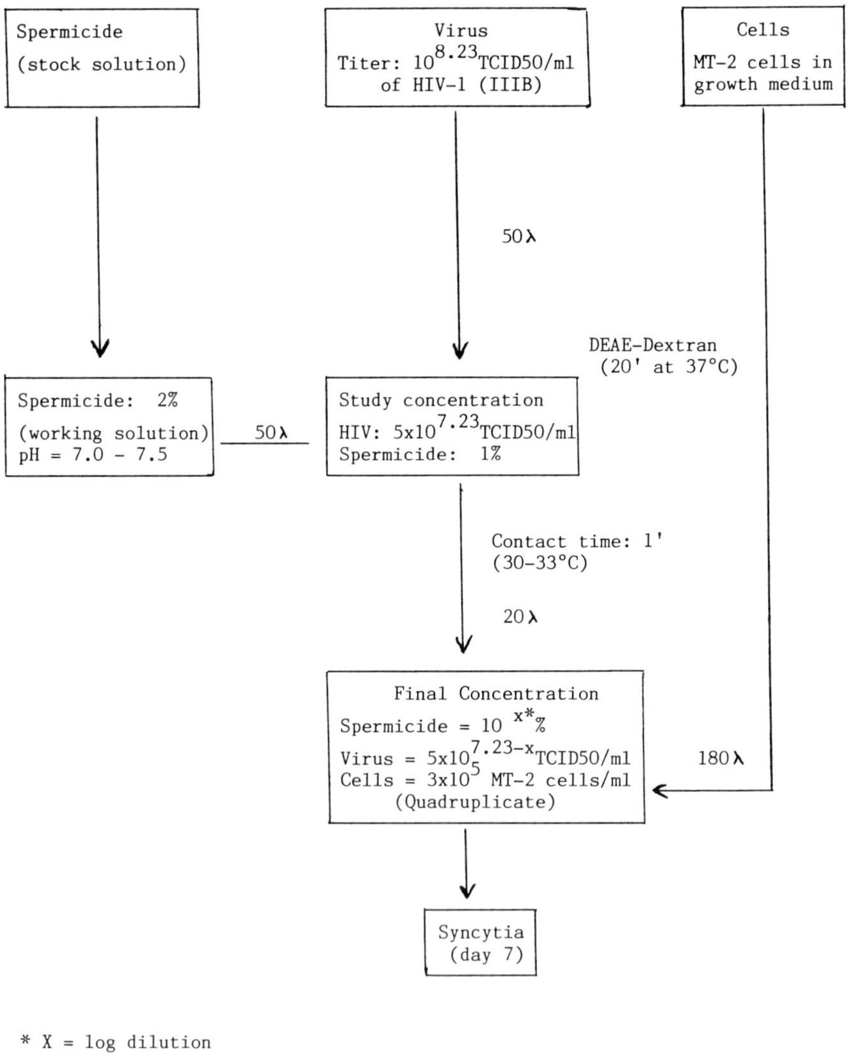

Fig. 5. Syncytium formation assay.

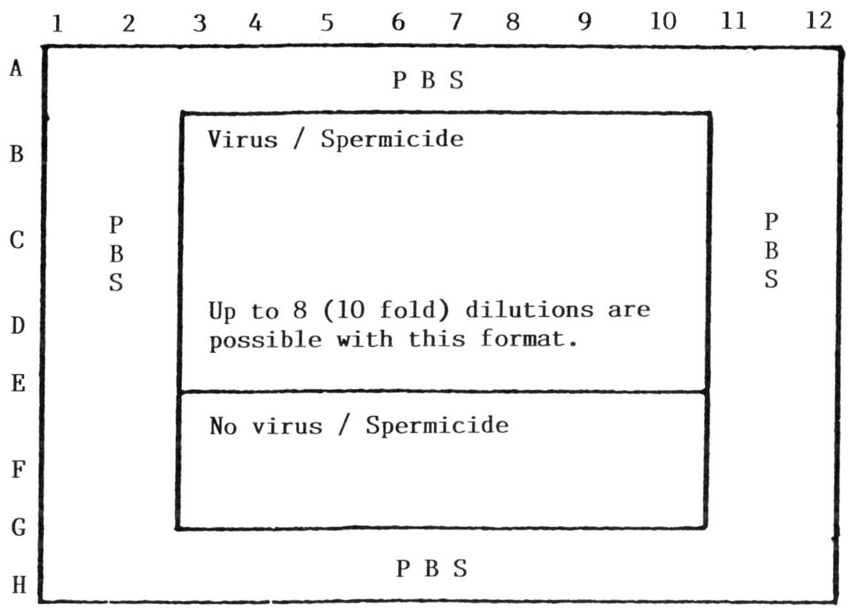

1. Current format provides for screening 1 spermicide in quadruplicate in rows B thru E.

2. Each spermicide dilution is tested in duplicate for normal cell sensitivity in rows F and G.

Fig. 6. Test plate format.

nucleated giant cells with more than five nuclei) are produced (Fig. 1) [17,18]. MT-2 cells do not spontaneously form syncytia and are susceptible to infection with the formation of syncytia by multiple laboratory isolates of HIV. The formation of syncytia results from an interaction of cells expressing the HIV envelope protein and the CD4 receptor, usually representing biologically active virus. Other measures of HIV expression, such as cellular fluorescence staining for HIV antigens, reverse transcriptase activity from supernatant fluids, cytopathology, and infectious viral yield, correlate with the formation of syncytia (Figs. 2,3), thereby validating the detection of syncytia as a parameter of HIV expression in vitro.

Inactivation of several orders of magnitude greater than the virus load that is likely to be found in seminal or cervical fluids is desirable. The transmission of HIV can occur via a cell-free or cell-associated route. Although the viral load in these fluids is unknown, our

1 - Virus/no spermicide (PBS) and no virus/no spermicide

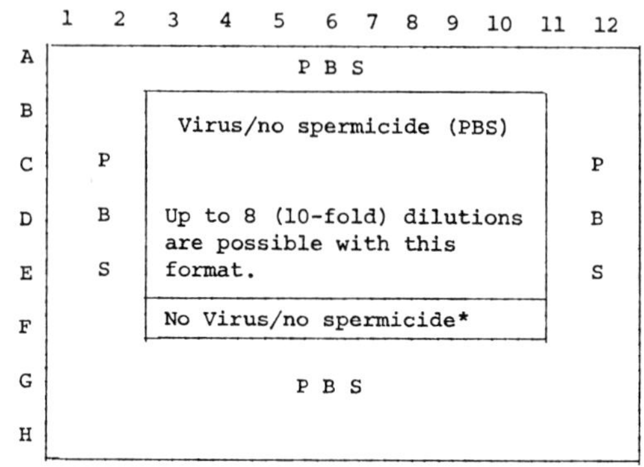

2 - Virus/1% nonoxynol-9

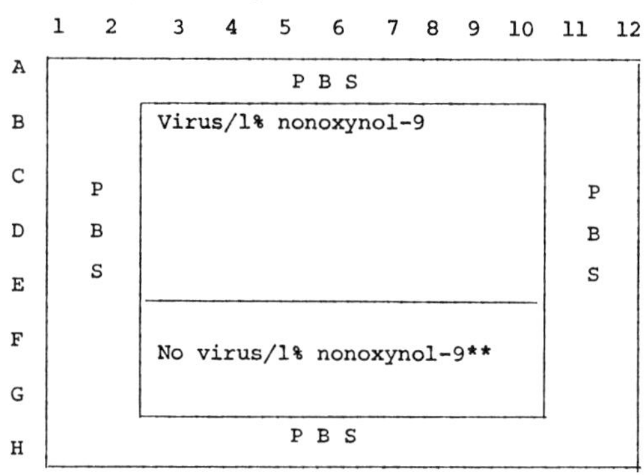

Current format provides for control virus titer and 1% nonoxynol-9 in quadruplicate (rows B thru E).

*Cell cultures without exposure to virus or spermicide are monitored on Row F.

**Each nonoxynol-9 dilution is tested in duplicate for normal cell sensitivity in rows F and G.

Fig. 7. Control plate format.

premise is that rapid (within 1 min) chemical inactivation of greater than 4–5 logs of infectious HIV (cell-free or cell-associated) in vitro represents a desirable level of virus kill. Therefore, a high-titer virus stock is necessary to perform these experiments. Agents that fail to

TABLE 4. Inactivation of HIV by Spermicidal Agents[a]

		Log titer reduction				
Compounds	Log $TCID_{50}$/ml	SE	A	*P*	B	*P*
DP-1	8.48	0.57	−0.25	NS	−4.98	<.0001
Encare	5.00	0.44	3.23	<.0001	−1.50	.008
Semicid	5.00	0.44	3.23	<.0001	−1.50	.008
Ortho-gynol jelly	7.48	0.57	0.75	NS	−3.98	<.0001
Ortho creme	7.50	0.41	0.73	NS	−4.00	<.0001

[a]For each experiment, the log $TCID_{50}$/ml (Reed and Muench method) is compared to the positive and negative controls for that experiment using the formula $Z = \text{Difference}/(Se_1^2 + SE_2^2)^{1/2}$, where the subscripts 1 and 2 refer to the test compound and the control, respectively. The one-tailed probability (*P*) is used since the test compound is expected to reduce the log virus titer and is not of interest if it raises the titer. "A" represents log $TCID_{50}$ control virus titer (8.23) − log $TCID_{50}$ compound virus titer. "B" represents log inactivation control (0.01% nonoxynol-9) virus titer (3.50) − log $TCID_{50}$ compound virus titer. SE, standard error; NS, not significant. The compounds were tested at a concentration of 0.1%.

TABLE 5. Secondary Evaluation: Experimental Parameters

Target cells: MT-2 cell line/normal peripheral mononuclear cells
HIV
  Cell-free (HIV-1 IIIB)
  Cell-associated (H9/HIV-1 IIIB)
Spermicide concentrations: 1%, 0.1%, 0.01%, 0.001%
Vehicle concentrations: 50%, 5%, 0.5%
Contact times: 10 min, 30 min, 1 hr

exhibit greater than 4–5 logs of HIV inactivation at standard concentrations may not be candidates for further study.

A precise way to measure the potency of a frozen virus stock is by estimating tissue culture infectious dose 50% ($TCID_{50}$) in a quantitative assay using replicate cultures of log 10 dilutions (Reed-Muench method) [19]. Tissue cultures were inoculated with serial tenfold dilutions (in quadruplicate) of the prototype HIV (IIIB) laboratory strain and were examined for 7 days for syncytium formation. Calculation of the highest dilution of virus that gave evidence of syncytia in 50% of the cultures, the endpoint determination, yielded a measure of the amount of infectious particles in the material. A $TCID_{50}$ is defined as the reciprocal of the dilution of HIV that was inoculated into microcultures containing MT-2 cells resulting in syncytia in 50% of the cultures by 7 days. In a representative set of

TABLE 6. HIV Inactivation by Spermicidal Agents

	$TCID_{50}/ml$[a]	
Concentration (%)	Octoxynol-9	Nonoxynol-9
1	$<10^2$	$<10^2$
0.1	$<10^2$	$<10^2$
0.01	$10^{4.23}$	$10^{3.76}$
0.001	$10^{6.33}$	$10^{5.49}$
0.0001	$10^{7.66}$	$10^{7.50}$
0.00001	$10^{8.23}$	$10^{8.23}$
Control	$10^{8.23}$	$10^{8.23}$

[a]Determined by Reed-Muench method (quadruplicate assays); $<10^2$ means no detectable syncytia.

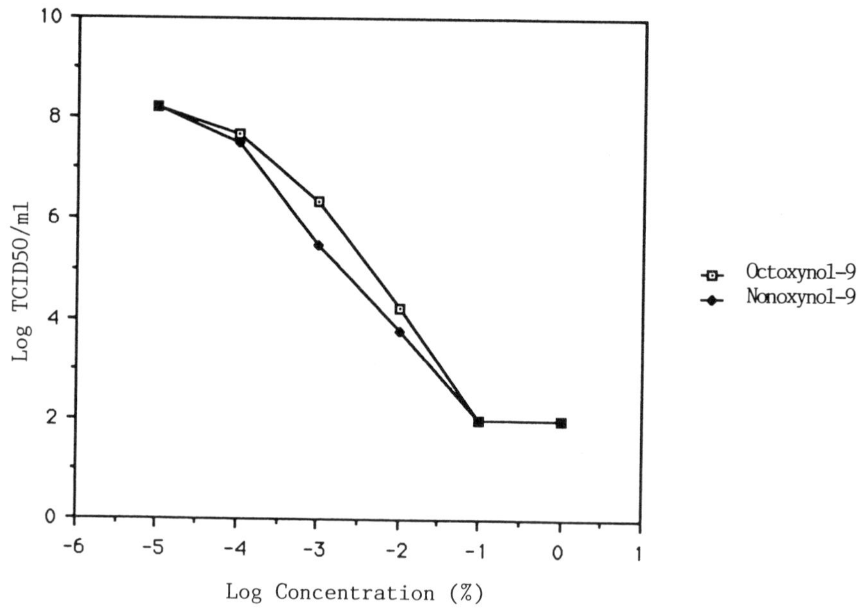

Fig. 8. Inactivation of HIV by spermicides.

experiments, the virus titer of our stock was calculated to be 8.23 log 10 $TCID_{50}/ml$ (Table 2). The higher the input dose of virus, the earlier the culture exhibited evidence of syncytium formation (Fig. 4). At lower input concentrations, virus expression was detected within 1 week.

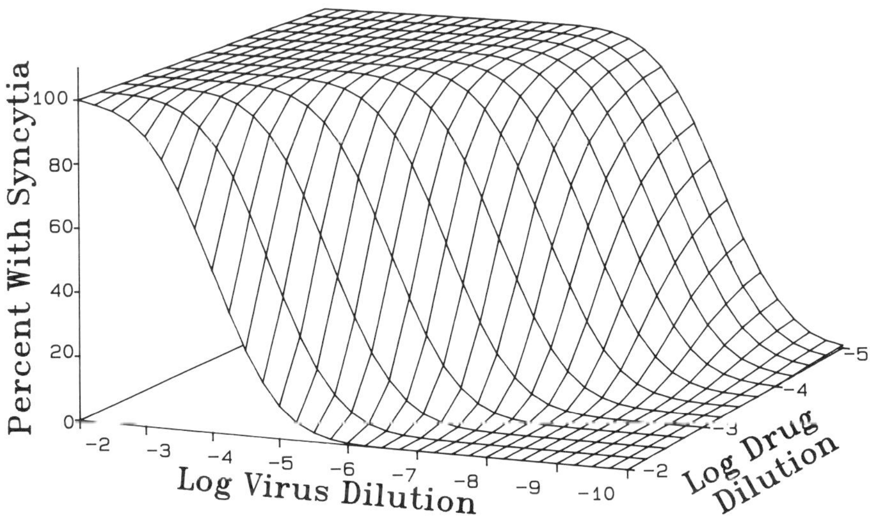

Fig. 9. Virus inactivation assay: syncytium formation.

The spermicide test concentration (1%) has been preselected in an attempt to prioritize active agents in comparision to N-9. The spermicide preparations are formulated in phosphate-buffered saline (pH = 7.4) or an appropriate solvent. The solvent must be evaluated for anti-HIV inactivating properties.

An outline of the syncytium-forming assay, the experimental controls, and the microtiter plate formats are shown in Figures 5–7 and Table 3. MT-2 cells (3×10^5 cell/ml) are incubated with serial tenfold dilutions (in quadruplicate) of treated HIV (IIIB) in microculture wells (6×10^4 cells/well/0.2 ml). Daily inspection of the culture for visual evidence of syncytia is undertaken. Because the assay can be performed with 0.2 ml of culture supernatant in a microtiter plate, HIV inoculation of target cell cultures can be monitored conveniently, and endpoint titrations of infectious HIV can be performed. No manipulation of the culture is necessary during the 7 day evaluation. The development and application of a $TCID_{50}$ syncytium-forming assay to spermicidal testing is ideally suited for inactivation experiments [20]. The $TCID_{50}$ assay can quantify infectious virus under conditions where virus input is limiting and a minimum number of cells can be used. Each set of experiments has four experimental controls. The inactivating potential of a compound cannot be

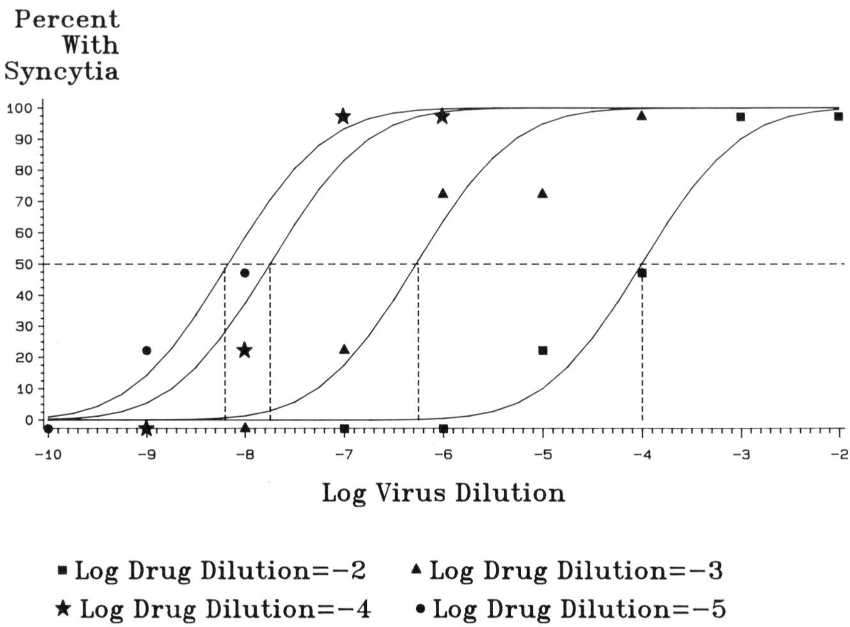

Fig. 10. Estimation of virus $TCID_{50}$/ml.

determined at concentrations that exhibit indicator cell cytotoxicity. In a representative experiment, N-9 (1% or 0.1%) inactivated greater than 4 logs of cell-free HIV after 1 min of exposure. Based on its potent inactivation profile, N-9 serves as the standard (inactivation control) to which candidate compounds are compared. Cytotoxicity was evident at concentrations of N-9 greater than or equal to 0.001%. A representative set of experiments evaluating candidate spermicides and vehicles is shown in Table 4. None of the compounds exhibited potent HIV inactivation properties.

Secondary Evaluation

The goal of the secondary evaluation studies is to provide a more comprehensive evaluation of the inactivation properties of the spermicide. The experimental design we selected is shown in Table 5. Normal peripheral blood mononuclear cells are compared with MT-2 cells as targets. The use of normal cells as targets requires evaluation by other measures of HIV expression. Quantitative determinations of the inactivation of cell-associated HIV must be performed. The spermicide and vehicle are tested alone and in combination. Spermicide/vehicle concentrations and contact time are varied and a series of concentration-kill and time-kill experiments are performed. The spermicidal preparation should exhibit maximum anti-HIV effects with concentrations well below those expected in vaginal mucus or the rectal vault. An obvious strategy to optimize therapeutic benefit while decreasing host toxicity is to use combinations of effective spermicidal agents. After secondary evaluation studies, spermicides can be prioritized and selected for animal toxicology.

A more detailed HIV-inactivation profile of N-9 and octoxynol-9 has been investigated. HIV was treated (1 min) with various concentrations of N-9 and octoxynol-9 (Table 6). Treated virus was serially diluted and inoculated into MT-2 cells, and the $TCID_{50}$/ml was determined by the Reed-Muench method (Fig. 8). The HIV-inactivation profile of a compound (octoxynol-9) can be represented in a three-dimensional model that takes into account variable drug and virus concentrations (Fig. 9). The fitted curves can be projected into a two-dimensional graph, and the 50% response can be interpolated (Fig. 10).

CONCLUSIONS

We have described a standardized, reproducible, and validated method for screening candidate spermicidal agents with anti-HIV inactivating properties. It is hoped that the anti-HIV screening technology that has been developed can aid in identifying and selecting a spermicidal preparation with maximum anti-HIV inhibitory effects.

ACKNOWLEDGMENTS

This paper was presented at the IV International Conference on AIDS, Stockholm, Sweden, June 12, 1988. We are grateful to R.C. Gallo, P.D. Markham, D.R. Hicks, and B. Voeller for providing valuable reagents and helpful discussions. We thank Maggi Mackle for technical assistance. Support for this project (CSA-88-034) was provided in part by the Contraceptive Research and Development (CONRAD) Program, Eastern Virginia Medical School, under a cooperative agreement with the U.S. Agency for International Development (U.S.A.I.D.) (DTE-3044-A-00-6063-00), which in turn receives funds for AIDS research from an interagency agreement with the

National Institute of Child Health and Human Development (NICHD). The views expressed by the authors do not necessarily reflect the views of U.S.A.I.D. or CONRAD.

REFERENCES

1. **Gallo RC, Salahuddin SZ, Popovic M, et al.:** Frequent detection and isolation of cytopathic retroviruses (HTLV-III) from patients with AIDS and at risk for AIDS. Science 224:500–503, 1984.

2. **Popovic M, Sarngadharan MG, Read E, Gallo RC:** Detection, isolation and continuous production of cytopathic retroviruses (HTLV-III) from patients with AIDS and pre-AIDS. Science 224:497–500, 1984.

3. **Stone KM, Grimes DA, Magder LS:** Personal protection against sexually transmitted diseases. Am J Obstet Gynecol 155:180–188, 1986.

4. **Conant MC, Hardy D, Sernatinger J, Spicer D, Levy JA:** Condoms prevent transmission of AIDS-associated retrovirus. JAMA 255:1706, 1986.

5. **Rietmeijer CAM, Krebs JW, Feorino PM, Judson FN:** Condoms as physical and chemical barriers against human immunodeficiency virus. JAMA 259:1851–1853, 1988.

6. **Pritchard JA, MacDonald PC:** Family planning. In Williams Obstetrics, 16th ed. New York: Appleton-Century-Crofts, 1980, p 1011.

7. **Katchadourian HA, Lunde DT:** Fundamentals of Human Sexuality. New York: Holt Rinehart & Winston, 1972.

8. **Jick H, Hannan MT, Stergachis A, Heidrich F, Pereramd DR, Rothman KJ:** Vaginal spermicides and gonorrhea. JAMA 248:1619–1621, 1982.

9. **Austin H, Louv WC, Alexander WJ:** A case-control study of spermicides and gonorrhea. JAMA 251:2822–2824, 1984.

10. **Louv WC, Austin H, Alexander WJ, Stagno S, Cheeks J:** A clinical trial of nonoxynol-9 for preventing gonococcal and chlamydial infections. J Infect Dis 158:518–523, 1988.

11. **Postic B, Singh B, Squeglia NL, Guevarra LO:** Inactivation of clinical isolates of herpes virus hominis types 1 and 2 by chemical contraceptives. Sex Transmitted Dis 5:22–24, 1978.

12. **Singh B, Postic B, Cutler J:** Virucidal effect of certain chemical contraceptives on type 2 herpes virus. Am J Obstet Gynecol 126:422–425, 1976.

13. **Hicks DR, Martin LS, Getchell JP, et al.:** Inactivation of HTLV-III/LAV-infected cultures of normal human lymphocytes by nonoxynol-9 in vitro. Lancet 2:1422–1423, 1985.

14. **Polsky B, Baron PA, Gold JWM, Smith JL, Jensen RH, Armstrong D:** In vitro inactivation of HIV-1 by contraceptive sponge containing nonoxynol-9. Lancet 1:1456, 1988.

15. **Malkovsky M, Newell A, Dalgleish AG:** Inactivation of HIV by nonoxynol-9. Lancet 1:645, 1988.

16. Goudsmit J, Paul DA, Lange JMA, et al.: Expression of human immunodeficiency virus antigen (HIV-Ag) in serum and cerebrospinal fluid during acute and chronic infection. Lancet 2:177–180, 1986.

17. Harada S, Koyanagi Y, Yamamoto N: Infection of HTLV-III/LAV in HTLV-I carrying cells MT-2 and MT-4 and application in a plaque assay. Science 229:563–566, 1985.

18. Nara PL, Hatch WC, Dunlop NM, et al.: Simple, rapid, quantitative, syncytium-forming microassay for the detection of human immunodeficiency virus neutralizing antibody. AIDS Res Hum Retroviruses 3:283–302, 1987.

19. Davis PD, Dulbecco R, Eisen H, Ginsberg HS: Microbiology, Vol. 3. Hagerstown, MD: Harper and Row, 1980.

20. McDougal JS, Cort SP, Kennedy MS, et al.: Immunoassay for the detection and quantitation of infectious human retrovirus, lymphadenopathy-associated virus (LAV). J Virol Methods 76:171–183, 1985.

27

Role of the Condom in Combatting Global AIDS: The Application of Sutton's Law to Public Health

James D. Shelton and Jeffrey R. Harris

When asked to explain why he robbed banks, the famous American bank robber Willie Sutton is alleged to have answered, "Because that's where the money is" [1]. Mr. Sutton's maxim has been applied many times in clinical diagnosis, but the emergence of the acquired immune deficiency syndrome (AIDS) pandemic gives rise to a need for its application to public health as well. Complete sexual abstinence is the only absolute means to prevent sexually transmitted AIDS. For those whose sexual behavior places them at risk of sexual transmission of the human immunodeficiency virus (HIV), however, the condom offers the best protection available. As described below, we believe the epidemiology of HIV, the sheer cost of condoms, and the particular role of the condom in HIV prevention mandate the prudent application of Sutton's Law to the public health strategy to prevent AIDS. We propose that, to be most effective, condom use must be focused where the need is greatest.

ROLE OF THE CONDOM IN THE MODERN WORLD

Since the dawning of the new contraceptive age a generation ago, the condom has taken a back seat to newer contraceptive methods. Condom use is unevenly distributed, with high use rates in only a few countries, primarily in the developed world [2]. Worldwide, condoms are used for contraception by only an estimated 6% of

Heterosexual Transmission of AIDS, pages 327–337

TABLE 1. Why Condoms May Fail

Leaks	Is taken off improperly or too soon
Breaks	Slips off
Is put on improperly or too late	Is not used

couples of reproductive age, with fully two-thirds of condom users residing in developed countries. Twenty-five percent of all users live in one country—Japan. China accounts for another 20% of the world total, but condom use in the rest of the developing world is low. Notably, in Africa, the partners of well under 1% of married women of reproductive age are estimated to use condoms [2].

The relatively low popularity of the condom can be attributed, in part, to negative attitudes toward it. These attitudes concern reliability, comfort, sensitivity, embarrassment, inconvenience (particularly regarding interruption of lovemaking), the poor image of condoms due to their traditional association with venereal disease and prostitution, and interference with sexual arousal and excitement [2,3].

Condoms have a high theoretical effectiveness against pregnancy: whereas method failures probably are less than 1% per year, use failures are substantially higher [2]. Table 1 lists the reasons why condoms may fail. Although leakage and breakage are probably real problems with condoms, a condom's poor performance in actual practice probably is due to inconsistent and inadequate use, especially nonuse. The ineffectiveness of condom use probably is related to the negative characteristics and attitudes mentioned above. On the positive side, if motivation can be increased or if negative perceptions can be reduced, the potential for increased effectiveness is excellent.

Although the condom's role as a contraceptive has been partly eclipsed by more modern methods, its traditional role in preventing sexually transmitted diseases (STDs) has remained robust. Indeed, that role has been reinforced by the emergence of newly recognized STDs and increasing evidence that condoms provide protection against STDs [2,4]. As can be verified through simple experimentation, neither water nor air molecules, which are less than 0.1 nm in diameter, readily pass through a correctly manufactured, modern latex condom. Neither can even the smallest virus pass through a latex condom. The relatively small HIV, approximately 120 nm in diameter, is no exception [5].

In addition to this straightforward evidence of mechanical effectiveness, epidemiologic evidence increasingly supports the view that the condom provides a high degree of protection against heterosexual HIV infection [4,6–12]. Data from six studies [7–12] on human heterosexual HIV transmission showed an important protective effect of condoms, including a notable dose-response effect (Table 2).

Thus the condom is an effective, albeit imperfect, tool to prevent HIV transmission. However imperfect the condom, the social, economic, demographic, and health impacts of the AIDS pandemic are likely to be so great [13–15], and the delay of condom use so costly, that we must rapidly apply our best technology against HIV in the most effective way possible.

COST CONSTRAINTS

Simple calculations illustrate the unacceptably high cost of unfocused condom distribution in the developing world. Even if we estimate a conservative price of $0.04 (U.S.) per condom and a coital frequency of 100 per couple per year, the cost of enough condoms for consistent use by any substantial portion of the population is prohibitive. For example, the cost for only 25% of the roughly one-half billion reproductive-aged men in the developing world (excluding China) would be one-half billion dollars per year for condoms alone. This may not seem like a huge amount of money to amass against a pandemic such as AIDS, but support for AIDS prevention is likely to be much more modest. Beyond the simple commodity cost, the cost of shipping, personnel, and other service-delivery components would undoubtedly multiply the cost severalfold. Use of commercial mechanisms might recoup some of these costs through sales revenue, but a strategy to achieve uniform availability of condoms clearly is impractical.

CONCENTRATION ON HIV INFECTION OR "WHERE THE MONEY IS"

From an AIDS public health intervention perspective, "where the money is" is "where the virus is." The epidemiology of HIV clearly indicates that the virus is concentrated in specific places and populations. This allows for concentration of public health efforts to prevent its spread.

Reliable population-based data on the prevalence of HIV infection are scarce. Still, enough data are available to demonstrate wide variations in prevalence [16]. First, wide variations exist from continent to continent, from country to country, and from region to region within countries. HIV-1 in Africa is largely concentrated in central and eastern Africa [13,15,16], but western Africa, Asia, and most of

TABLE 2. Human Studies on Condom Efficacy in Preventing HIV Transmission

Study	Subjects	Methodology	Results	
Fischl et al. [7]	Miami partners of HIV-positive individuals	Prospective	Seroconversion Without barrier contraception	86%
			With barrier contraception	10%
Mann et al. [8]	Prostitutes, Zaire	Cross-sectional	Seropositive No condom use	26%
			Up to 25% use	35%
			26% to 49% use	32%
			50% to 74% use	0%
			75% to 100% use	0%
Ngugi et al. [9]	Prostitutes, Kenya	Prospective	Approximate seroconversion No condom use	72%
			Less than 50% use	56%
			50% or more	33%
			100% use	0%
CDC [10]	Prostitutes United States	Cross-sectional	Seropositive No or some condom use	11%
			100% condom use	0%
Padian [11]	Female partners of HIV-infected men, California	Cross-sectional	Relative risk of seropositivity 0.6 (95% CI = 0.3–1.3) (Much condom use likely to have begun after seroconversion)	
Curran and Fish [12]	Female partners of sero-positive hemo-philiacs	Prospective	Seroconversion No or some condom use	17%
			100% condom use	0%

Latin America appear to have much lower rates of HIV-1 infection [17]. Marked urban-rural differences are also present in many countries [14,16]. For example, HIV seroprevalence among reproductive-aged adults in Kinshasa, Zaire, is approximately 7–8% [17], but, in at least one area of rural Zaire, the seroprevalence appears to be below 1% and may have been stable for the last decade [18].

Of great importance, the prevalence of HIV infection varies markedly with the level of sexual activity. In Africa, HIV seroprevalence is strikingly higher among the most sexually active groups [13]. Prostitution is a particularly high-risk activity. In 1985, 65% of low socioeconomic status prostitutes in Nairobi, Kenya, had antibodies to HIV [19], but only about 2% of pregnant Nairobi women had antibodies [17]. By early 1987, the antibody prevalence in this same cohort of prostitutes had risen to about 85% [19]. Similarly, in Burkino Faso, the seroprevalence in prostitutes was 14.6%, whereas seroprevalence in pregnant women and healthy controls was 1.7% and 0.0%, respectively [20].

With HIV infection as concentrated in definable subpopulations as it appears to be, simple public health sense mandates that prevention efforts (including use of the condom) focus on areas of high virus concentration and on behaviors highly associated with HIV transmission. Particularly for poor countries, prevention resources are scarce and must be directed where the impact will be the greatest. Accordingly, intervention among individuals who practice high-risk behaviors for sexual HIV transmission is critical to stemming the tide of AIDS in the world.

OPPORTUNITIES FOR FOCUSED INTERVENTION WITH THE CONDOM

Specific opportunities for intervention will vary from place to place. Public health strategies should be based on good epidemiologic information and on the practical ability to reach specific populations at risk. Persons practicing high-risk behaviors—including prostitutes, their clients, and many homosexual and bisexual men—should receive high priority for intervention. Others who should be considered include: single urban men and women, patients attending STD clinics, long-distance truck drivers and traders, intravenous drug users, the military, prisoners, and other sexually active individuals residing in areas of high prevalence of infection.

Providing condoms through channels and mechanisms directed against other STDs may be particularly advantageous in preventing HIV transmission and may have other benefits. HIV transmission appears significantly linked to sexually transmitted genital ulcers, such as those produced by chancroid, syphilis, and herpes [21,22]. Thus the use of condoms may prevent HIV infection directly by inhibiting the transmission of HIV and indirectly by preventing other STDs. Furthermore, the health delivery infrastructure in many developing countries is fragile, grossly overburdened, and ill-equipped to take on the major burden of AIDS prevention, yet programs against STDs do exist in some developing countries as well as in developed countries. These programs may serve as an appropriate institutional framework for condom promotion against HIV and other STDs.

CAN A FOCUSED CONDOM STRATEGY WORK?

Modifying sexual behavior among highly sexually active people is a formidable challenge at best, and the unpopularity of condoms in the developing world does not give rise to optimism. Nevertheless, some basis for hope exists. Prostitutes in the developed world appear to be rapidly adopting condom use [23,24]. Furthermore, a modest condom promotion effort among low socioeconomic status prostitutes in Nairobi, Kenya, has been remarkably successful [9]. Before the intervention, 7–10% of prostitutes reported occasional use of condoms. After the intervention, 70–80% of prostitutes in the active intervention groups reported using condoms at least some of the time, and condoms were used in 35–38% of all encounters in those groups. Programs aimed at the sexual behavior of homosexual men in the developed world likewise appear to have been successful [25–27]. These examples provide encouragement that a focused condom approach can work, and they support the rationale for further focused efforts.

The motivation to prevent AIDS appears to differ dramatically from the motivation to prevent pregnancy. Anecdotal reports of increased condom use and condom shortages in developing countries suggest that motivation can be high. AIDS is a particularly devastating and frightening disease; unlike pregnancy, it puts both males and females at risk of death.

A focused condom strategy may be useful in areas with either a high or a low prevalence of HIV infection. In high-HIV-prevalence areas, AIDS represents a widely recognized public health crisis, and individuals may have friends or acquaintances with AIDS. Motivation to use condoms is likely to be high. Even in high-prevalence areas, large segments of the population may be relatively free of HIV infection and can be protected. Moreover, since infections with other STDs may hasten the development of clinical AIDS among seropositive individuals, preventing such STDs with condoms may hinder this progression. In low-prevalence areas, providing condoms to those at highest risk of HIV infection may be the most important tool to prevent the infection from ever "taking off" and becoming well established in that population.

In either case, programs must consider innovative, sensitive, and specific service-delivery techniques to promote condom availability and acceptability among individuals at high risk of sexual transmission. They will need to take advantage of lessons learned from successful social marketing of contraceptives, oral rehydration solution, and other health interventions in the developing world.

FOCUSED USE OF CONDOMS AS PART OF A LARGER HIV PREVENTION EFFORT

In our view, the ideal AIDS prevention strategy must go well beyond focused condom promotion. A prevention strategy should also emphasize fidelity, abstinence, fewer partners, and avoidance of high-risk partners as well as the promotion of blood transfusion screening, sterile injection practices, and, when appropriate, specific approaches to intravenous drug users. A comprehensive AIDS prevention strategy should extend beyond high-risk groups to include a major education and communication component directed toward the general population. To avoid inappropriate fear and to protect themselves, members of the general population must understand how HIV does and does not spread. Individuals should be enabled to identify whether they themselves or their potential sexual partners are at high risk of infection. However, general communication, by itself, may have little or no impact on changing high-risk sexual behavior, as witnessed by one evaluation of the major national AIDS health education campaign in the United Kingdom [28]. Rather, promotional efforts focused on high-risk behaviors appear to be essential in changing such behaviors.

CONCLUSIONS

On the one hand, the high cost, logistic difficulties of distribution, and low acceptability of the condom in the developing world make the condom appear to be a less-than-formidable public health weapon against AIDS. On the other hand, the condom appears to be the best technology at hand for those at risk of sexual transmission of HIV and other STDs. Because HIV infection is highly concentrated, it makes good public health sense to focus condom availability and promotion efforts selectively toward sexually active individuals at high risk of HIV transmission. General communication efforts that fail to reach high-risk individuals may expend significant resources but have little impact on HIV transmission. Optimism for the success of focused efforts comes from early experience and the sense that the devastating morbidity and mortality of HIV infection can result in strong personal motivation for prevention.

Whatever the ultimate success of condom intervention strategies and programs, we must put forth our best efforts as soon as possible. We must begin now, document our efforts, evaluate them carefully, and learn from our successes and failures. The future course of the international AIDS pandemic, for us and for future generations, may depend on our actions today.

ACKNOWLEDGMENTS

Support for this work came from the U.S. Agency for International Development. The views expressed herein are solely those of the authors and do not necessarily represent those of the U.S.A.I.D.

REFERENCES

1. **Sutton WF, Linn E:** Where the Money Was. New York: Royal Production Corporation, 1976.

2. **Sherris JD, Lewison D, Fox G:** Update on Condoms—Products, Protection, Promotion. Population Reports, Series H, Number 6. Baltimore: Johns Hopkins University, Population Information Program, 1982, p H-129.

3. **Chapman S, Hodgson J:** Showers in raincoats: Attitudinal barriers to condom use in high-risk heterosexuals. Comm Health Stud 12:97–105, 1988.

4. **Feldblum PJ, Fortney J:** Condoms, spermicides, and the transmission of human immunodeficiency virus: A review of the literature. Am J Public Health 78:52–53, 1988.

5. **Van de Perre, Jacobs D, Sprecher-Goldberger S:** The latex condom, an efficient barrier against sexual transmission of AIDS-related viruses. AIDS 1:49–52, 1987.

6. **Wellings K:** AIDS and the condom. Br Med J 293:1259–1260, 1986.

7. **Fischl MA, Dickinson GM, Scott GB:** Evaluation of heterosexual partners, children, and household contacts of adults with AIDS. JAMA 257:640–644, 1987.

8. **Mann J, Quinn TC, Piot P:** Condom use and HIV infection among prostitutes in Zaire. N Engl J Med 316:345, 1987.

9. **Ngugi EN, Plummer FA, Simonsen JN, et al.:** Prevention of transmission of human immunodeficiency virus in Africa: Effectiveness of condom promotion and health education among prostitutes. Lancet 2:887–890, 1988.

10. **Centers for Disease Control:** Antibody to human immunodeficiency virus in female prostitutes. MMWR 36:157–161, 1987.

11. **Padian N:** Male-to-female transmission of HIV, in reply. JAMA 258:3386–3387, 1987.

12. **Laurian Y, Peynet J, Verroust F:** HIV infection in sexual partners of HIV-seropositive patients with hemophilia [letter]. N Engl J Med 320:183, 1989.

13. **Quinn TC, Mann JM, Curran JW, Piot P:** AIDS in Africa: An epidemiologic paradigm. Science 234:955–963, 1986.

14. **Anonymous:** AIDS in Africa. Lancet 2:192–193, 1987.

15. **Piot P, Plummer FA, Mhalu FS, Lambouray J, Chin J, Mann JM:** AIDS: An international perspective. Science 239:573–579, 1988.

16. **Torrey BB, Way PO, Rowe PM:** Epidemiology of HIV in Africa: Emerging issues and social implications. Miller N, Rockwell R (eds): AIDS in Africa: The Social Impact and Policy Implications. Lewiston/Queenston: Edwin Mellen Press, 1988.

17. **Liskin L, Blackburn R, Maier JH:** AIDS—A Public Health Crisis. Population Reports, Series L, Number 6. Baltimore. Johns Hopkins University, Population Information Program, 1986.

18. **Nzilambi N, De Cock KM, Forthal D, et al.:** Stability of HIV infection prevalence over 10 years in a rural population of Zaire. N Engl J Med 318:276–279, 1988.

19. **Plummer FA, Simonsen JN, Ngugi EN, Cameron DW, Piot P, Ndinya-Acholu JO:** Incidence of human immunodeficiency virus (HIV) infection and related diseases in a cohort of Nairobi prostitutes. Abstract M8.4: III International Conference on AIDS, Washington, DC, 1987.

20. **Kanki PJ, M'Boup S, Ricard D, et al.:** Human T-Lymphocytic virus type 4 and the human immunodeficiency virus in West Africa. Science 236:827–831, 1987.

21. **Simonsen JN, Cameron DW, Gakinya MN, et al.:** Human immunodeficiency virus infection among men with sexually transmitted diseases: Experience from a center in Africa. N Engl J Med 318:274–278, 1988.

22. **Stamm WE, Handsfield HH, Rompalo AM, Ashley RL, Roberts PL, Corey L:** The association between genital ulcer disease and acquisition of HIV infection in homosexual men. JAMA 260:1429–1433, 1988.

23. **Krogsgaard K, Gluud C, Pedersen C, et al.:** Widespread use of condoms and low prevalence of sexually transmitted diseases in Danish non-drug addict prostitutes. Br Med J 293:1473–1474, 1986.

24. **Smith GL, Smith KF:** Lack of HIV infection and condom use in licensed prostitutes. Lancet 2:1392, 1986.

25. **Doll LS, Darrow W, O'Malley PO, Bodecker T, Jaffer H:** Self-reported behavior change in homosexual men in the San Francisco city clinic cohort. Abstract F.8.1: III International Conference on AIDS, Washington, DC, 1987.

26. **Eijrond BDF, Van Der Hoek JAR, Emsbroek JA, Schoonhoven FJ:** Declining incidence of sexually transmitted diseases as a result of an AIDS-prevention campaign. Abstract F.8.5: III International Conference on AIDS, Washington, DC, 1987.

27. **Fineberg HV:** Education to prevent AIDS: Prospects and obstacles. Science 239:592–596, 1988.

28. **Sherr L, Green J:** Evaluation of health education in Britain. Abstract T6.2: III International Conference on AIDS, Washington, DC, 1987.

DISCUSSION

DR. CAMERON: I would like to comment on the slide that you showed of Elizabeth Ngugi's article showing protection from HIV in women using condoms. The data that I presented from Frank Plummer's study this morning, and other data presented at Stockholm, have shown that efficacy correlates with the impact of condom use on genital ulcer disease.

DR. SHELTON: Then your hypothesis is that the condoms protect against genital ulcer disease?

DR. CAMERON: Yes. The majority of the protection seen in Elizabeth Ngugi's slide is indirect through prevention of genital ulcer disease.

DR. SHELTON: Well, I remember your multivariate analysis, but I guess I did not think that it ruled out the hypothesis that a condom could be preventing straightforward mechanical transmission in the presence of ulcers, and that it is effective not just because it was preventing ulcerative disease.

Also, I think I remember that the *P* value for the residual effect, even after allowing for an effect through genital ulcerative disease, was something like 0.056, which certainly does not rule out some additional effect.

DR. CAMERON: Of course. I believe as an article of faith that condoms do prevent direct transmission. I believe that condoms do have an impact, but there is a secondary impact, and that is as a control measure against chancroid.

DR. JOHN: Is there any information on condom use in male homosexuals in terms of preventing transmission? This question is not specifically addressed to you, Dr. Shelton, but to anyone. When I get home next week, people will want to know the state of the art and they will definitely ask me about the vaginal condom. Is it licensed?

DR. SHELTON: I think Dr. Tanquary is going to talk about the vaginal condom. With respect to your first question, I tried to find information on HIV transmission in homosexual men. I have a recollection of seeing one article. Mostly, gay men have not used condoms much in the past, so it has been difficult to study whether there has been HIV transmission prevention. Prospective studies have been difficult. So, the answer to your question is that I do not know; maybe someone else here does.

DR. HODGEN: Would you comment on condoms not made of

latex? What is the prevalence of other types of condoms used and do they work as well?

DR. SHELTON: Well, I guess there is the natural skin condoms but, other than that, latex is pretty much universal. People have tried other materials, and there are other kinds of materials under development.

I think the interesting thing about the natural skin condom is that aesthetically they operate under a different principle. They have one fixed size providing something of a "loose fit"; they do not fit everybody tightly. Nevertheless, they are extremely popular among some. I think this points to the fact that other concepts for condoms may be useful besides our general picture of a male condom.

28

Condoms: Overview of Technology, Materials, and Development

A. Charles Tanquary and Julie Hull Witte

Better condoms have been needed since the first products appeared several thousand years ago. A major technological advance occurred in the mid-1800s, when crepe rubber condoms were developed soon after vulcanization was discovered. In further advances 60 years ago, latex was substituted for crepe, and mechanized dipping was introduced [1,2]. Although the industry has considerably improved quality and reliability in recent decades, improvements are still needed, especially since condoms are the first line of defense against acquired immune deficiency syndrome (AIDS).

Condoms should be free of defects, stable during storage and use, easy to use, comfortable, safe, and effective. Condoms also should resist deterioration on exposure to sunlight, ultraviolet light, atmospheric pollutants, and lubricating oils. To the extent possible, condoms should enhance sexual pleasure, or at least detract little from sensation.

Where needs are not fully met by commercial products, or where use is low and potential consumption is high, opportunities exist for introducing new and better products that are manufactured at lower costs or are sold at higher prices. Since present condom manufacturing processes are capital-, energy-, and labor-intensive, the best route to new products is through the application of technologies now foreign to this industry.

Historically, mature industries such as the condom industry are wedded to raw materials and processes and do little to create their own obsolescence. Condom manufacturers are expected to resist

Heterosexual Transmission of AIDS, pages 339–354

change for many reasons. One is the perception that the present products are unique and can never be matched by alternative means. Another is that the market has scarcely been tapped, and shortages are projected. A third is the increasing concern about product liability actions. In a litigious society, continuing with an old line of products whose deficiencies are well known to the public is safer than embarking on something new that may create unrealistic expectations of safety and efficacy. Major changes in concepts and practices are likely to originate outside the condom industry or at its fringes. Indeed, a number of new condom products, most of which originated elsewhere, are at various stages of development.

HISTORICAL BACKGROUND

Innovators will find the past instructive for assessing the present state of the art and predicting trends. Figure 1 depicts some milestones in the history of condoms. Condoms may have been used in

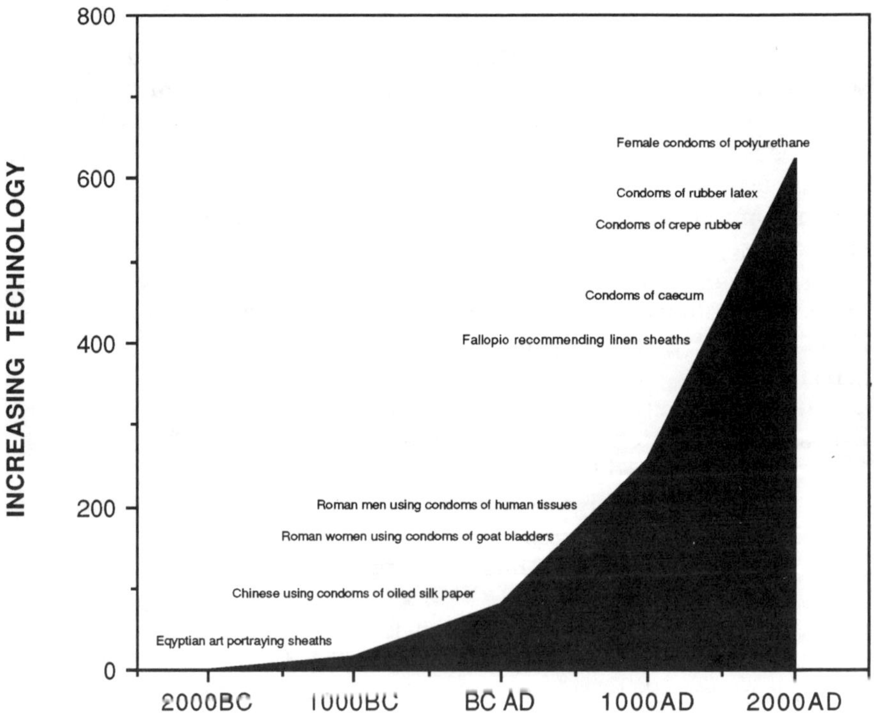

Fig. 1. History of the technology of condoms.

Egypt as early as 3000 years ago. Egyptian art of the time portrayed men wearing sheaths [3,4], but the purpose served by the sheaths is not clear. That the sheaths were dyed various colors to denote social status suggests adornment rather than function [5].

Three thousand years ago, the Chinese made condoms using oiled silk paper according to their ancient medical treatises [4]. Both Greek and Roman mythologies include tales of gods and mortals using condoms of goat bladders to protect women. These condoms probably were worn by women, since the Romans prescribed the use of goat bladder for forming a pouch that was placed in the vagina to receive the penis and trap semen [4,5]. In recent times, a primitive New Guinea tribe was found to be using a large, flexible plant pod as a female condom. This pod was cut off at one end to form a long pouch [5].

In the 1500s, Fallopius described a linen sheath that was intended to prevent syphilis. By the 1700s, the only material commonly used for condoms was derived from animal intestines [3]. Although ox caecum was used at first, lamb caecum soon predominated because of its greater softness. The advent of natural rubber condoms a century later did not totally displace these "natural skin" products.

Shortages of natural rubber during the early 1940s led to the use of nylon as a replacement, but the products were unacceptable. Other efforts in the 1960s to develop condoms from alternative materials, including films of ethylene copolymers, were unsuccessful. A polyurethane condom made by dipping was promising, except for its high cost [6].

PRESENT COMMERCIAL PRODUCTS

It is not surprising that condoms have been made of animal membranes for thousands of years, since these materials had long been used as containers for various purposes. What is surprising is that the natural condom made of caecum remains a viable commercial product, retaining up to 5% of the market, even at premium prices. Most users choose them because of their combination of comfort and increased sensation. These qualities are believed to derive from the higher heat transmission and the exchange of fluids during intercourse. One patent, a decade ago, suggested perforating rubber condoms with arrays of 2 μm holes, sufficient to permit fluid exchange while retaining sperm. This product obviously was not intended for prophylaxis. Other patents have described the use of collagen and other hydrogels for improved heat transmission. The use of hydro-

TABLE 1. Comparison of Commercial Products

	Natural rubber	Natural skin
Source	Latex of tree	Caecum of sheep
Chemical composition	Polyisoprene	Proteinaceous membrane
Polymer class	Hydrocarbon elastomer	Hydrogel
Mechanical properties	High strength	Low strength
	High elongation	Low elongation
	Low modulus	High modulus
	High toughness	Low toughness
	High tear resistance	Moderate tear resistance
	High puncture resistance	Good puncture resistance
Mechanical behavior	Elastic	Limp
Size	49–52 mm	62–80 mm
Fit	Tight fitting	Loose fitting
Permeability	Impermeable to sperm	Impermeable to sperm
	Impermeable to viruses	Permeable to HIV

gels has been proposed as a route to superior condoms that possess some of the qualities of natural skin [6].

The existence of dissimilar products that serve the same market demands attention. Analyses of their relative merits may suggest ways to combine their best qualities in new products. A comparison of natural rubber and natural skin condoms follows, and the large differences between them are shown in Table 1.

Natural rubber is hydrophobic, a hydrocarbon, whereas natural skin is hydrophilic, a hydrogel. Their mechanical properties appear to be totally different, except for resistance to puncture and tear. Table 2 lists typical values of tensile and tear properties and contrasts the rubbery behavior of natural rubber with the leathery behavior of natural skin. These values are normalized to unit thickness and cross-sectional area. The wall thickness of the skin condom is 150 μm, three times the thickness of the rubber condom. Figure 2, which is a graph of tensile force vs. strain, shows that the breaking forces are approximately the same due to the differences in thickness (Russell DD, personal communication), but the force required to stretch the natural skin condom is 20 times that for rubber. This means that a natural skin condom stretches hardly at all. Therefore, different widths must be available to allow for the lack of stretching.

Figure 3, which is derived from data from the Kinsey study [4],

TABLE 2. Tensile and Tear Properties of Commercial Products (Russell DD, personal communication)

	Tensile strength psi (MPa)	Elongation at break (%)	Stress at 20% strain psi (MPa)	Tear strength pli (kN/m)
Natural rubber latex	3,300 (22.8)	710	35 (0.24)	287 (50.2)
Natural skin, wet	970 (6.7)	25	205 (1.41)	166 (29.1)
Natural skin, dry	1,450 (10.0)	26	1,080 (7.44)	233 (40.8)

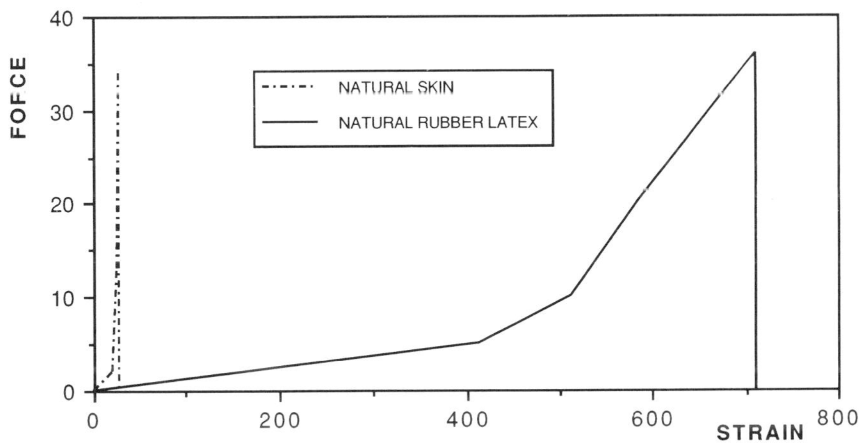

Fig. 2. Force vs. strain for commercial condom products.

shows the distribution of penis circumference for white U.S. males. Natural skin condoms range in size from 62 to 80 mm in layflat width (124–160 mm in circumference). Therefore, a 62 mm condom is large enough to fit 70% of this population, and an 80 mm condom fits 100%. A 52 mm rubber condom must stretch 20–50% to cover the same range. A rubber condom is held in place by the retractive forces of the condom itself, while a skin condom is held by an elastic band at the open end.

This comparison leads to the conclusion that the properties of a synthetic material need not match those of natural rubber for the synthetic material to merit consideration. The latitude permitted depends on other factors, including whether the condom is designed for a man or a woman. Therefore, a wide range of materials can be considered and choices made using the criteria of process cost, raw materials cost, and product quality and performance.

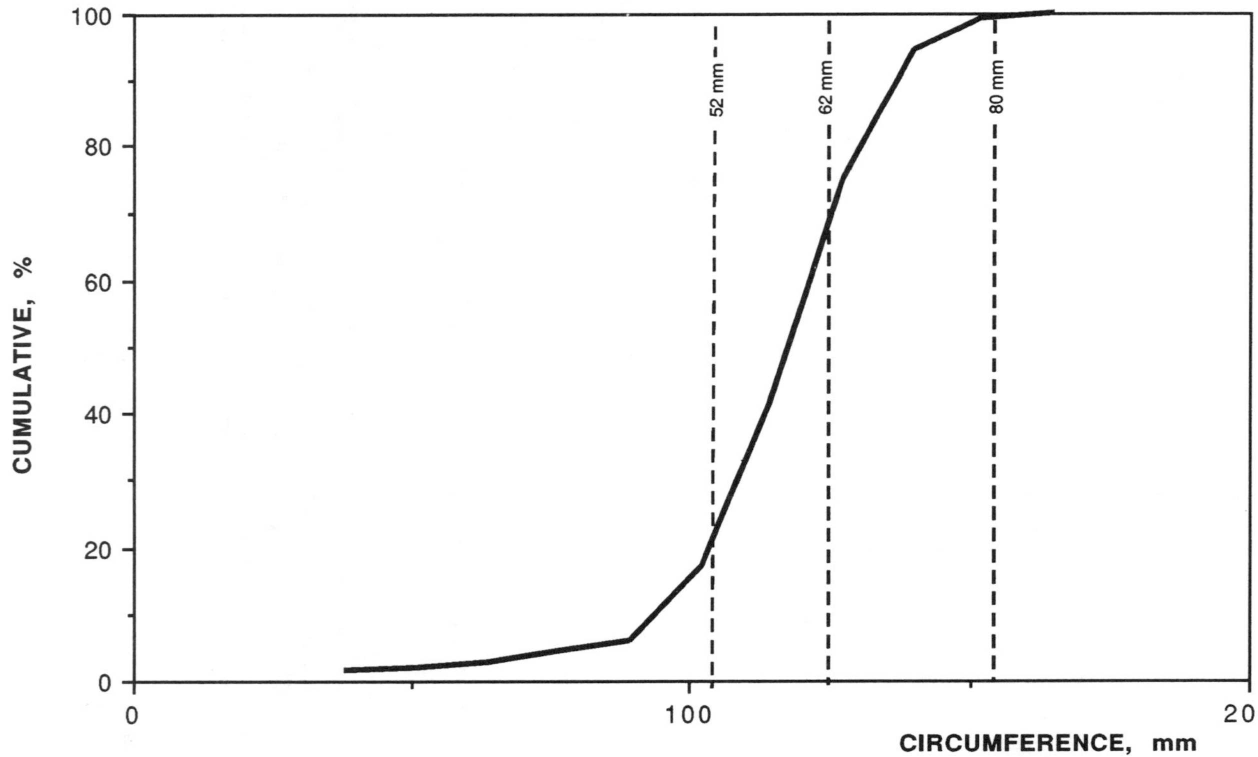

Fig. 3. Erect penis circumferences of U.S. white males [4], with vertical lines showing the sizes of commercial condom products: Rubber latex, 52 mm (104 mm circumference); and natural skin 62 and 80 mm (124 and 160 mm).

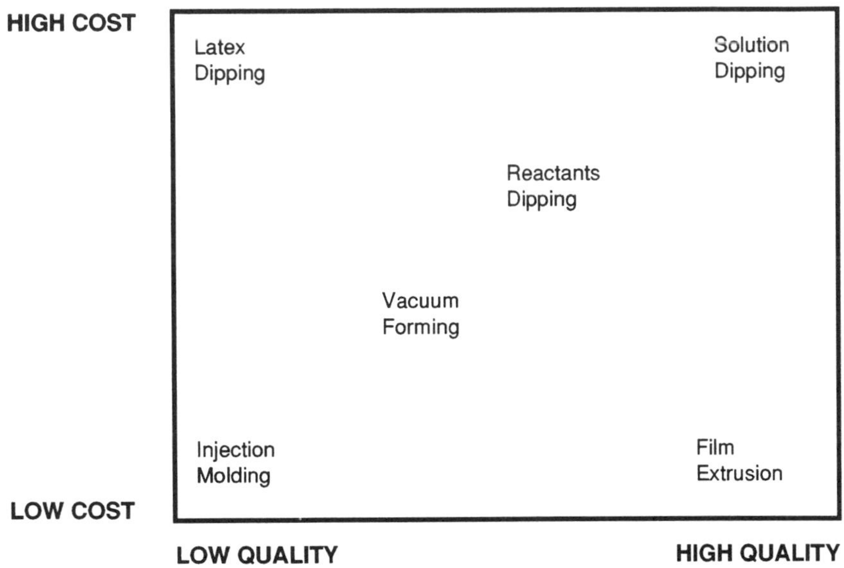

Fig. 4. Process cost vs. product quality.

SELECTION OF PROCESSES

Figure 4 shows some processes that have been used for condom manufacture. Injection blow molding, the process commonly used for making bottles, was proposed many years ago, and equipment was promoted for this purpose, but the products were crude. Thin, uniform walls were difficult to achieve. Vacuum forming requires the extrusion of a thick film, or billet, and then the deep drawing of the material into a cavity. This process is being explored in Europe as a way to make a female condom. The use of reactive prepolymers to form polyurethanes is the basis of a number of patents, and one product appears to be on the verge of being introduced. The problem here is the necessity to remove extractables to avoid toxicity.

Solution dipping (tried in the 1960s) resulted in high costs, because most effective solvents for polyurethane are toxic and carcinogenic and must be removed by heating and washing processes. Adding further to the cost is the necessity of removing these pollutants from air and water effluents. This process, nevertheless, is feasible and should prove attractive for premium products that are likely to appear soon, according to industry sources.

Film extrusion appears to offer the best properties at the lowest cost. The failures to achieve satisfactory products in the 1960s were due mostly to the lack of appropriate raw materials. Today, the thermoplastic elastomers (TPEs) that are available can be extruded into film and fabricated into shapes by heat sealing, welding, and other processes common in the plastics industry.

SELECTION OF MATERIALS

The major classes of TPEs are ranked by performance and cost in Figure 5 and compared in Table 3 [7]. The cost refers to raw materials only and does not include potential savings in process costs. The best performance is obtained from the polyamides, polyesters, and polyurethanes.

The cheaper materials are notably deficient in strength, tear resistance, and resistance to oils [8]. Resistance to oils is an important criterion in view of the catastrophic deterioration of natural rubber on exposure to many common household lubricants [9]. Although offering advantages in many industrial applications, the polyamides and polyesters appear to be poorly suited to condoms, since they are hard materials, intermediate between rubber and plastics. The thermoplastic polyurethanes (TPUs) offer the best combination of properties, and both the polyester- and the polyether-based materials have been used extensively for biomedical purposes [8,10]. Of the

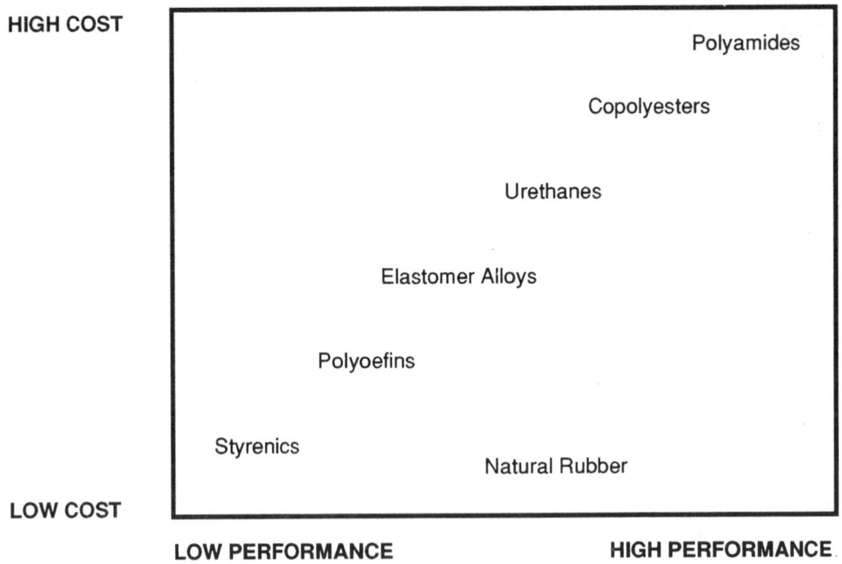

Fig. 5. Materials cost vs. performance of thermoplastic elastomers.

TABLE 3. Characteristics of Thermoplastic Elastomers

	Retention of properties on exposure to								
TPE class	Oils	Water	Oxygen	Ozone	Light	Softness	Tear strength	Tensile strength	Implant studies
Styrenics	P[a]	E	P	P	P	E	P	F	Few
Polyolefins	P	E	P	P	P	G	F	P	Few
Elastomer alloys	P	E	P	P	P	E	P	P	Few
Polyester urethanes	E	P	E	E	E	G	E	E	Numerous
Polyether urethanes	G	G	G	G	F	G	E	E	Numerous
Copolyesters	E	P	G	G	P	P	F	G	Few
Polyamides	E	E	G	G	E	P	G	G	Few
Natural rubber[b]	P	G	P	P	P	E	F	G	Numerous

[a]Scale: E, excellent; G, good; F, fair; P, poor.
[b]Control.

two, the polyether-based material is superior because of its hydrolytic stability.

Two biomedical TPUs are compared with natural rubber in Table 4. Since each is twice as strong as rubber, film half as thick could be used to provide the same breaking force. Figure 6 shows the stress-strain behavior at low extensions, in the range of interest for most condom products. The top two curves are for the same material, first as produced by the extrusion process, and then as changed by stress-softening. Stress-softening, also called the Mullins effect, is a well known phenomenon that occurs when thermoplastic elastomers are stretched [10,11] (Wheeler RG, personal communication). The hard segments are disrupted to create a fine-grained structure, which is more elastic. The result is a substantial drop in tensile modulus to values less than half that of the untreated material.

Similar decreases in modulus can occur when polyurethanes are plasticized, and two effective plasticizers are water and nonoxynol-9 (Russell DD, personal communication; Wheeler RG, personal communication). It should thus be possible to make TPU condoms that approach the modulus of rubber while retaining good strength and tear resistance. However, plasticizers are known to decrease resilience, which for the polyurethanes is already low. If the resilience becomes too low, the condom may fit snugly at first but become loose during intercourse due to the slow recovery from cycling

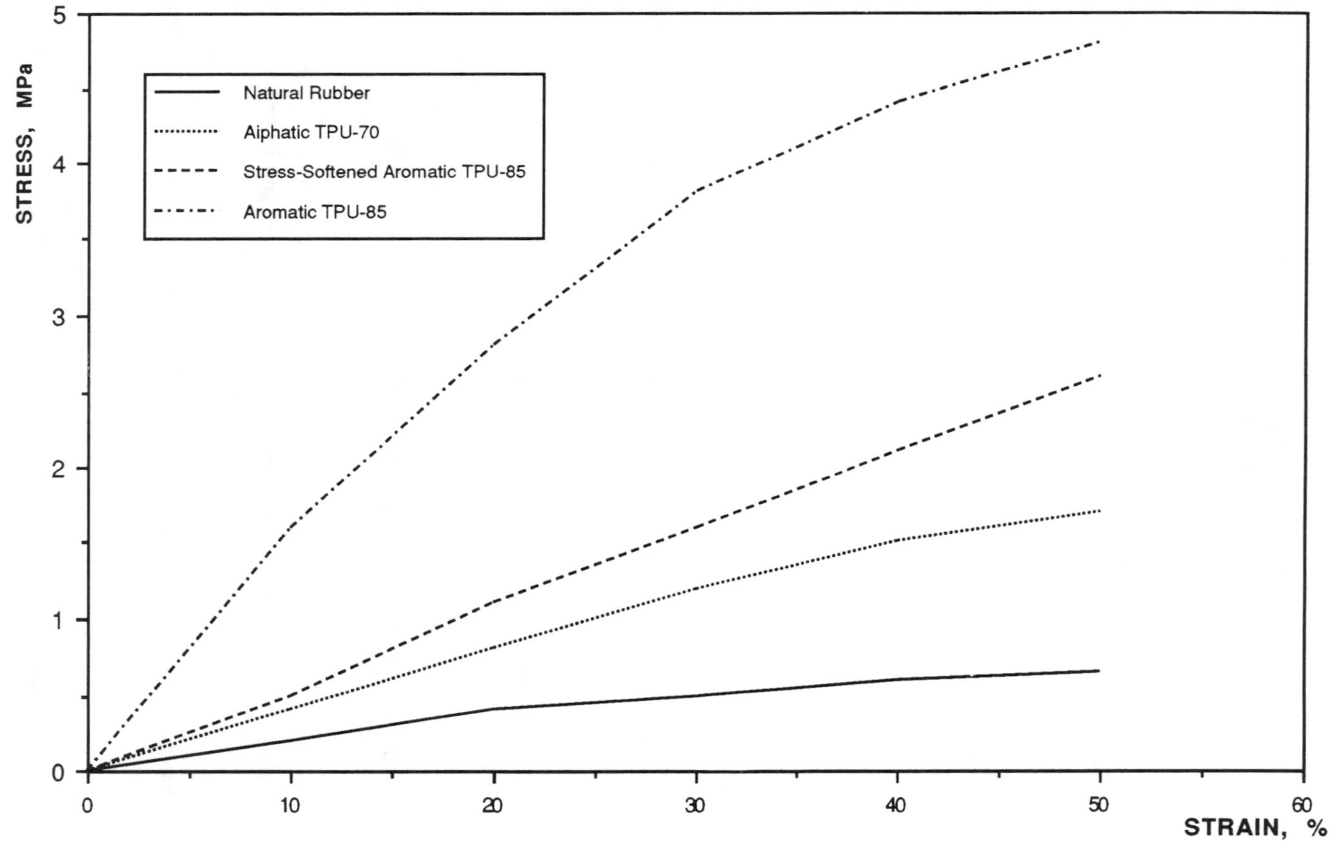
STRESS, MPa
5
4
3
2
1
0
Natural Rubber
Aiphatic TPU-70
Stress-Softened Aromatic TPU-85
Aromatic TPU-85
0
10
20
30
40
50
60
STRAIN, %

TABLE 4. Tensile and Tear Properties of Biomedical Polyether Thermoplastic Polyurethanes (TPUs) (Russell DD, personal communication)

TPU	Tensile strength psi (MPa)	Elongation at break (%)	Stress at 50% strain psi (MPa)	Tear strength pli (kN/m)
Aromatic (80A)	6,500 (45)	580	600 (4.1)	400 (70)
Aliphatic (70A)	7,200 (50)	460	245 (1.7)	410 (72)
Natural rubber[a]	3,300 (23)	710	100 (0.7)	290 (51)

[a]Control.

stresses. This engineering design problem can be solved in several ways, the simplest of which is to offer a range of sizes.

NEW PRODUCTS

Industry innovators are focusing on polyurethanes, especially the polyether-based polyurethanes, for condoms. Most condoms under development are being made of these materials. Wisconsin Pharmacal is introducing a female condom of a polyether-based TPU [12] (Fig. 7). The film is made of a biomedical material, Estane (from BF Goodrich), and the inner ring is fabricated from a harder TPU. Early versions of the condom had seams, which showed that the device had been made from film by heat sealing, but recent versions are seamless, perhaps through the use of vacuum forming. The narrowest portion of the condom, below the outer ring, is 80 mm in layflat width, which is the same as the largest natural skin condoms (Fig. 7). Thus it should be equally accommodating. This female condom has been tested extensively in Europe, where it is called the "Femshield," and it is being tested in the United States and elsewhere in preparation for approval for marketing. However, the National Women's Health Network (NWHN) is challenging the approval process, contending that any device bearing the name "condom" should be proved effective against STDs through trials of appropriate duration [13]. In its petition, the NWHN is questioning the approval of a female condom of natural rubber latex. The outcome may affect the introduction of other condoms that differ significantly in design from conventional rubber condoms.

Fig. 6. Stress-strain behavior of elastomers at low extensions.

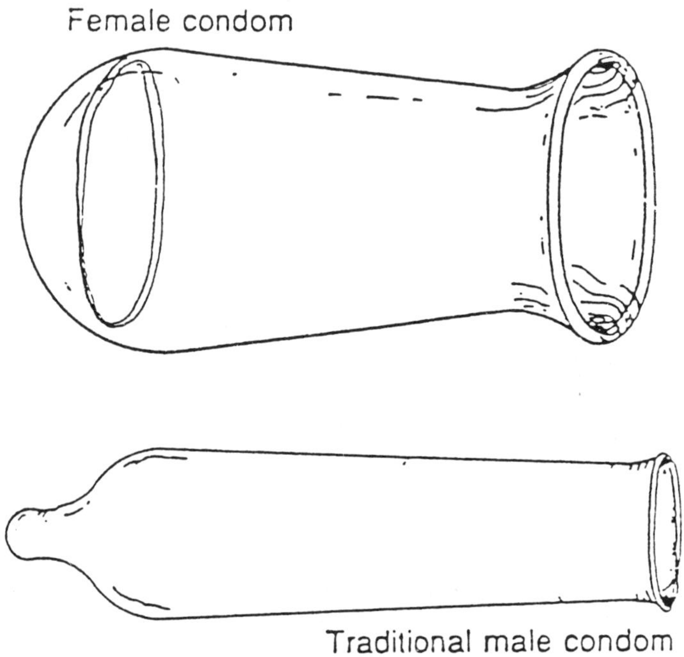

Fig. 7. Comparison of Wisconsin Pharmacal's female condom with typical male condom. (Courtesy of Margaret Pyke Centre, London.)

ACKNOWLEDGMENTS

This project was funded by Family Health International (FHI) under a Cooperative Agreement with the U.S. Agency for International Development. FHI is an international not-for-profit organization that conducts research and provides technical assistance in health, family planning, STDs, and AIDS. It is based in Research Triangle Park, North Carolina. The views expressed are solely those of the authors.

REFERENCES

1. **Quinn JJ:** Condoms: Manufacturing perspectives and use. In Zatuchni GI, Sobrero AJ, Speidel JJ, Sciarra JJ (eds): Vaginal Contraception: New Developments. Hagerstown, MD: Harper & Row, 1979.

2. **Update on Condoms—Products, Protection, Promotion. Population Reports,** Series H, No. 6. Washington, DC: George Washington University, 1982.

3. **Everett J, Glanze WD:** The Condom Book. New York: New American Library, 1987.

4. **Brackett JW:** Condom Info Guide. New York: Essential Medical Information Systems, 1988.

5. **Finch BE, Green H:** Contraception Through the Ages. Springfield, IL: Charles C. Thomas, 1963.

6. **Discussion:** Improving condoms: Problems and possibilities. In Redford MH, Duncan GW, Prager DJ: The Condom: Increasing Utilization in the United States. San Francisco: San Francisco Press, 1974.

7. **Rader CP:** Elastomeric alloy thermoplastic vulcanizates. In Walker BM, Rader, CP (eds): Handbook of Thermoplastic Elastomers, 2nd Ed. New York: Van Nostrand Reinhold, 1988.

8. **Williams JL:** Medical applications of thermoplastic elastomers. In Walker BM, Rader, CP (eds): Handbook of Thermoplastic Elastomers, 2nd Ed. New York: Van Nostrand Reinhold, 1988.

9. **Voeller B, Coulson AH, Bernstein GS, Nakamura RM:** Mineral oil lubricants cause rapid deterioration of latex condoms. Contraception 39:95, 1989.

10. **Lelah MD, Cooper SL:** Polyurethanes in Medicine. Boca Raton, FL: CRC Press, 1986.

11. **Halper WM, Holden G:** Styrenic thermoplastic elastomers. In Walker BM, Rader CP (eds): Handbook of Thermoplastic Elastomers, 2nd Ed. New York: Van Nostrand Reinhold, 1988.

12. **Thermoplastics elastomers.** Mod Plastics 66 (1):98, 1989.

13. **NWHN Petitions FDA to halt sale of the micro condom.** Medical Devices Rep, Vol 17, No. 51, 1988.

DISCUSSION

DR. PHANUPHAK: Besides the physical specifications or physical testing of the condoms, do we know anything about acceptability by clients or by those who tested the condoms? For example, would the color or texture of the condom make a difference in terms of more people using it? We find that the acceptance of condoms depends a lot on the psychology of the one who uses it. Also, ethnic groups may have different reasons for not using condoms. For example, people in the Middle East were reluctant to use condoms.

We think about the males who will refuse to use them, but at the same time women are also sometimes reluctant to use them. For example, consider that when a man uses a condom, he will reach climax much slower than when not using a condom. So, the prostitute may favor not using condoms because she can then serve more clients. Also, some women complain that it hurts when men use condoms. Do we, then, know anything about the psychological and physical acceptance of condoms?

DR. TANQUARY: You have asked an excellent question. Not nearly enough is known. When I entered this field a brief time ago, I was expecting to find answers easily to many of these kinds of questions, but I find that very little work has been done in trying to assess what I would call consumer preference for various products.

We know that natural skin condoms, for example, appeal much more to men than to women. Women dislike the product because it is messy and smells bad, but men consider it comfortable. Also, some women prefer the rubber condom because they enjoy the sensation. So there are very definite differences and preferences. I do not think we are doing enough to enhance the sexual pleasure associated with condoms. If we could, we would make condoms addictive.

MR. SPIELER: In the table comparing cost and quality, you showed latex having the highest cost and the poorest quality. I can understand highest cost if you are looking at technologies that are less expensive than latex, but do you also think latex is the lowest quality, particularly in light of what Dr. Shelton said about how remarkable it is that latex condoms work so well, given all the adversities of clinical trials, etc.?

DR. TANQUARY: Yes, I think it is remarkable that they work so well. We have a project at Family Health International (FHI) assessing the quality of condoms in developing countries. We have looked extensively at natural rubber condoms, and I think they are excellent products overall. The problems come, as you know, in the peculiar circumstances of condom storage in the developing countries, where they are sometimes stored in hot conditions for several years. So, what we are really looking for in new materials is stability. When I talk about quality, I am really talking about a lot of things, but one important criterion, as far as I am concerned, is stability. The condom has to be stable under long-term storage.

MR. SPIELER: So the baseline for your table comparing cost and quality of different materials starts with the assumption that you want to develop a product of higher quality and lower cost than latex?

DR. TANQUARY: Yes. However, there is a reverse side to that coin, which we all should recognize. If we develop synthetic materials that last for years and years, that are very stable in storage, that are not attacked by ozone, sunlight, and so on, how are we going to get rid of them? We are very worried about that. Dr. Potts tells me that we have a more important problem to worry about, forget about the environmental contamination. I agree, but I still worry about billions of condoms that might be piled to the ceiling.

These new condoms also are heavier than water and do not readily float. So, we also have a problem of contaminating lakes and streams.

DR. RIETMEIJER: Some in vitro studies claimed to have evaluated synthetic membrane or synthetic skin condoms. Do you have any idea what these products might be?

DR. TANQUARY: In terms of a synthetic skin, it is very possible that they are referring to a hydrogel. I am not sure. I know that one material that has received very extensive examination is the Biomer material of Johnson & Johnson that has been made into condoms. Whether it is that to which they are referring I do not know.

DR. WILLIAMSON: I just wanted to respond to the question on acceptability. I agree that we need to know more about acceptability, and there is some research going on in that area. We at FHI have been doing research on the acceptability of spermicidally lubricated condoms. We did a study last year in five countries and found that condom users liked the spermicidally lubricated condoms. This was quite encouraging. Now we are doing a test of stronger latex condoms to see whether some people are willing to trade off a slightly thicker condom for greater strength, and that study is going to be done in three countries.

The point about acceptability is that a number of delivery systems and social marketing projects have shown that you can increase acceptability of condoms by offering a great variety in color and size, and so forth, with a good delivery system and good advertising.

Japan has had excellent success in packaging condoms and delivering good products with very widespread household distribution. So I think even the condoms we have could be delivered much, much better.

DR. ROSENFIELD: You mentioned the linen condoms of the Middle Ages. I have visions of a condom tailor. I wonder whether they got involved with measuring and such things? This leads me to a question.

At one point, in Thailand, Meachi's sister was a columnist, and she wrote a series of rather scathing articles against the U.S. Agency for International Development about the condoms being distributed, which the Thais were having to tie on with a string because they were too large. Do we decide the right sizes of condoms for distribution? Is one condom the right size for all people in mass distribution programs, or should there be further research in this area?

DR. TANQUARY: Well, there definitely are differences in sizes. The size that is used most frequently in Asia is 49 millimeters rather than 52, and there have been some complaints in North America,

Europe, and Africa about 52 millimeters being too small. There is one approach to finding the appropriate size, and that is a social marketer's task. Give several sizes to the salesmen and see which products they can sell. This is a very direct approach. However, it does not answer your question. I do not know what the sizing should be, but I think we should have a greater variety of sizes than we have now.

29

In Vitro Testing of Condoms for Prevention of HIV Infection: A Review

Cornelis A.M. Rietmeijer and
Franklyn N. Judson

Condoms increasingly are viewed as an important means of preventing spread of the human immunodeficiency virus (HIV). Consequently, use of condoms has been recommended in the report by the Surgeon General of the United States [1] on the acquired immune deficiency syndrome (AIDS) and by many other public health authorities worldwide. Based on physical properties alone, undamaged latex condoms should provide an effective barrier against all known sexually transmissible agents, including HIV. Quality control measures by the condom manufacturer, as recommended by the American Society for Testing Materials Standard D3492-83 for latex condoms and the International Organization for Standardization, include tests for electric current conductivity, water leakage, and air burst, which detect holes many times smaller than the 120 nm size of an HIV particle. These measures should result in an acceptable quality level (AQL) for condoms.

The U.S. Food and Drug Administration (FDA) requires failure rate due to water leakage to be less than four condoms per 1,000 in any given batch [2]. To evaluate quality control by condom manufacturers, repackagers, and importers, the FDA expanded its testing program early in 1987. In the water-leak test used in this program, a condom is filled with 300 ml of water and checked for leaks. Of 165 different U.S. manufactured batches, 38,000 condoms were tested by February, 1988. Nineteen batches (12%) had leakage rates exceeding four per 1,000. In contrast, the failure rate of 265 imported batches

Heterosexual Transmission of AIDS, pages 355–363

was 21%. So far, this program has resulted in 16 condom recalls by four domestic manufacturers, and automatic detention of condom shipments from seven foreign manufacturers who failed the AQL more than once [2].

Recently, Nakamura and coauthors [3] tested 31 brands of locally purchased condoms according to several standard in vitro procedures, including measurement of dimensions, water leakage, tensile strength, ultimate elongation, air burst test (volume and pressure at burst), package integrity, and pinhole electrical conductivity. A total test score was calculated for each condom on a scale of 0 to 100. Eight brands scored higher than 80, 22 brands scored between 50 and 79, and one brand scored a low 21. Although the water leakage test appeared to be the most discriminating, it was concluded that no single parameter evaluated condoms adequately.

Given the incurable and deadly nature of HIV infection, the significant slippage and breakage rates of condoms (which probably are highest in anorectal intercourse), and the difficulty of establishing infection rates in open populations, these results underscore the need for in vitro testing models that more closely approximate anorectal and vaginal intercourse. Both the permeability of condoms to HIV and the efficacy of back-up virucidal chemicals in case of condom breakage should be evaluated. In vitro models have been developed to test the impermeability of condoms to various sexually transmitted pathogens including *Neisseria gonorrhoeae* [4], *Chlamydia trachomatis* [5], herpes simplex virus type 2 [4–6], cytomegalovirus [7], and hepatitis B virus [8]. This review focuses on recent studies of in vitro models used to evaluate the permeability of condoms to HIV.

MATERIALS AND METHODS

Conant and coauthors [9], Van de Perre and coauthors [10], and Scesney and coauthors [11] used syringe models similar to the one originally described by Conant and coauthors [6]. A syringe plunger was placed inside a condom, to which an HIV-containing suspension was added. The condom-fitted plunger then was inserted into the syringe barrel and brought into contact with HIV-negative culture medium through the tip of the syringe during a series of vigorous aspiration and expulsion cycles.

This model was further modified by Blair and Drew [12] after Katznelson et al. [7]. The tip was removed from 30 ml syringes and the outer surface smoothed. A condom containing HIV suspension was stretched over the outer surface, and a second condom containing HIV-negative medium was unrolled over the first condom. Then the syringe was inserted into a coated centrifuge holder and plunged up and down 50 times. A similar model was used by Voeller et al. [13].

Rietmeijer and coauthors [14] used a different model, originally described by Judson and coauthors [5]. Each condom was mounted on a hollow dildo and inserted into a tight-fitting glass cylinder. HIV suspension and HIV-free medium were placed on opposite sides of the condom. Then the dildo was pumped up and down 100 times and otherwise agitated in the cyclinder for 5 min. Subsequently, samples from cylinder and condom tip were taken for HIV culture before and after deliberate condom rupture.

Virologic Methods

At a concentration of at least 0.5×10^6 infectious HIV particles per milliliter, titers of HIV suspensions used in all studies were considerably higher than HIV concentrations likely to be found in infected blood, semen, or vaginal fluid. Four studies did not identify the composition of the HIV suspension. In one study [14], both cell-associated and cell-free HIV were used; in another [13] study, the suspension contained cell-free HIV only.

The presence of HIV in previous HIV-negative media was determined by direct antigen detection in one study [12]. In the other five studies, samples were cocultured with stimulated human peripheral mononuclear cells, H9 cells, or other HIV-permissive cell lines and assayed for reverse transcriptase, HIV antigen, and/or viral RNA (Table 1).

RESULTS

Conant et al. [9] tested three latex condoms ('Trojan ENZ,' both lubricated and unlubricated, and 'Ramses Extra' with additional unspecified spermicide), one natural membrane condom ('Fourex'), and one synthetic membrane condom ('Skinless Skin'). None of the condoms leaked HIV. This study found similar results for high concentrations of mouse retrovirus. Van de Perre et al. [10] tested two each of six different condoms, five of which were latex condoms: three lubricated without spermicide ('Durex Coral,' Durex, Belgium; 'Ortho Shields,' Cilaq, Belgium; 'Prime,' Ansell Inc., U.S.), one with additional spermicide ('KLU,' Ansell Inc., U.S.), and one recommended for male homosexual use ('Man-To-Man,' Johnson Enterprises, U.S.). In addition, a natural membrane condom ('Kling-Tite Naturalamb,' Young Rubber Corporation, U.S.) was also tested. All

TABLE 1. In Vitro Studies of Condoms as Physical and Chemical Barriers Against the Human Immunodeficiency Virus (HIV)

Study reference	Model	HIV detection	Condom type	Number of brands	Number of replicates	Back-up viru-cidal	Effective
Conant et al. [9]	Syringe	RT-essay	Latex antigen	3	1	+	Yes
			Membrane (natural)	1	1	−	Yes
			Membrane (synthetic)	1	1	−	Yes
Van de Perre et al. [10]	Syringe	RT-essay	Latex antigen	4	2	−	Yes
			Latex	1	2	+	Yes
			Membrane (natural)	1	2	−	No
Scesney et al. [11]	Syringe	RT-essay	Latex RNA-blot	1	?	−	Yes
			Latex	1	12	N-9[a]	66%
Rietmeijer et al. [14]	Dildo	RT-essay	Latex	1	10	−	Yes
			Latex	1	20	N-9	Yes
Voeller et al. [13]	Piston	RT-essay	Latex antigen	8	10	−	Yes
			Latex	3	10	−	90%
			Latex	1	25	+	76%
			Membrane (natural)	1	20	−	Yes
Blair and Drew [12]	Syringe	Antigen	Latex	5	3	−	Yes
			Membrane (natural)	1	12	−	Yes
			Membrane (synthetic)	1	12	−	Yes

[a]N-9, nonoxynol-9.

latex condoms were impermeable to HIV, but the natural membrane condom showed significant passage of the virus. In addition, HIV inactivation of more than 50% occurred after incubation of HIV for 10 min in two of the condoms, whereas complete inactivation followed in three condoms after 1 hr, suggesting that HIV may be inactivated by chemical compounds other than spermicides in condoms.

Rietmeijer and coauthors [14] tested 20 latex condoms containing N-9 ('Lifestyles Extra,' Ansell, U.S.) and 10 similar condoms without

N-9 ('DUO,' Ansell, U.S.). No condom without N-9 leaked HIV in outside medium after intercourse was simulated. After deliberate rupture of the condom, HIV could be detected outside seven condoms without N-9. In none of 20 condoms containing N-9 could HIV be detected in outside medium after deliberate rupture. These condoms contained 0.45 ml of 6.6% (vol/vol) N-9 ointment in the condom tip and 0.45 ml of 6.6% (vol/vol) N-9 in silicone lubricant evenly distributed over the inside and outside condom surfaces, yielding an N-9 concentration of 0.25% in the outside medium after rupture.

Comparable results with similar condoms were obtained by Scesney, Gantz, and Sullivan [11]. Again, no leakage occurred from condoms without N-9, whereas condoms containing N-9 inactivated HIV after condom rupture in eight of 12 condoms tested. Although N-9 killed HIV at concentrations exceeding 0.005% in a separate experiment, these concentrations may not have been reached in their condom investigations. Blair and Drew [12] found no evidence of HIV leakage from three each of five different types of latex condoms, nor from 12 replicates of a natural membrane condom and 12 replicates of a synthetic membrane condom (brands not specified). However, significant inactivation of HIV was noted inside the condoms, resulting in a decrease of HIV antigen concentration in latex condoms greater than 75% after 30 min of exposure and complete inactivation in both types of skin condoms. Preliminary results from a separate study by these investigators suggested that the propylene glycol- and paraben-containing lubricant present in these skin condoms denatures at least 75% to 90% of HIV after 30 min.

Of 31 unspecified latex condom brands tested and ranked by Nakamura and associates [3] (see above), ten each from the eight highest rated brands and five lowest were compared for HIV leakage by Voeller et al. [13]. The highest rated brands did not leak, but in three of the five lowest-ranked brands leakage occurred in one of the ten replicates. In the lowest rated brand, leakage was visible from 10 of 25 replicates. However, the spermicide contained in this condom inactivated the high HIV titre in five of the ten replicates and reduced activity in the other five. Oil-based lubricants, particularly those containing mineral oil, caused visible blistering of some brands within 5 min. Water-based lubricants did not affect the condom latex.

DISCUSSION

The results of these studies indicate that, even when subjected to unrealistic physiological forces, the great majority of latex condoms tested so far are impermeable to HIV. Moreover, condoms containing N-9 may inactivate HIV when the condoms break or slip, given sufficient N-9 concentrations. However, these encouraging results should not be overinterpreted. First, these studies used small samples and are no substitute for on-line quality control, which is the responsibility of the industry and the FDA. Second, the experiments required extensive manipulation in an unsterile environment that, when combined with the potential toxicity of materials used in model components, could have inhibited HIV. Indeed, several studies noted such inhibition. This factor is unlikely to have biased the overall outcome significantly for latex condoms, but the permeability results for membrane condoms probably were influenced by the toxicity of the lubricant to HIV. In vivo, the undefined inhibition of HIV caused by condom components or lubricants could even provide an additional measure of protection.

Although the number of natural membrane condoms tested in these studies was too small to allow conclusions to be drawn, other investigations suggest that the pores in these condoms allow passage to small viral particles, such as a 22 nm hepatitis B virus surface antigen [8], or the bacterial virus OX174 [13,15], but not to larger viruses, such as 180 to 200 nm herpes simplex virus [6]. This difference offers a plausible explanation for the conflicting results regarding HIV, which at 80 to 120 nm is of intermediate size. It would appear that natural condoms should not be relied on to prevent HIV or other sexually transmitted infections.

Although never firmly established, a condom failure rate in vivo of 10% is often cited [16]. In a small field study, an in vivo failure rate of 7% was found [17]. Even if the majority of latex condoms do not meet the AQL of fewer than four condom failures per 1,000, defective manufacturing is unlikely to be the major cause of overall condom failure. An additional cause may be inadequate condom storage and handling, during which condoms may be exposed to known harmful conditions, such as ultraviolet light [17], high temperatures and humidity [17], ozone [18], oil-based lubricants [13], and other possibly corrosive substances. However, many researchers believe that most condom failures in vivo are caused by improper use rather than by product defects [16]. Therefore, the most important way to improve condom effectiveness is to inform the public in detail about how to use condoms.

The addition of virucidal substances to condoms as a back-up measure for rupture may be another way to improve the effectiveness of condoms as barriers against HIV infection. In three studies reviewed here [11,13,14], N-9 in condoms was shown to kill HIV after deliberate condom rupture when the concentration exceeded 0.25%.

However, it is not clear whether condom rupture in vivo results in adequate concentration of N-9 in the vaginal vault or rectum. An additional concern is that these virucidal substances probably will not affect intracellular virus, so that an HIV filled "Trojan horse" may still cause infection after the antiviral agent has dissipated [19].

CONCLUSIONS

Condoms even in combination with N-9 probably do not provide absolute protection against HIV transmission. The best advice for persons with HIV infection is still to abstain from vaginal or anorectal intercourse, and for those at risk for HIV infection to have a mutually monogamous relationship with a known HIV-negative partner. For those who do not practice sexual abstinence or monogamy, the proper use of latex condoms in combination with N-9 or with another latex-compatible, HIV-neutralizing agent that may become available is highly recommended.

REFERENCES

1. **Koop CE:** Surgeon General's report on acquired immunodeficiency syndrome. JAMA 256:2784–2789, 1986.

2. Condoms for prevention of sexually transmitted diseases, Leads from the MMWR. JAMA 259:1925–1927, 1988.

3. **Nakamura NM, Coulson AH, Voeller B, et al.:** In vitro condom testing. Abstract 6510: IV International Conference on AIDS, Stockholm, June, 1988.

4. **Smith L, Oleske J, Cooper R, et al.:** Efficacy of condoms as barriers to HSV-2 and gonorrhea: An in vitro model. Abstract 077: First Sexually Transmitted Diseases World Congress. San Juan, Puerto Rico, Congress of the Latin American Union Against Veneral Diseases, 1981, p 29.

5. **Judson FN, Bodin GF, Levin MJ, Ehret JM, Master HB:** In vitro tests demonstrate condoms provide an effective barrier against *Chlamydia trachomatis* and herpes simplex virus. Abstract 176: Fifth International Meeting of the International Society for Sexually Transmitted Diseases Research, Seattle, 1983, p 208.

6. **Conant MA, Spicer DW, Smith CD:** Herpes simplex virus transmission: Condom studies. Sex Transmitted Dis 11:94–95, 1984.

7. **Katznelson S, Drew WL, Mintz L:** Efficacy of the condom as a barrier to the transmission of cytomegalovirus. J Infect Dis 150:155–157, 1984.

8. **Minuk GY, Bohme CE, Bowen TJ:** Condoms and hepatitis B virus infection. Ann Intern Med 104:584, 1986.

9. **Conant MC, Hardy D, Sernatinger J, Spicer D, Levy JA:** Condoms prevent transmission of AIDS-associated retrovirus. JAMA 255:1706, 1986.

10. **Van de Perre P, Jacobs D, Sprecher-Goldberger S:** The latex condom, an efficient barrier against sexual transmission of AIDS-related viruses. J AIDS 1:49–52, 1987.

11. **Scesney SM, Gantz NM, Sullivan JL:** Impermeability of condoms to HIV and inactivation of HIV by the spermicide nonoxynol-9. Abstract WP171: III International Conference on AIDS, Washington, DC, 1987, p 138.

12. **Blair M, Drew WL:** Condom model for evaluating HIV transmission. Abstract 6512: IV International Conference on AIDS, Stockholm, June, 1988.

13. **Voeller B, Hicks D, Coulson AH, et al.:** Testing HIV leakage through condoms. Abstract 6508: IV International Conference on AIDS, Stockholm, June, 1988.

14. **Rietmeijer CAM, Krebs JW, Feorino PM, Judson FN:** Condoms as physical and chemical barriers against human immunodeficiency virus. JAMA 259:1851–1853, 1988.

15. **Lytle CD, Vohra S, Carney PG, Cyr WH:** Natural membrane condom leakage using viral probes. Abstract 6511: IV International Conference on AIDS, Stockholm, June, 1988.

16. **Goldsmith M:** Sex in the age of AIDS calls for common sense and "condom sense." JAMA 257:2261–2266, 1987.

17. **Free MJ, Hutchings J, Kubis S:** An assessment of burst strength distribution data from monitoring quality of condom stocks in developing countries. Contraception 33:285–299, 1986.

18. **Baker RF, Sherwin RP, Bernstein GS, Nakamura RM:** Precautions when lightning strikes during the monsoon: The effect of ozone on condoms. JAMA 260:1404–1405, 1988.

19. **Levy JA:** The transmission of AIDS: The case of the infected cell. JAMA 269:3037–3038, 1988.

DISCUSSION

Dr. VOELLER: In the Van de Perre study, the authors looked at only two natural skin condoms. They found leakage in one and not in the other. The one that leaked, however, was peculiar in that they found complete inactivation of the virus within the condom but found virus on the outside, which raises the question of what on earth they were seeing.

This is the sole example, I think, of leakage of HIV, in contrast to hepatitis B, through skin condoms. In our studies, in which we looked at a great many more natural skin condoms, and in the studies of Larry Drew and his group in San Francisco, and in some FDA-simulated studies, natural skin condoms seemed to be really rather effective, if one ignores the hepatitis B problem. With respect to HIV, I think skin condoms may have gotten something of a bad rap.

DR. RIETMEIJER: I think that is a good point. The way that I look at this is that the pores, if they exist in natural condoms, may be in the size range of 100 nm, so that would explain the conflicting results with HIV. It has been shown that they permit the passage of smaller viral particles; for example, the hepatitis B-associated antigen. On the other hand, larger viruses, such as herpes simplex virus, have been shown not to go through these types of condoms, so I think maybe it is the pore size that determines whether the HIV virus passes through.

DR. LEFTWICK: I would like to expand on what Dr. Voeller has just said. We found that many of the actual in vitro models are not suitable for use with skin condoms. They are fine for latex but not for skin. In fact, the actual pumping up and down does produce minute holes, and that may sometimes explain why we find these different results in the literature. Continuing from that, we have also done some studies looking at nonbiologic particles to see how they go through condoms, and, certainly, particles the size of the HIV virus do not pass through natural skins.

DR. RIETMEIJER: Let me comment on the first point that you made. Actually, our model was designed to simulate anal intercourse perhaps more than vaginal intercourse. I think that condoms are put under stress when they are used, and so if little pores might be caused by that, I think we have another reason not to use the membrane (skin) condoms.

DR. LEFTWICK: Is hard surface to hard surface contact the cause of it?

DR. RIETMEIJER: That is correct. It is hard to get a very good model, that I would concede.

DR. FOLDESY: I would like to ask a question of the representatives of the condom manufacturers. My understanding is that skin condoms are almost uniquely a U.S. phenomenon. Second, approximately what percentage of condoms sold are skin condoms?

DR. RIETMEIJER: I do not know.

Dr. STAAB: I am from Shmid Laboratories, and I just looked over at Bill Vander Haar from Carter-Wallace, another manufacturer, and we are in agreement. It is a couple of percent; it is not 20%.

30

Relevance of Condom Testing

Bruce Voeller

In an act of vaginal or anal coitus, use of virtually any type of condom as a barrier against sexually transmitted diseases (STDs) or impregnation reduces the associated risk. Too often, however, promoters of condom use are unaware that different brands, or even production lots, of condoms vary in their strength and related characteristics, including their susceptibility to degradation by lubricants and to deterioration induced by air pollutants, ultraviolet radiation, and other storage variables.

Little but anecdotal data has been published about the clinical efficacy of condoms against any virus, including the human immunodeficiency virus (HIV). HIV efficacy trials are urgently needed, inasmuch as we know that condoms are useful HIV barriers but do not know how effective. Unfortunately, adequate clinical trials for HIV protection may be hazardous to subjects, are extremely costly, and are very time-consuming. Unwittingly to select an inferior or a mediocre condom, then conduct an otherwise model clinical efficacy trial and draw world-watched conclusions about the level of HIV protection afforded by condoms, would be unfortunate.

In our zeal to stop AIDS, we must not lose sight of another important distinction. Although a mediocre brand of condom might be good enough to reduce the national rate of sexual spread of HIV substantially, and lead to an important public health advance, the brand might still leave considerable risk for individuals using it during intercourse. Wide public distribution, for instance, of an 80% (or even a 50%) effective condom might bring about an important reduction in the public burden of AIDS. Such a level of efficacy would

Heterosexual Transmission of AIDS, pages 365–378

be unacceptable to most of us, however, in our own lives or in the lives of individuals we counsel.

For these reasons, we would like to know how good various brands of condoms are in comparison to one another and on some absolute scale. Testing condoms should allow us to make these comparisons and evaluations and to suggest manufacturing and design improvements. These suggestions might even include abandoning latex condoms and moving toward the ultimate condom, multilayered films of synthetic materials, resistant to oil-based lubricants and aging, slippery on the outside and adhesive inside, biodegradable, burst-proof, and having a high coefficient of heat transfer, which has been linked to heightened sensation.

Ideally, knowledge of the strength and other properties of condoms, as measured in physical tests, should allow prediction of the failure rates of condoms (method failure) in providing contraceptive and STD protection, at least in the hands of highly motivated and knowledgeable users. Rates should be predictable for breakage of condoms during use and for leakage of HIV through the condom wall during the stresses of anal or vaginal coitus. These goals are probably realizable eventually. However, several troubling assumptions undermine faith that an optimal condom can be designed and produced at the present time, during the AIDS crisis. These assumptions are that

1. one or more physical tests of condoms exist that correlate with coital breakage or leakage;
2. the physical and frictional stresses to which condoms are subjected during coitus are known, and can be simulated in the laboratory and used to establish how many "safety nets," or orders of magnitude of protection, users need from a condom;
3. the form and quantity of the infectious units are known with respect to whether they are free HIV, sperm-bound virus, or cell-enclosed virus, or some combination thereof; and
4. latex condoms are basically latex condoms; that is, data from one brand are generally applicable to other brands.

Virtually none of these assumptions, nor their numerous subsets, is accurate. This lack of accuracy is true even for clinical surveys of condom breakage and of failure during coitus, the yardsticks by which the significance of testing must be measured. With the exception of the Wigersma and Oud [1] exploration of breakage rates of several brands of condoms used by 17 couples during anal intercourse, a few conference abstracts, the Richters et al. study of breakage by Australian prostitutes [2], and that of Free and Hutchings (see Chapter 31, this volume), virtually no data have been published on the incidence of breakage during vaginal or anal coitus, the location of breaks, whether they were "blow-out" breaks or longitudinal tears, whether sexual lubricants were used (and which ones), what brands were used, how old the condoms were and how they had been stored, when during intercourse breakage occurred, or what act was engaged in at breakage. Almost no published information bears on these issues, never mind weighing their relationship to the various physical tests for condom strength.

As was extensively explored at the Kinsey Institute's 1987 Conference on Sexuality and AIDS [3], many of the scientific aspects of human sexuality critically needed to cope with the AIDS crisis are unknown or ill established. Because of AIDS, some scientists have come to realize how little sound information exists about the range and incidence of various sexual practices in the United States. Fewer appreciate yet how little knowledge we have about sexual physiology or about anatomical variability relevant to AIDS. Alfred Kinsey collected well over 1,000,000 specimens of the esoteric group called gall wasps and recorded in minute detail the size of their diverse appendages, yet, for the somewhat more familiar and accessible species *homo sapiens,* we have almost no frequency distribution data for penis length and girth—data of some relevance to condom breakage.

In short, condom testing relevant to predicting device efficacy is in its infancy, albeit a promising infancy. The discussion that follows reviews some of what we know, and need to learn, to make condom testing relevant to controlling unwanted pregnancy and the spread of STDs.

COMPARISON OF BRANDS OF LATEX CONDOMS

Only a few studies have compared brands of condoms to determine if one differs from another. Each study has reported important distinctions in the strength and other characteristics of various brands sold to the public. A decade ago, the Consumers Union ranked U.S. brands after testing their physical differences [4]. More recently, because of the AIDS crisis, the College of Health in London conducted the British government's survey of three dozen brands marketed in the United Kingdom [5]. Brands varied widely in strength, five brands actually failing the British standards. Similar results were found in a recent study funded by the Australian Consumers' Association [6]. Over the past 2 years, the U.S. Food and Drug Administration has repeatedly mandated or negotiated recall of entire production lots of condoms from the four U.S. manufacturers as well as impounding lots of imported brands [7].

In an NIH-funded study, our own group [8] purchased approximately 1,000 condoms from each of 31 brands at local distributors. The condoms were tested for their physical characteristics and ranked on a 100-point scale. The test scores ranged from a high of 98.9 to 50.9, with an outlier at 21.3. Eight brands had a score of 80 or above, and excluding the outlier, 22 brands had scores between 50 and 79 [8]. Two additional lots, each comprising 1,000 condoms from each of the top eight of 31 brands, have now been tested, and the new data are being compared with the results reported above.

The results of the NIH study and of a new Consumers Union study of three dozen brands of condoms are being prepared for publication in 1989. The brands tested in the two studies overlap 60%. Results from the two studies will be compared in detail. The questions naturally arise, what are the physical tests the several research groups employed? what were the viral leakage tests? and what is the significance of these various tests for condom use during actual coitus?

PHYSICAL TESTS OF CONDOMS

All the comparative studies cited above employed one or more of the standard U.S. (ASTM) and international (ISO) procedures for testing latex condoms [9]. These tests were originally designed as quality control measures by the manufacturers of the products. The key tests in these protocols are used to detect defects or deficiencies in the physical characteristics of large production lots (batches) of condoms. Although the condom characteristics tested may also include various gauges such as shelf life (measured after artificially induced aging) and the integrity of the condom's packaging, the two principal classes of properties monitored are

1. the physical strength of the condoms, to ensure that a lot meets or exceeds standards agreed upon by the industry (and more recently by some regulatory agencies),
2. the absence of holes—whether the condoms contain pores or imperfections that might leak sperm (in the case of contraception) or STD agents, including HIV.

The number of condoms sampled for any lot is determined by the size of the lot, according to the Military Standard-105D (MIL-STD-

105D. Sampling Procedures and Tables for Inspection by Attributes) [10]. The tables in the MIL-STD-105D are the basis for almost all the sampling protocols for quality control used by industry in general. Lots of condoms exhibiting more than a set percent of failures in the various ASTM tests may not be sold.

The chief test of physical strength in the ASTM protocol is the Tensile and Elongation Test (T&E), which measures the breakage tension and the percent increase in length of a section cut from the test condoms. Its counterpart test in the ISO protocol is the Air Burst Test, which measures the burst volume and the burst pressure of a condom inflated at a standard rate.

To measure leakage through the condom wall, condoms are loaded with water and examined for leaks. In addition, they are usually tested electronically for holes. When the condom is loaded with a standard volume of water, which stretches it to about 400% its initial size, this test is also a physical strength test.

Clearly these diverse tests are based on fundamental characteristics necessary for an effective condom. Intuition tells us the tests should, thus, be reasonable predictors of breakage and leakage (i.e., condom deficiencies) during sexual intercourse. As a first approximation, this is true. However, these tests were developed only as reasonable quality control measures, for which they are quite stringent, and they may not be as directly relevant to actual coitus as might seem initially true. One of several possible examples may make this more clear. From interviewing of "habitual condom breakers," it was found that most breakage appeared to occur in the tipmost 25–35% of the condom, rarely further back [11]. Unpublished industry data agree with this localization [12]. In the ASTM's T&E strength test, the test sample is cut not from this principal breakage area but further back (80 mm from the open end). Moreover, the test sections (rubber bands) are transections of the condom, not longitudinal ones. Differences in longitudinal and transectional strength and of different regions of the condom could result during the dipping process by which condoms are produced.

The number of different ASTM or ISO tests performed has varied from study to study. Because of the vast extent of FDA monitoring, their routine work is limited to one test, the water leak test. The other groups have used a combination of three to five tests.

In our own comparison of 31 brands of latex condoms, all of the usual ASTM and ISO tests were conducted [8]. A particular brand could rank high in one test but low in another. Of the individual ASTM and ISO tests, the water leak test appeared to be the most discriminating, but examples of brands with good water leak test results and poor tensile strength and other poor test results were also found. We concluded that the use of any single parameter from the list of standard tests could not be used to evaluate condoms [8].

Even separating out water leak (pin hole) tests from the other measures of physical strength, lack of concordance among tests is seen within some brands. This discordance may arise in part from applying a set standard with narrow permissible thickness tolerances to condoms ranging more widely in thickness. In response to public concern about HIV transmission and condom strength, several manufacturers have produced thicker brands. Other much thinner brands are also now being marketed. They were developed to overcome users' dissatisfaction with the reduced coital sensitivity attributed to the usual condoms.

Each new class of condoms exhibits substantially different results when its tensile strength (T) values are compared with its elongation (E) values—so too when air burst values for pressure (P) and volume (V) are compared. Thin condoms, for example, tend to inflate to impressive volumes, but burst at low pressures. These P and V properties tend to be reversed with thicker-than-usual condoms (depending also on manufacturing formulation).

Roger Stube at the Consumers Union has proposed a possible method to unify test comparisons and overcome problems due to such brand differences as thickness. He points out that the mathematical product of pressure and volume is work. Thus the work required to attain burst of the condom takes both P and V values into account and can be readily calculated. A similar argument using Young's modulus, the mass (weight) of a condom, and a suitable coefficient pertains to bringing concordance to T&E values in the ASTM test. Evaluation of these proposed solutions is now being made at the Consumers Union and by our group.

CONDOM LEAKAGE OF HIV

In the absence of adequate clinical evaluation of the HIV barrier efficacy of condoms, laboratory evaluation of HIV leakage through condoms assumes considerable importance. Because this virus is vastly smaller and more life-threatening than the cellular agents causing pregnancy and STDs such as gonorrhea and syphilis, the standards for assessing leakage must be more stringent and more carefully considered than has been tolerated for the cellular agents, for which clinical efficacy has been fairly well evaluated [13].

HIV leakage should be tested under conditions that subject condoms to tough, but reasonable, demands. These conditions include the use of high virus titers, frictional and stretching forces (and durations) comparable to vigorous coitus, assay methods of enough sensitivity to detect leaked HIV, and leakage conditions free from potential false-positive or false-negative values. As will become apparent, we do not always have sound sexual and physiological data to know whether we are conducting tests within realistic physiological conditions. It seems better to err on the side of excessive demands on the condom than too lenient ones. If viral leakage is found in sound experiments, further study can evaluate whether the effective endpoints are relevant to protection.

Some of these test conditions are being met little by little. As was noted above, virtually any condom reduces the risk of HIV infection during coitus. As a crude first approximation of condom efficacy, Voeller and Potts [14] noted early in the AIDS crisis that condoms hold air or water, with molecular weights under 40, orders of magnitude lower than that of HIV.

Better approximations were made in two widely cited notes [15,16] on condoms' in vitro efficacy with free, cultured HIV. The studies introduced physical stressing of condoms by pistoning the virus-loaded condom within a small syringe. Each group tested several brands of condoms but did not indicate how brands were selected, nor did they test multiple replicates within brands to see if some fraction leaked.

The methodologies used began to put HIV leakage testing on the right track, but the authors, who studied a combined total of fewer than 20 individual latex condoms, somewhat overstepped the limits of their data, one group stating that their studies "conclusively indicate that retroviruses cannot pass through the condom membranes" [15].

In elegant studies of the effect of nonoxynol-9 on leakage of HIV from a single brand of condom supplied by the manufacturer, Rietmeijer et al. [17] used ten replicate control condoms, adding to the evidence that condoms can restrict dispersal of HIV in suspension.

As reviewed elsewhere in this volume, Dr. Deborah Anderson and her colleagues (Chapter 14) and Dr. Virginia Scofield and her colleagues (Chapter 12) have been evaluating whether HIV in semen exists as free virus, as HIV within T4 lymphocytes and macrophages, or as HIV bound to motile sperm. We, too, are surveying 20 HIV-seropositive men and a group of HIV-seropositive women for HIV localization in semen or vaginal secretions, respectively, as reported in this volume by Dr. Gerald Bernstein (Chapter 18). If all seminal or vaginal-secretion HIV is restricted to microscopically visible cells, the problem of condom leakage is greatly reduced compared with HIV's presence entirely or in part as free virus, which is far smaller.

Inasmuch as these issues were unresolved when we began our own HIV leakage studies, we adopted the "worst case" possibility, that the infectious unit is free HIV. If no free virus exists in sexual fluids, detection of HIV leakage in studies such as ours could be of less interest. In our research, we selected the eight highest-scoring brands of condoms from among the 31 extensively tested in the ASTM and ISO protocols, as well as the lowest scoring five brands [8]. Comparing 10 replicates per brand, no leakage of very-high-titer HIV [$TCID_{50} = 10^{-9}$)] was observed from any of the highest scoring eight brands [18], nor from 10 replicates tested by us from each of the two similarly highest-ranked brands among 3 dozen brands evaluated by the British College of Health [4,19]. However, we found leakage in four of the five lowest-scoring brands (all of U.S. manufacture) [18]. The single lowest scoring brand leaked HIV extensively, but this particular lot was visibly faulty and was probably atypical of the brand [20]. Of the other three brands that exhibited leakage, one of the 10 replicates leaked HIV for each of the brands [18]. Thus 120 condoms from among 12 brands with high test scores were leak-free, whereas (setting aside the faulty, lowest brand) three condoms of the 40 tested from the four other lowest-scoring brands leaked.

These results appear to indicate that the physical differences seen among various brands of condoms have potential as predictive indices of viral leakage through condoms. However, funding limitations restricted us to looking at only a single production lot of each brand tested and only the highest- and lowest-ranked brands. Confirmation of the initial results with additional lots is critically important. Leakage studies of the untested, intermediate-ranked brands may reveal where a cut-off point in physical scores separates leaking condoms from ones with full integrity.

SEXUAL PHYSIOLOGY AND CONDOM TESTING

If condoms are to be tested for their ability to prevent HIV transmission across the latex film, they should be subjected to stretching, physical pressures, frictional abrasion (and durations of these) similar to those during vaginal or anal intercourse. Indeed, the ability of a condom to serve as a barrier should not be tested merely under "average" conditions but under more demanding ones.

The two published notes discounting leakage of HIV from latex condoms [15,16] stressed the test condoms by loading them with a suspension of HIV, then placing them over the head of a small (12, 20 ml) syringe plunger and reciprocating it within the syringe barrel. Drew and his colleagues [21,22] developed a hand-operated piston-receptacle model more realistically approximating human sex organ dimensions. The test condom was loaded with HIV and unrolled over the dildo-piston. A second standard receptor condom containing culture medium was then unrolled over the test condom. This was further refined by Voeller and Hicks [19] and Voeller et al. [18]. Both the Drew group and our own loaded the test condom with volumes of HIV concentrate comparable to average ejaculate volumes (2–3 ml) and subjected it to 50 piston strokes within the vagina-simulating cylinder. The strokes were intended to stress the test condom as in coitus. However, inasmuch as the condom was already loaded with HIV, the effect was comparable to 50 postejaculatory strokes, an unrealistic event for most people. Moreover, each of the models is but limitedly reproducible because they are not machine-standardized. The syringe model and the piston/receptacle model are only rough, best guess approximations of actual coital stresses and conditions.

Scholarly information relevant to many of the physical attributes of sexuality needed to simulate coitus are largely unknown or ill documented. Review of the published scientific literature and numerous meetings with sex-research authorities, including Drs. Wardell Pomeroy, C.A. Tripp, and Paul Gebhard, research colleagues of the late Alfred Kinsey; Dr. June Reinisch, Director of the Kinsey Institute; and Drs. William Masters and Virginia Johnson, make clear that few data exist.

There are a few exceptions. Although the data are now nearly half a century old, Kinsey and his colleagues [23] reported that "For perhaps three-quarters of all males, orgasm is reached within two minutes after the initiation of the sexual relation, and for a not inconsiderable number of males the climax may be reached within less than a minute or even within ten or twenty seconds after coital entrance." Data for penile thrust distances, rates, and durations are scant, as are frictional resistance values during vaginal and anal intercourse. For the most part, data bearing on vaginal and rectal pressures during coitus are anecdotal or unknown, although some rectal and vaginal manometric readings linked with surgery or pregnancy exist. All these deficiencies severely limit appropriate conditions for condom testing. Little by little, however, we are piecing together some of the needed data.

By reviewing unedited pornography video "rushes," we have collected data on stroke rate (as high as 210 per minute over a 5 sec period, 150 per minute during 120 sec.), ejaculation distance (>38 inches vertically), and duration of uninterrupted coital thrusting (10.4 min).

My colleagues, Drs. Bernstein and Nakamura, at the USC Medical Center, have collected over 1,000 semen samples for artificial insemination. Volumes range as high as 13 ml and average just under 3 ml. Combining ejaculation distances with the ejaculate volumes allows calculation of the ejaculation "muzzle velocity," and thence the momentum transfer at the tip of a condom (the region of the condom most stressed during coital penetration and where most breaks are reported). These average ejaculate volumes just match the volume of the teat (3 ml) of the "tip"-type condom promoted by many AIDS groups. However, inasmuch as ~3 ml is the statistical mean ejaculate volume, it follows that about 50% of males exceed the capacity of that tip.

We have also found funding and volunteers to study the vaginal pressures operative against a condom during intercourse. This work will be conducted using life-sized dildos fitted with embedded high-quality pressure sensors connected to electronic recording devices. With these we expect to measure vaginal and rectal pressures from coital penetration through orgasm and withdrawal.

These various pieces of information are helping us to set more realistic standards for stressing condoms in HIV leakage studies and in thinking about just how many margins of strength a condom should possess in order to cope with actual coitus under quite diverse conditions.

Through funding from CONRAD, we have also obtained a prototype Simulated Coital Instrument from Fuji Latex Co. in Tokyo and are awaiting another commissioned from London International and its U.S. subsidiary, Schmid Laboratories. These machines are fully automated, eliminating the technician-generated variation in stroke pace, depth, and torque implicit in the hand-operated devices we and others have used heretofore. The instruments have a soft, life-like receptacle (vagina), which can be adjusted in size and shape. The dildo-piston, too, is made of soft plastic to life-like size. Both elements can be operated at a range of temperatures. The frictional forces between the two elements can be varied, as can the thrust rate, depth, and duration. The physical sexual data being collected will assist us in refining the simulated coital values we use to standardize our testing of condoms. This is true for further HIV leakage testing, development of less time-consuming and costly surrogate leakage tests, evaluating the relationship between physical test of condom strength and user needs, and the effects of lubricants.

OTHER FACTORS

As was noted above, there are few clinical data concerning condom breakage or failure during use. A part of the breakage that occurs may not be due to manufacturing deficiencies, condom aging, possible differences in vaginal or anal friction, or the more familiar mistakes made by users, such as puncturing the condom during unpackaging it or applying it to the penis.

Our interviews with 25 men who consistently broke latex condoms (>10% of occasions used) during postpenetration sexual intercourse indicated that 23 of the 25 men regularly used either Johnson's Baby Oil or Vaseline Intensive Care or Nivea hand lotions to facilitate sexual intercourse, substances widely used for this purpose. Mineral oil is a common denominator in each of these lubricants. When our persistent condom breakers were interviewed, it became evident that the probable source of their breakage was that they mistakenly thought lubricants such as Vaseline Intensive Care, Nivea, and Johnson's Baby Oil were water-based, because they washed off fairly readily with water compared with Vaseline or Crisco. Only the latter were perceived as proscribed oil-based lubricants. Air burst tests revealed that 60 sec of exposure of condoms to mineral oil caused approximately 90% decrease in their burst volumes. Vaseline Intensive Care and Johnson's Baby Oil, each containing mineral oil, also affected condom integrity [24].

REFERENCES

1. **Wigersma L, Oud R:** Safety and acceptability of condoms for use by homosexual men as a prophylactic against transmission of HIV during anogenital sexual intercourse. Br Med J 295:94, 1987.

2. **Richters J, Donovan B, Gerofi J, Watson L:** Low condom breakage rate in commercial sex. Lancet 2:1487–1488, 1988.

3. **Voeller B, Reinisch JM, Gottlieb M (eds):** AIDS and Sex: An Integrated Biomedical and Biobehavioral Approach. New York: Oxford University Press, 1989 (in press).

4. **Consumers Union:** Condoms: A report based on laboratory tests and on detailed questionnaires filled out by nearly 1900 readers. Consumer Reports 583–588, 1979.

5. **College of Health:** It's only condom sense. Self-Health: The Journal of the College of Health 16:10–15, 1987.

6. **Condoms revisited.** Choice, 42–45, 1989.

7. Condom recalls reported after inspections by FDA. The Wall Street Journal, June 19, 1987; U.S. Health and Human Services News, June 19, 1987; **Parachini A:** Condoms and AIDS: How safe is 'safe'? Los Angeles Times, August 18, 1987; **Parachini A:** Condoms may

get warning labels, Los Angeles Times, August 24, 1987; F.D.A. seeks to destroy 45,000 flawed condoms, The New York Times, Sept. 8, 1988.

8. **Nakamura RM, Coulson AH, Voeller B, Bernstein GS, Browdy B, Hicks D, Detels R, Perlman J:** In vitro condom testing. Abstract 6510: IV International Conference on AIDS, Stockholm, June, 1988.

9. **ASTM (American Society for Testing and Materials) and ISO (International Standards Organization).**

10. **U.S. Department of Defense:** Military Standard: Sampling Procedures and Tables for Inspection by Attributes. M11-STD-105D. Washington, D.C.: U.S. Government Printing Office, April 29, 1963.

11. **Voeller B:** In: Minutes of the Roundtable Meeting on New Condom Design, National Institute of Child Health and Human Development, April 20, 1988. Bethesda, MD: National Institutes of Health, p 7.

12. **Ansell Laboratories:** In: Minutes of the Roundtable Meeting on New Condom Design, National Institute of Child Health and Human Development, April 20, 1988. Bethesda, MD: National Institutes of Health.

13. **Stone KM, Grimes DA, Magder LS:** Primary prevention of sexually transmitted diseases: A primer for clinicians. JAMA 255:1763–1766, 1986.

14. **Voeller B, Potts M:** Has the condom any proved value in preventing the transmission of sexually transmitted viral disease—for example, acquired immune deficiency syndrome? Br Med J 291:1196, 1985.

15. **Conant M, Hardy D, Sernatinger J, Spicer D, Levy J:** Condoms prevent transmission of AIDS-associated retrovirus. JAMA 255:1706, 1988.

16. **Van de Perre P, Jacobs D, Sprecher-Goldberger S:** The latex condom, an efficient barrier against sexual transmission of AIDS-related viruses. AIDS 1:49–52, 1987.

17. **Rietmeijer CAM, Krebs JW, Feorino PM, Judson FN:** Condoms as physical barriers against human immunodeficiency virus. JAMA 259:1851–1853, 1988.

18. **Voeller B, Hicks D, Coulson AH, et al.:** Testing HIV leakage through condoms. Abstract 6508: IV International Conference on AIDS, Stockholm, June, 1988.

19. **Voeller B, Hicks D:** Testing condom leakage of HIV. Los Angeles; Mariposa Occasional Paper 8, 1987.

20. **Bernstein GS, Baker R, Coulson AH, et al.:** Detection of a defective lot of condoms medicated with Nonoxynol-9. Abstract 6522: IV International Conference on AIDS, Stockholm, June, 1988.

21. **Katznelson S, Drew WL, Mintz L:** Efficacy of the condom as a barrier to the tranmission of cytomegalovirus. J. Infect Dis 150:155–157, 1984.

22. **Blair M, Drew WL:** Condom model for evaluating HIV transmission. Abstract 6512: IV International Conference on AIDS, Stockholm, June, 1988.

23. **Kinsey AC, Pomeroy WB, Martin CE:** Sexual Behavior in the Human Male. Philadelphia; W.B. Saunders Company, 1948.

24. **Voeller B, Coulson AH, Bernstein GS, Nakamura RM:** Mineral oil lubricants cause rapid deterioration of latex condoms. Contraception 39:95–102, 1989.

DISCUSSION

DR. VANDER HAAR: I am from Carter-Wallace. Reference was made earlier to the fact that no studies correlate the kind of stresses involved in sexual intercourse with the models used to test condoms. Are you aware of any of the correlations or of anybody who has tried to make those correlations in the development of the in vitro testing models?

DR. VOELLER: Do you mean, for example, in the sense of the things that I was suggesting, such as number of pelvic thrusts, pace, and frictional forces?

DR. VANDER HAAR: More along the lines of frictional forces.

DR. VOELLER: As far as we are aware, and that applies to everyone we have talked to in and out of the industry—The FDA, Masters and Johnson, the Kinsey Institute—there are precious few data, and those that exist are not very reliable. We are about to begin some studies using remote probes on dildos, pressure sensors, and a recording device. I have also been looking at raw pornographic film footage so that we could get better data on the number of pelvic thrusts, the rate, the duration, etc. It is very different from what I have been told by everybody I have talked to, including many sex experts. The rates can be as high as 210 thrusts per minute, which is quite extraordinary, and the total number is immense. There are all kinds of factors like this that we are beginning to look at.

Under grants from CONRAD, London Rubber Company, Schmid, and Fuji Latex, we have purchased two simulated coital machines. Once you have this physiological and physical information, these machines allow you to reproduce it and to test condoms in a variety of ways, including the use of oil- and water-based lubricants. We are beginning such studies.

DR. MAYER: Do you think that the scale you have developed to evaluate condoms is sufficient to take into account different kinds of intercourse, such as vaginal vs. anal, or do you think you are going to have to revise it? Some of the top eight and the bottom five condoms might perform differently under different circumstances.

DR. VOELLER: I think that different weightings will give different rankings, but I do not think there would be a major shift in rankings; however, that remains to be proved. As I indicated, there has been a bit of controversy over a *Los Angeles Times* article that gave the rankings without our permission, and to our considerable dismay, because they were based on a single lot of condoms. This was unfair to everyone involved. From our point of view, it is essential that we have the additional two lots of each condom tested to see if the rankings remain the same, and to do the comparison with the Consumers Union studies. They looked at three to five lots per brand, using a much smaller range of tests than ours, but we want to make those comparisons. There was a 60% overlap in the brands that we tested. Once that is done and the data are compared, we will be in a much better position to say whether the rankings are relevant and what they are.

31

Condom Quality Management

Michael J. Free and Jane Hutchings

If latex condoms are properly designed, have ample and uniform elastic properties, and are free from pinholes, they can significantly reduce the risk of transmission of disease organisms through penile contact. However, use of condoms cannot eliminate that risk. The natural latex rubber from which condoms are made may vary from batch to batch. In addition, differences in manufacturing technology, manufacturing practices, and prevailing standards can produce considerable differences in the quality of condoms. Although condom storage in tropical and developing country environments is known to accelerate deterioration of the latex, inexperience or lack of interest by many manufacturers has impeded the development of product formulations better able to withstand environmental hazards.

A condom quality management program addresses some of these issues by ensuring that condoms are suitable for use when they reach the user. Two major considerations with respect to condom suitability are quality of design and conformance to specifications. To ensure quality of design, the purchasing authority responsible for selecting condoms takes into account the physical environment and level of infrastructure in which they will be stored and used, the characteristics of the target population, and the system of condom marketing and distribution. Some design criteria are related to condom integrity, for example, uniform high strength and elasticity and the absence of holes. Other criteria may be selected to enhance acceptability or improve shelf life. Ensuring conformance to specifications requires vigilance by purchasing authorities and program managers in the field, and the use of a few simple product tests at key points in the procurement and logistics management process.

Heterosexual Transmission of AIDS, pages 379–397

QUALITY MANAGEMENT THROUGH ISSUANCE AND CONTROL OF APPROPRIATE PROCUREMENT SPECIFICATIONS

Most published condom standards, certification schemes, or regulatory reviews by various national or international bodies do not guarantee suitability for use. Standard tests for condoms have focused on the incidence of pinholes. Although this focus has led to a reduction in the frequency of pinholes, it has not effectively controlled the attributes that affect condom breakage: high and uniform elasticity and strength and shelf stability.

Failure of condoms from pinholes or pores is a function of the size and location of the holes, viscosity of semen, size and critical number of disease organisms required for infection, and extent of coital activity following ejaculation. Therefore, the presence of a pinhole does not automatically equate with condom failure. However, condom breakage, undetected until after ejaculation, almost always results in a major exchange of body fluids and a risk of exposure to disease organisms comparable to using no condom. Although pinholes are difficult for users to detect, clinical evidence suggests that breakage occurs at a much higher frequency than pinholes [1–9]. Therefore, controlling and minimizing the factors that lead to condom breakage are the principal objective of condom quality management.

By developing and issuing appropriate specifications and through testing to ensure the specifications are met, the purchasing authority plays a major role in influencing condom suitability. Procurement specifications and compliance procedures can draw upon the various published standards but also must incorporate the available published [2,3,10–13] and unpublished information on condom quality, stability, efficacy, and acceptability. In this way, specifications development can circumvent the lengthy process of assimilating new data that marks the development of standards. (International standards for latex condoms are still being approved approximately 15 years after initiation of discussions.)

Current information can lead to the development of design specifications for latex condoms that will ensure delivery of a high level of efficacy and the ability to withstand to some degree suboptimal conditions during transport and storage. In its guidelines for condom procurement, the World Health Organization (WHO) Global Programme on AIDS (GPA) has recognized the crucial role played by the purchasing authority. The GPA guideline includes a set of recommended specifications for latex condoms [14].

Research is underway in several countries to study condom resistance to breakage and the effect of environmental factors. These studies may provide data that will allow the development of specifications for latex condoms stored in difficult environments or used by special target groups. In the longer term, condoms made from plastic [15] (some of which are already approaching the market) and latex blended with other elastomeric materials may become affordable to donor agencies and developing country programs. These plastic or blended products should set new standards of uniformity, resistance to breakage, and stability.

QUALITY MANAGEMENT THROUGH MONITORING CONDOMS IN THE DISTRIBUTION SYSTEM

Even though they are purchased according to appropriate design specifications and independently tested, condoms remain perishable goods. Condom shelf life depends on a mixture of adverse conditions acting in various combinations and to differing degrees to bring about deterioration of the latex. Ozone, temperature, humidity, ultraviolet light, abrasion, mechanical loads, and animal pests all can contribute to the process of condom deterioration. Currently, little is known about the interaction of these factors with condom packaging materials, lubricants, powders, processing chemicals, color dyes, and other design features.

Stages of Distribution

Three stages in the interval between manufacturer and consumer bring distinctly different conditions to bear on the process of deterioration. These stages are 1) transport to and storage in warehouses, 2) storage and display in retail or clinic outlets, and 3) transport or storage by the consumer prior to use. During warehouse storage, condoms are packaged in cartons or crates and are adequately protected from light but not from heat. Humidity and ozone (or chemical pollutants) may also factor into deterioration at this stage if the primary packaging is permeable to these agents or if package seals are broken. Poor warehousing practices or cartons unable to withstand the weight of stacking under damp conditions may crush some condoms.

The retail or distribution stage is usually shorter in length than warehouse storage. During this period, condoms remain exposed to the hazards of heat and humidity, but also face the added factors of mechanical damage from handling and deterioration due to ultraviolet (UV) light from sunlight or fluorescent lamps. Condoms also are more likely to be exposed to damaging levels of temperature, humidity, ozone, and chemical pollutants during this stage than during the warehouse stage. UV light, an ozone generator, can be especially degrading. The strength of condoms exposed to UV light may be reduced dramatically (by 60–80%) after 1 day's exposure [10].

At the consumer stage, condoms probably are less prone to damage from exposure to light. However, compression and damage from improper storage, such as in pocket, can interact with the type and strength of packaging in determining the effect of this stage on suitability for use.

Little can be done within the scope of condom supply systems to improve the conditions at the retail and consumer stages. However, purchasers can specify improved packaging for protection against rough handling and exposure to light and other environmental hazards. To ensure condom integrity at the user stage, program managers in the field must make certain that the condoms are in the best possible condition when they reach the retailer. To be sure of a high reserve of strength and elasticity at the retail end of the supply chain, a field system of quality management is needed.

A Condom Quality Monitoring System for Field Use

A condom quality monitoring system for countries with low infrastructure and extreme environments was first described in 1979 [16]. The system includes local sampling and local testing of condom stocks and the generation of simple test reports. Based on the level of deterioration indicated by the data, a limited number of interventions can be recommended within the scope of the system. The test equipment for such a system must be low-cost, simple, and rugged and require no special skills to operate, calibrate, or maintain. The quality tests selected for use in the field testing program should apply to the whole condom and, if possible, be drawn from tests recognized by international standards organizations or authorities. In the system described above, heavy emphasis is placed on a monitoring approach whereby the quality of condoms aging in storage is continually related to the quality of the same condoms at time of arrival in country. This relative testing approach provides information on rate of deterioration, sudden changes in strength or uniformity of a batch of condoms, the weak points in the storage and distribution system, and the relative or overall quality of different condom stocks.

In selecting sensitive and appropriate monitoring approaches, several tests of condom strength and elasticity have been developed or reviewed, including a tear test, a biaxial tension test, a tensile test, and the standard air inflation test [16]. The tear test and biaxial tension test correlate highly with air inflation data. In condoms uniform throughout their length, air inflation results also correlate highly with tensile test properties [10]. Such results are not surprising because burst volume depends principally on ultimate elongation and the initial size of the condom [11]. The problem of the tear, biaxial, and tensile tests for monitoring purposes, however, is that all are carried out on small sections of latex film taken from the shaft portion of the condom and are incapable of detecting flaws or deterioration throughout the condom. Unique among the tests for strength, the air inflation test tests the entire condom, a necessary feature since deterioration is not uniform throughout the condom under normal field conditions. Further research to improve test methodology is underway in several laboratories. Meanwhile, the air burst test has been shown to be a sensitive and cost-effective means of testing and monitoring condoms for quality management.

During the past 10 years, condom quality management laboratories, such as those described in this paper, have been installed in Bangladesh, Guatemala, Indonesia, Mexico, Pakistan, the Philippines, and Thailand. Additional facilities are scheduled for Egypt, the People's Republic of China, and 10 African countries. Establishment of these facilities during the past 10 years has been sponsored by a number of agencies and foundations, including the U.S. Agency for International Development (U.S.A.I.D.), the WHO, and the Andrew W. Mellon Foundation.

The Nature of Condom Deterioration: The Basis for Current Quality Monitoring Practice

The selection of testing and reporting methods for the quality management system was based on several observations that have been further validated through more recent experimental findings.

1 Pinholes are a manufacturing defect and are not a result of deterioration of the latex. Condoms that are extremely degraded may exhibit an increased number of perforations, but these condoms are well past the end of their useful life and usually will break even during normal handling. Therefore, tests for leakage are carried out only as part of predelivery quality checks during procurement and the in-coun-

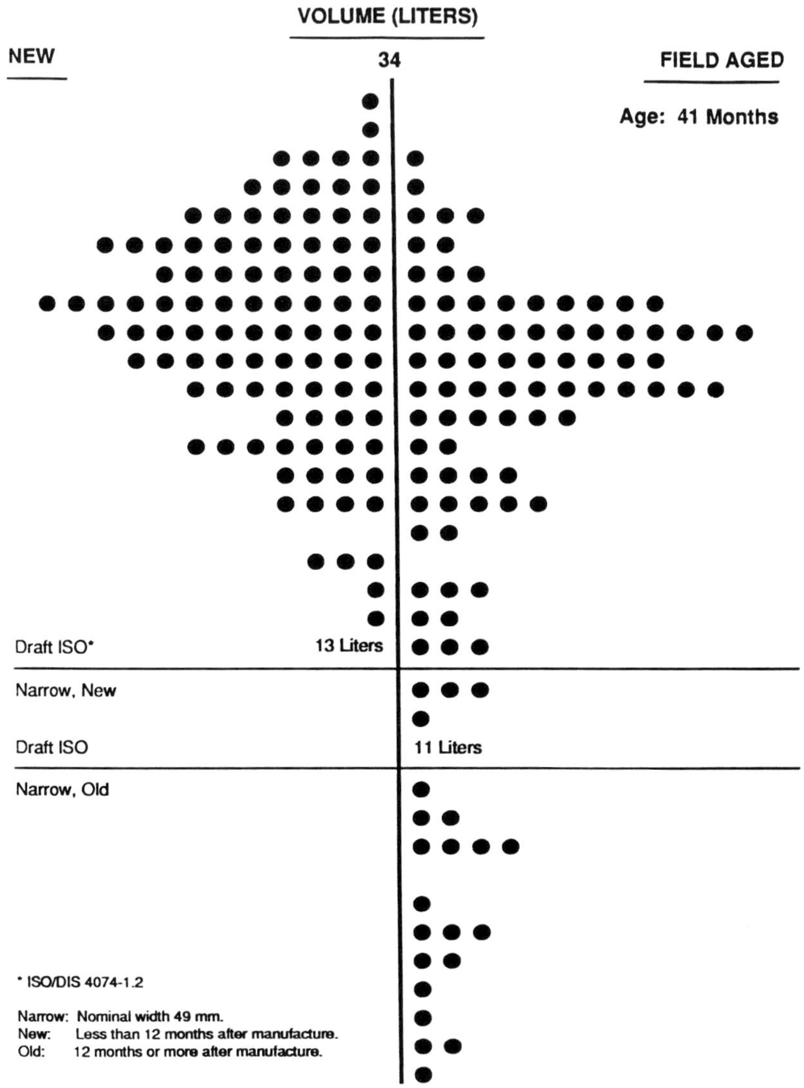

Fig. 1. Burst volume data distribution for new and field-aged condoms.

try receipt checks. No further tests for pinholes are required.

2 Deterioration trends are reflected in the elastic properties of the latex film [3]. Condoms become less elastic with age.

3 Condoms within a production lot tend to be heterogeneous with respect to their elasticity and ultimate strength prop-

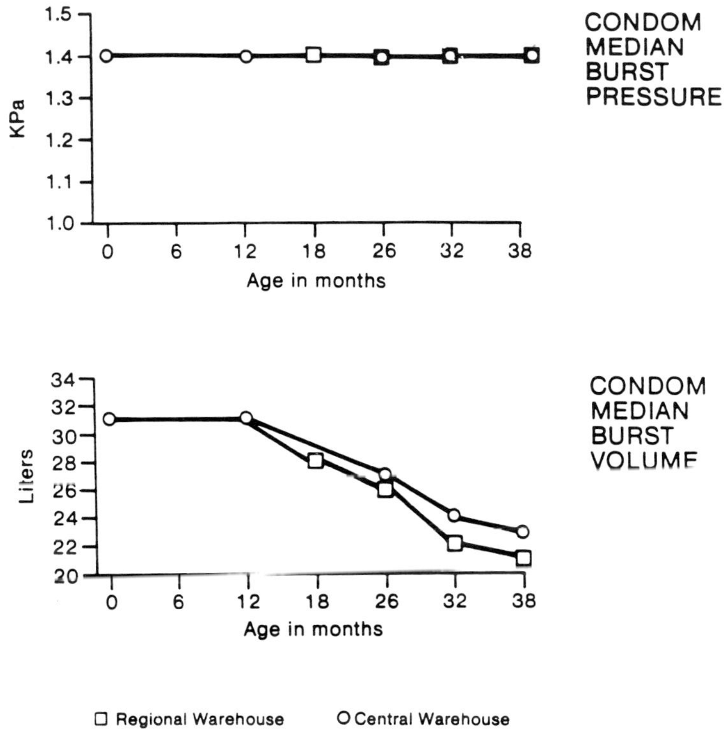

Fig. 2. Loss of condom elasticity over time. The burst volume of this aging lot of condoms declines over time, indicating a loss of elasticity. The burst pressure, however, remains constant [3].

erties as well as their response to agents that cause deterioration. Therefore, as condoms age, burst volume data become progressively more widely distributed around the mean, compared with distribution of data typical of good-quality new condoms [3]. Typically, batches of condoms that have undergone some deterioration consist of individual condoms with elasticity and strength properties similar to new condoms as well as condoms exhibiting a 50–80% reduction in these properties.

4 The elasticity and strength of condoms in a production batch often are not normally distributed around the mean; they have a strong tendency to skew severely downward or even to split into a bimodal population as deterioration progresses [3,10]. Therefore, careful sampling must be undertaken. Data are best expressed as median and lower quartile rather than as mean and standard deviation.

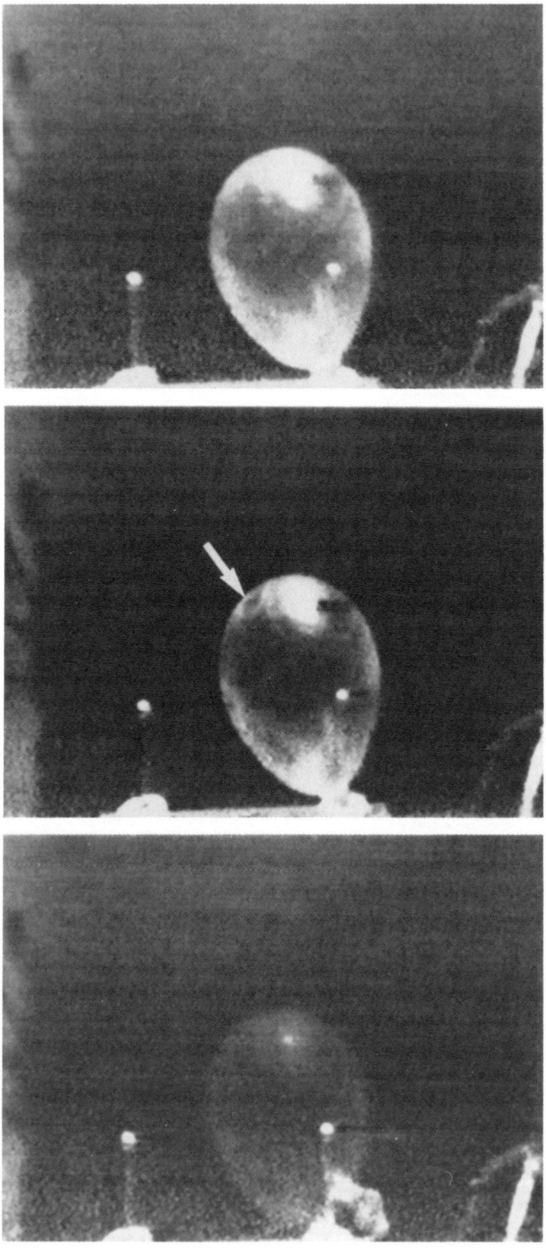

5 Individual rolled condoms deteriorate in a nonuniform fashion. The reservoir (closed) end of the condom that remains unrolled and unprotected by overlying layers of latex film generally exhibits the most significant deterioration. Therefore, testing this portion of the condom is of paramount importance in assessing the effects of deterioration on the condom's mechanical properites.

6 Reduced elasticity and a reduction in the ultimate strength of a condom result in an increased probability of breakage during use [2,3,5]. In one study, a marked increase in the frequency of breakage of artificially or naturally aged condoms during clinical use occurred when elastic properties fell below 50% of normal values (below 15 liters burst volume for condoms of 100 mm circumference, using a 150 mm test length according to ISO/DIS 4074-1.2) [3].

The data characteristic of condom deterioration in tropical countries are illustrated in Figures 1–3 and Table 1. Figure 1 shows the characteristic distribution of burst volume data in field-aged vs. new condoms. Figure 2 demonstrates the progressive reduction in elastic properties (burst volume) over time, even in the face of relatively unchanging ultimate stress (burst pressure). In this case, the loss of elasticity appeared sensitive to different storage conditions: storage at the peripheral warehouse accelerated the trend compared with the central warehouse storage. Table 1 demonstrates the lack of uniformity in the deterioration of the rolled, packaged condom in storage [17]. The samples tested represent 3–3.5-year-old condoms. The results of the tensile test, which evaluates the stress and strain values of a 20-mm-wide ring cut from the shaft portion of the condom, indicate satisfactory values. None of the samples had a mean tensile value of less than 17 megapascals, and no single specimen had a

---

Fig. 3. Field-aged condom at moment of burst. The three images, from top to bottom, show a field-aged condom bursting while being inflated with air at a constant flow rate of 24 standard liters per minute. A high-speed video system filming at 200 fields per second and a 1/50,000th of a second strobe were used to capture the moment at burst. The three images were reproduced from the video tape. The top frame shows the condom filling with air. In the second frame a hole due to a weak spot on the condom surface has developed near the top left side of the condom and appears as a dark spot (see arrow). Much like a balloon popping, the hole continues to expand until, by the third frame, all of the air has escaped from the condom. The dim outline of the condom in the third image is a ghost or latent image retained for a split second by the video camera after the condom has burst. Remnants of the condom can be seen as a dark mass just to the right of the ghost image.

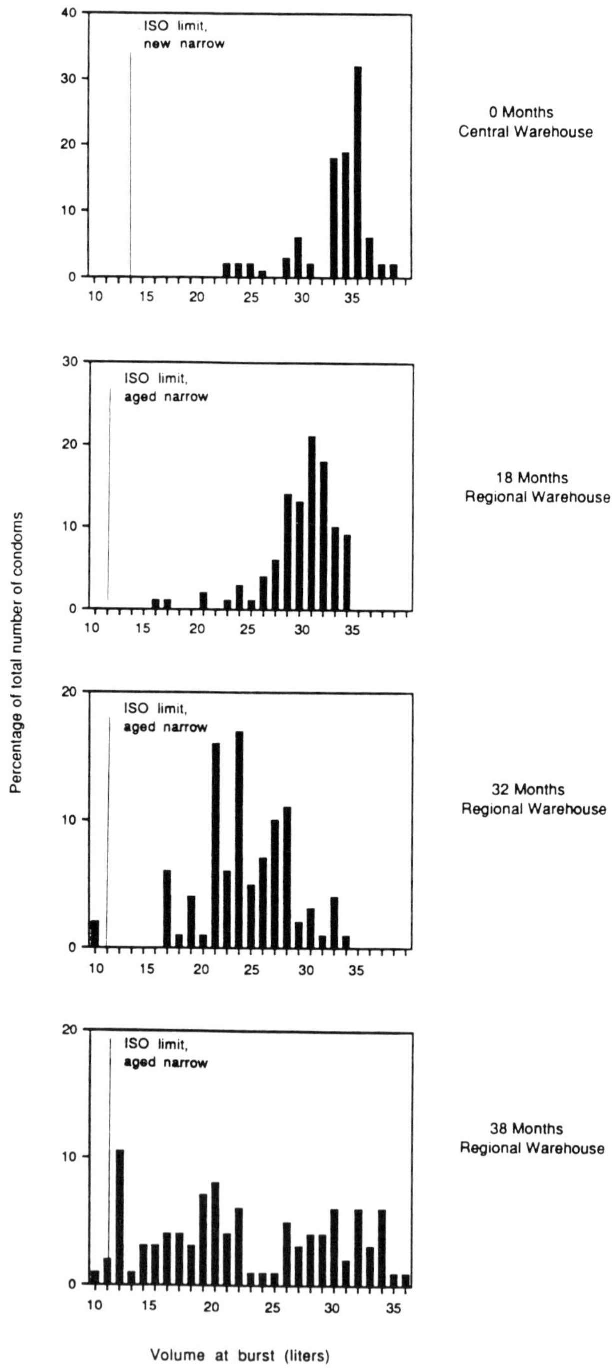
ISO limit,
new narrow
0 Months
Central Warehouse
ISO limit,
aged narrow
18 Months
Regional Warehouse
ISO limit,
aged narrow
32 Months
Regional Warehouse
ISO limit,
aged narrow
38 Months
Regional Warehouse
Percentage of total number of condoms
Volume at burst (liters)

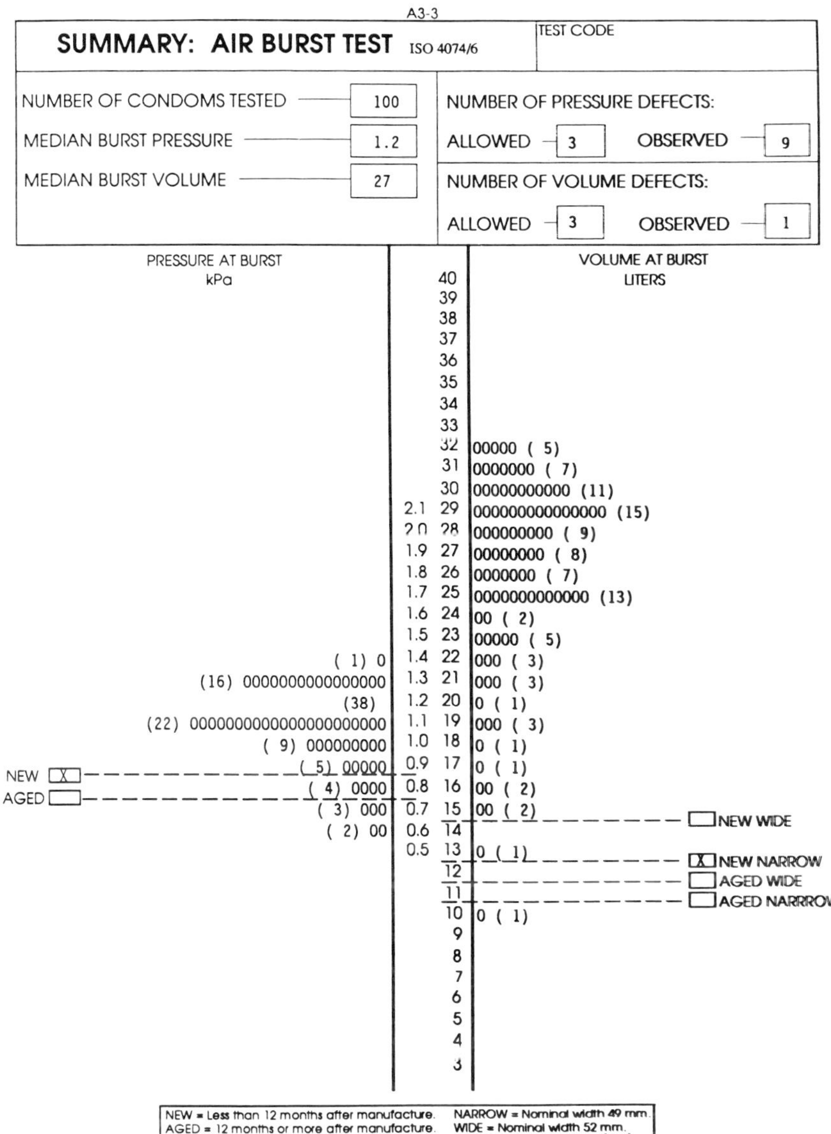

Fig. 5. Lot plot.

Fig. 4. Changes in burst volume distribution for one lot of stored condoms tested at four time intervals.

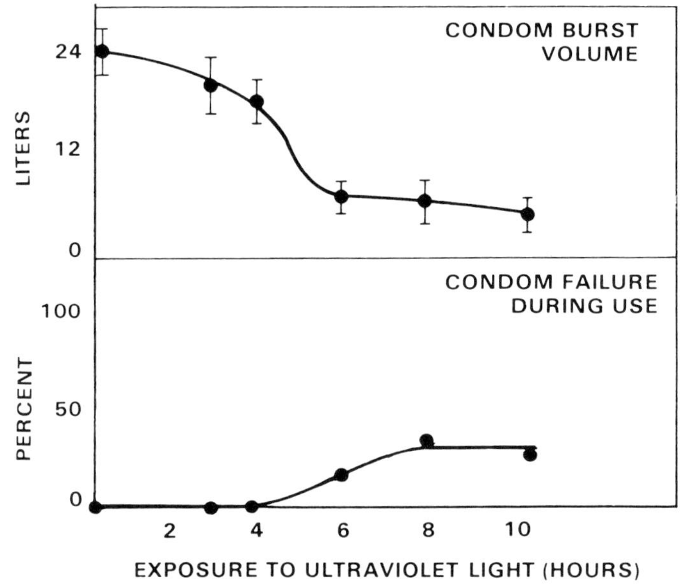

Fig. 6. Relationship between condom strength and failure during use. The decline in burst volume of a sample of condoms exposed to ultraviolet light parallels the increase in breakage during actual use that occurs in condoms that were exposed to ultraviolet light for varying periods of time prior to their use. Note the sharp decline in burst volume and the parallel increase in breakage during use that occur with six hours of exposure to ultraviolet light.

tensile value of less than 15 megapascals. All samples displayed acceptable elongation values, with no specimens failing to stretch less than 625%.

Based on these test results alone, these samples would have been deemed acceptable. Notably, however, in each group tested, individual samples failed to meet the ISO/DIS 4014-1.2 proposed minimum limit for burst volume. In this test series, condoms burst at low volumes while retaining normal tensile test values in the midregion of the shaft. The zone from which the tensile samples were taken (approximately 85 mm from the closed end) is within the rolled, and therefore more protected, portion of the condom. Characteristically, these condoms, when inflated, burst at the closed end, indicating deterioration in the unrolled portion. A severely deteriorated field-aged condom at the moment of burst is shown in Figure 3. Consistent with this result are the samples that failed the water breakage test. When filled with 300 ml of water, the condoms did not display pinholes but rather burst under the pressure of the water. Such

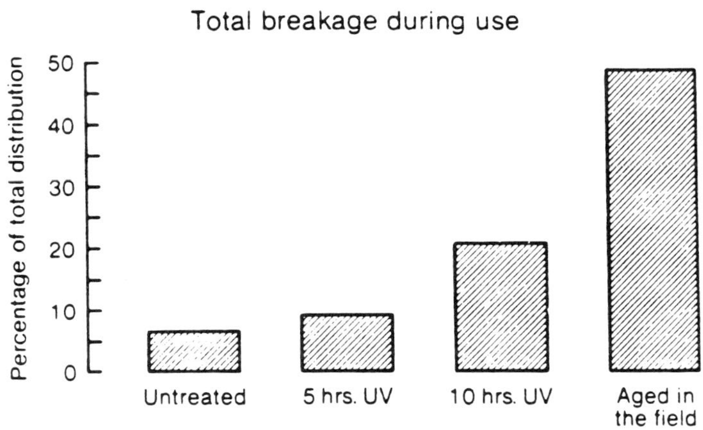

	Untreated	5 hrs. UV	10 hrs. UV	Aged in the field
Median volume	25	25	11	14
Median pressure	1.9	1.7	1.1	1.3
Number under ISO volume limit	2	2	45	44
Number under ISO pressure limit	0	0	8	10

Fig. 7. Relationship between condom strength and breakage during use in a developing country setting.

breakage suggests deterioration in the tip (closed end) of the condom.

Quality Management Using Field Test Data

During the past 10 years, numerous examples of advanced deterioration have been found in condoms stored in developing countries. Sometimes deterioration is apparent within 12–18 months after

TABLE 1. Results From Condoms Tested by PIACT/Bangladesh in 1981 (Akwell, May 1982)[a]

Lot No. PIACT/ Bangladesh[b]	Number	Tensile strength at break: Mean <17 MPa[c]	Tensile strength at break: No. specimens <15 MPa	Tensile strength at break: No. low liers <20 MPa	Percent elongation at break: Mean <700	Percent elongation at break: No. specimens <625	Air burst: No. 11: liters (0.388 ft^3) or less	Water test (No. of): Leaks	Water test (No. of): Breaks
11a 12-78 Tahiti	25	OK	0	0	OK	0			
11b	50						12		
11c									
12a 3-79 Tahiti	25	OK	0	0	OK	0			
12b	50						4		
12c	25								5
13a 3-79 Tahiti	25	OK	0	0	OK	0			
13b	50						4		
13c									2
14a 3-79 Tahiti	25	OK	0	0	OK	0			
14b	50						9		
14c									8
15a 4-79 Tahiti	25	OK	0	0	OK	0			
15b	50						10		
15c									3
17a 4-79 Tahiti	25	OK	0	0	OK	0			
17b	50						1		
17c									7
18a 4-79 Tahiti	25	OK	0	0	OK	0			
18b	50						14		
18c	25								5

[a]Adapted from Belsky [17].
[b]The manufacturing date of these condoms is shown (e.g., 12-78 = December 1978).
[c]MPa, mega pascals.

arrival in a country. As noted, some condoms within a batch more readily succumb to deterioration and form a subpopulation of weak outliers in an otherwise strong lot. Fortunately for monitoring purposes, these critical changes in condom elastic properties are preceded by a characteristic shift in the burst volume distribution within a given lot, batch, or shipment (Fig. 4). Downward changes over time in the distribution of burst volume data provide an early warning of condom instability. These telltale shifts in data distribution can be detected by sampling condom stocks, using a statistically appropriate sample size, inflating the samples with air until they burst, and plotting the distribution of burst volume data. When the early, predictive changes are observed over time, program managers can take appropriate action to distribute stocks before the risk of breakage during use increases significantly.

If the rate of deterioration is found to be rapid, appropriate action can be taken to improve the storage and distribution system to extend the local shelf life of condoms. Examples of appropriate action are to

1 speed up customs clearance and ensure that the product is not left exposed on the dock at the port of entry;
2 improve central warehouse conditions, emphasizing proper stock rotation;
3 adjust regional inventories and distribution practices to ensure rapid turnover;
4 request from the suppliers improved formulations or better grades of packaging material, for example, aluminum foil laminated with plastic rather all plastic film; and
5 test condoms systematically at different levels in the supply line to determine where in the distribution system the condoms are being stressed.

All condom testing field stations should be linked to a network of audit and calibration checks to ensure uniformity and consistency of results. Stocks should be sampled and tested upon receipt in country, and thereafter at 6 month intervals, following the stock as far into the peripheral warehouse system as is practical. Data from the testing can be conveniently displayed in "lot plot" fashion (Fig. 5), and the medians for volume and pressure at burst plotted on a monitoring graph, as illustrated in Figure 2. In addition to median burst volume as a measure of condom integrity and thus suitability for use, other parameters are being explored. These parameters include weighted quotients sensitive to the number of low outliers, and measurements relating force (pressure) and expansion (volume), that is, work required to burst the condom.

Specific limits for burst volume and pressure can be defined below which certain actions are elicited. Typical actions include 1) increasing the distribution rate for condoms that show early signs of instability and 2) removing from the supply system severely deteriorated condoms. Intermediate actions can involve more intensive testing, and sorting of sublots. The limits can, to some extent, be defined locally based on experience and using as a guideline the limits and quality levels described by the International Organization for Standardization in its draft standard ISO/DIS 4074-1. A reference also can be made to clinical data [2,3] that suggest a significant increase in risk of failure during use when the burst volume falls below a level ranging from 10 to 15 liters, depending on the circumference of the condom (Figs. 6, 7). In addition to quality monitoring of stored condoms, field testing stations are also being used to

1. qualify potential condom suppliers,
2. carry out predelivery and receipt checks of procured condoms,
3. check the quality of condoms transferred from other programs, and
4. carry out independent quality audits of products from local manufacturers.

REFERENCES

1. **Sherris JD, Lewison D, Fox G:** Update on condoms—products, protection, promotion. Population Rep 10:H121–H156, 1982.

2. **Free MJ, Skiens EW, Morrow MM:** Relationship between condom strength and failure during use. Contraception 22:31–37, 1980.

3. **Free MJ, Hutchings J, Lubis F, Natakusuma R:** An assessment of burst strength distribution data for monitoring quality of condom stocks in developing countries. Contraception 33:285–299, 1986.

4. **Wigersma L, Oud R:** Safety and acceptability of condoms for use by homosexual men as a prophylactic against transmission of HIV during anogenital sexual intercourse. Br Med J 295:94, 1987.

5. **Chapman S, Hodgson J:** Showers in raincoats: Attitudinal barriers to condom use in high-risk heterosexuals. Community Health Stud 12:97–105, 1988.

6. **Cohn DL, Gourley PJ, Cole VJ, Judson FN:** Condom usage for anal intercourse in a longitudinal cohort of gay and bisexual men. Abstract 6540: IV International Conference on AIDS, Stockholm, June, 1988.

7. **Gotzsche PC, Hording M:** Condoms to prevent HIV do not imply truly safe sex. Scand J Infect Dis 20:233–234, 1988.

8. **Ross MW:** Problems associated with condom use in homosexual men. Am J Public Health (in press).

9. **Potter LS, Clarke K:** Multi-Country Study of Acceptability of Spermicidally Lubricated Condoms: Summary Report. Research Triangle Park, NC: Family Health International, 1988.

10. **Free MJ, Budic KA:** Relationships Between the Air Burst and Tensile Test Parameters Used to Determine Condom Strength. A Report on Laboratory Trials Designed and Conducted by Program for the Introduction and Adaptation of Contraceptive Technology in Collaboration with Akwell Industries, Inc. under the Sponsorship of United States Agency for International Development Order Number SF-147-PE-77, 1980.

11. **Cahoon JR, Thornton-Trump AB:** Testing and stress analysis of condoms. Abstract: Society for Experimental Stress Analysis Meeting, Hawaii, 1982.

12. **Budic KA:** Interlaboratory study of tensile test methods for condoms. ASTM Subcommittee D-11.40, 1981.

13. **Baker RF, Sherwin RP, Bernstein GS, Nakamura RM, Voeller B, Coulson AH.** Precautions when lightning strikes during the monsoon: The effect of ozone on condoms. JAMA Vol 260, 1988.

14. **World Health Organization Global Programme on AIDS:** WHO Specifications and Guidelines for Condom Procurement. Geneva: WHO (in press).

15. **Report of the Roundtable Meeting on New Condom Design:** Bethesda, MD: Contraceptive Development Branch, Center for Population Research, NICHD, 1988.

16. **Free MJ, Duncan GW:** Quality assessment of barrier contraceptives. In Zatuchni GI, Sobrero AJ, Speidel JJ, Sciarra JJ (eds): Vaginal Contraception: New Developments. Hagerstown, MD: Harper & Row, 1980, pp 208–218.

17. **Belsky RL:** An Assessment of Reported Condom Deterioration in Bangladesh. A report supported by United States Agency for International Development (ADDS) AID/DSPE-C-0053, 1982.

DISCUSSION

DR. BERNSTEIN: I would like to ask you to comment on two things. First, what significance do you see in the fact that many lots of condoms have been recalled by the FDA because their testing using the pinhole or water leak test does not meet the standards that were supposedly met at the manufacturing point? Second, what do you have to say about problems that might occur from condom storage in the United States as opposed to the much more extreme conditions that exist in some of the other countries in the world? Both of us have seen deterioration in some condoms that, as far as we know, never got out of this country.

DR. FREE: We do not know whether it was due to deterioration or was a defect from the start. Regarding your first question, as far as I know, the FDA has in its history only tested for pinholes and, as far as they are concerned, condoms that have lower than 0.4% pinholes are okay. If they have 0.5%, they are not. They use a rather more severe sampling plan, but, nevertheless, it is a snapshot and it is a bit of a roulette game for a manufacturer, I imagine. But, certainly, I am not perturbed that condoms may have a 0.5% incidence of pinholes. I am much more perturbed about condoms that have a severely skewed downward distribution of strength at the start, or have a subpopulation of very weak ones.

With respect to the United States, I am sure the situation is much, much better than in the developing world, but the FDA in combination with U.S.A.I.D., Program for Appropriate Health and Technology (PATH), and a number of other groups, and with the cooperation of the Health Industry Manufacturers' Association (HIMA) is about to start a longitudinal study in the United States and in the developing world of factors that affect deterioration. This study is going to be valuable for improving the product and for specifying the product and could lead to a product adapted for the developing world, but it is going to be 3–5 years before those data are available.

DR. WILLIAMSON: I know there has been interest, and Bruce Voeller talked about building a coital machine that tries to more closely simulate actual use conditions. It strikes me that there are many things that are going to be hard to simulate, including jewelry, fingernails, teeth, rolling them on backwards, and so forth. I think you cannot really get around the need to do some studies on real people, watching how they actually use them. Whether it is a Masters and Johnson kind of study or not, I think we need to know much more about how people are actually using them.

DR. FREE: We must differentiate between research and quality assurance.

DR. WILLIAMSON: Right. Lubricants are another area of concern. I think this coital machine sounds great, but there are so many more variations in human behavior that are not going to be captured by a coital machine.

DR. FREE: Quite right.

DR. VALLEROY: I had something to add to the comments of Dr. Williamson. In one of the studies in the Dominican Republic, we found that prostitutes will take condoms and unroll them before actually putting them on, the way you would with a pair of stockings. None of us had anticipated that behavior.

We have just heard an excellent series of papers on whether condoms work, and we found out that condoms will work if they are used properly. I have a question on whether condoms are being used at all. It has been over 2 years since the U.S. Surgeon General published his report and told the American public that, barring abstinence, the greatest protection would be afforded by the use of a condom, used properly from start to finish. Since we have representatives of condom manufacturers here, I just wanted to ask them what the effect of the Surgeon General's publicity on the sale of condoms has been since 1986? If condom use is not increasing in the United States, where we have a barrage of information on the television, through advertising, what can we expect in other countries?

MR. FREED: That was an excellent question. Let us go back to October, 1986, when the Surgeon General made his quite revolutionary and valid statement, and from the end of 1986 take it 1 year later. By the end of 1987, condom sales were up about 50% in units, so there was a dramatic growth, but since that time they have flattened out and there has been almost no growth. So if you go from the end of 1987 to the end of 1988, it has been totally flat, and that is a trend we see continuing.

DR. FREE: The new bottleneck, of course, is latex supply, and the price of latex has shot up considerably, more than 200% in the last year, and inevitably is going to rise further. This is going to affect the price of this commodity and is a matter of concern at the present time.

32

Role of Condoms in Preventing HIV Transmission in Developing Countries

Jeffrey R. Harris, Lenni W. Kangas, and James D. Shelton

As we begin to deal with the reality that most transmission of the human immunodeficiency virus (HIV) in developing countries is through sexual contact, the role of condoms assumes new meaning. Many persons do not confine themselves to the mutually faithful relationships that are the only certain protection against sexual transmission of HIV. Condoms, therefore, represent the most promising technology available for intervention.

That condoms have an important role to play in the prevention of HIV transmission is not universally accepted. Even in developing countries where condom use is accepted, ensuring sufficient supplies of condoms is being acted upon only slowly. In this paper, we support the role of condoms in the prevention of acquired immune deficiency syndrome (AIDS) by examining their effectiveness for preventing HIV transmission, reviewing the reasons that prevention has failed, and discussing current alternatives. We then present our data on condom supply and demand worldwide. We end by discussing the behavioral, logistical, and technological challenges that must be faced if condoms are to assume an important role in the prevention of HIV transmission in developing countries.

Heterosexual Transmission of AIDS, pages 399–413

EFFECTIVENESS OF CONDOMS

Four types of data support the effectiveness of condoms for preventing HIV transmission: in vitro data and in vivo data on prevention of pregnancy, of sexually transmitted diseases (STDs), and of HIV transmission. Feldblum and Fortney [1] recently reviewed these data, which are briefly summarized here.

In vitro studies, including those that simulate sexual intercourse, have shown that an undamaged latex condom provides an effective physical barrier against HIV transmission [1,2]. This finding is not surprising, given that the HIV particle, at approximately 120 nm in diameter, is more than 1,000 times as large as air or water molecules. Condom quality control tests, some testing for impermeability to air or water, detect holes many times smaller than HIV [2,3].

In vivo data show that condoms are effective for pregnancy prevention, but the level of effectiveness depends on the motivation and knowledge of the user. When a typical new user uses a condom, first-year failure rates average 10–12% [4–6]; the lowest reported failure rate among first-year users is 4% [7–9]. Older, experienced condom users have achieved 2 year failure rates as low as 2.1% with spermicidal condoms [6,9,10]. Three studies [7,11] in the United Kingdom revealed only one pregnancy per 100 married couples using condoms consistently and correctly for 1 year.

A number of in vivo studies [2] have demonstrated the effectiveness of condoms in preventing STDs. These data are even more significant in light of recent studies demonstrating an increased risk of HIV transmission among persons with ulcer-producing STDs [12–15].

Two in vivo studies [16,17] provide the best direct evidence that condoms are effective in preventing HIV transmission. In a study in the United States of heterosexual HIV transmission among patients with AIDS and their spouses, seroconversion occurred in 14 (82%) of 17 discordant couples who did not use condoms or used them irregularly but in only three (17%) of 18 couples who reported using condoms consistently [16]. In a prospective study [17] in Nairobi, Kenya, condom use and incidence of HIV infection among female prostitutes were assessed after a program of education about AIDS. Seroconversion occurred in 20 (71%) of 28 women who did not use condoms and in 23 (46%) of 50 women who reported some use. The level of protection increased significantly with the frequency of condom use. Recognizing the role condoms can play in preventing HIV transmission, the U.S. Food and Drug Administration (FDA) [18] in April, 1987, notified manufacturers, importers, and repackagers of condoms that their labels could state "for prevention of sexually transmitted diseases, including . . . AIDS."

REASONS FOR CONDOM FAILURE

The reasons that condoms fail to prevent HIV transmission are not well known but are probably similar to those in pregnancy prevention: failure to use, improper use, and breakage. Failure to use is thought to occur primarily because condoms reduce glans sensitivity and male pleasure. A small minority of men have difficulty maintaining an erection while wearing a condom [3,19]. Condoms also fail because of improper use, such as allowing semen spillage into the vagina by not holding the base of the condom as the penis is withdrawn after ejaculation.

Considerable concern has been expressed recently about condom breakage, but most reports do not include the number of times the study participants actually used condoms. Three recent studies provide such a condom use denominator. In a retrospective, recall-dependent study [18] of attendees at four reproductive health and family planning conferences in the United States, 282 individuals who had used condoms were asked about condom breakage. Overall, respondents reported that condoms broke in 244 (0.62%) of more than 39,000 acts of intercourse. In another study [20] in Sydney, Australia, the incidence of condom breakage in one female and two male brothels was monitored for 4 months. Condoms broke in three (0.5%) of 664 uses for anal intercourse and in five (0.8%) of 605 uses for vaginal intercourse. Finally, a small study in Denmark [21], in which 40 female prostitutes and hospital staff members each tested 10 latex condoms, recorded a rupture rate of 5%. Thus, although condom breakage appears to be a variable phenomenon, the two larger studies indicate that breakage is relatively infrequent.

A large proportion of condom breakage is preventable. Breakage can be reduced by educating users to leave empty space at the tip when putting on condoms or by manufacturing only condoms with reservoir tips to capture ejaculate. Breakage can also be reduced by avoiding oil-based lubricants that cause deterioration of latex [20,22]. In the developing world, breakage can be reduced by improving storage conditions to avoid prolonged exposure of condoms to excessive heat or light.

ALTERNATIVES TO CONDOMS

Although condoms are not 100% effective at preventing HIV transmission, no alternative barrier methods have been shown to be more effective in preventing HIV transmission. Spermicides, such as nonoxynol-9 (N-9), have been proposed as alternatives because of their demonstrated virucidal properties [1] and efficacy in reducing gonorrhea and chlamydia infection [23]. Preliminary in vivo results are disappointing, however. A continuing trial of N-9-impregnated vaginal contraceptive sponges has shown no reduction of HIV transmission to Nairobi prostitutes using them, even though gonorrhea and chlamydia infections were reduced (Kreiss J, personal communication). Further research is clearly needed on other formulations of N-9 and on other virucidal spermicides. At present, spermicides cannot be considered a safe alternative to condoms for the prevention of HIV transmission.

Another alternative to the traditional male condom is a female condom. One such device, manufactured in the United Kingdom from a high-grade polyurethane, has a ring at each end connected by a thin cylinder shaped much like a condom. The lower ring is fitted in the vagina similar to fitting a diaphragm; the upper ring rests at the entrance to the vagina. An acceptability trial [24] has been completed in the United Kingdom, and the World Health Organization (WHO) is presently overseeing acceptability studies in four developing countries. An acceptability study and an assessment of durability are underway in New York and Wisconsin, respectively. Acceptability studies should be followed by effectiveness studies. The female condom, if proved acceptable and effective, could greatly facilitate prevention of HIV transmission by allowing women protection without active male cooperation.

SUPPLY OF CONDOMS IN DEVELOPING COUNTRIES

Regardless of their effectiveness, condoms will not prevent HIV transmission unless adequate supplies are available. Since 1987, the U.S. Agency for International Development (U.S.A.I.D.) has been the leading and virtually exclusive provider of condoms for AIDS-control programs in developing countries, directly and through the WHO Global Programme on AIDS. From fiscal year (FY) 1987 through FY 1989, U.S.A.I.D. provided $8.6 million for condom purchases for AIDS prevention; $5.0 million is projected for FY 1990.

Although these budgets appear substantial and represent about 16% of all U.S.A.I.D. condom purchases (the rest are primarily for family planning/contraception), the average yearly allocation of condoms for AIDS prevention, $3.0 million, buys only 60 million condoms. Sixty million condoms provide 600,000 "couple-years of pro-

TABLE 1. Estimated Annual Condom Requirements to Supply 10% of Urban Males Aged 15–49 Years in Nine Countries in Africa With High Prevalence of HIV Infection

Country	Male population (thousands)	Urban (%)	Urban male population (thousands)	Annual condom requirement (thousands)
Burundi	1,100	5	55	550
Central African Republic	616	42	259	2,590
Congo	410	48	197	1,970
Malawi	1,664	12	199	1,990
Rwanda	1,369	6	82	820
Tanzania	4,480	18	806	8,060
Uganda	3,500	10	350	3,500
Zaire	7,005	34	2,382	23,820
Zambia	1,508	43	648	6,480
Total	21,652		4,978	49,780

tection," assuming 100 acts of intercourse with condoms per couple per year.

Illustrative calculations provide perspective on the inadequacy of current supply. If the annual U.S.A.I.D. allocation of 60 million condoms were distributed only in Nigeria, a country of 112 million population, with 22 million sexually active males aged 15–49 years, it would supply less than 3% of these men with condoms for 1 year. Table 1 provides estimates of the number of condoms required annually to supply 10% of urban males aged 15–49 years in nine of the most heavily HIV-infected countries in Africa. Even this limited requirement amounts to 49.8 million condoms per year, almost equal to the global supply that U.S.A.I.D. makes available. Worldwide, U.S.A.I.D. shipped 73 million condoms during the 2 year period ending December, 1988. Of this total, 33 million went to Africa, 18 million to Asia, and 22 million to Latin America and the Caribbean.

DEMAND FOR CONDOMS IN DEVELOPING COUNTRIES

The major reason that U.S.A.I.D., until now, has responded positively to all requests for condoms is that condom use in developing countries is quite low. Table 2 shows the prevalence of condom use for major regions of the world. Although in 1987 an estimated 46 million couples worldwide used condoms [18], in all developing

TABLE 2. Contraceptive and Condom Use Among Married Couples of Reproductive Age by Geographic Region, 1987[a]

	Contraceptive use prevalence (%)	Condom use prevalence (%)
World total	51	5
Developing countries	45	3
Africa	14	0.5
East Africa	74	3
South Asia, Oceania	33	3
Latin America	54	2
More developed regions	70	13

[a]Source: World Contraceptive Use in 1987, Chart by Population Division, United Nations, New York.

countries only 3% of reproductive-aged adults used condoms, and in Africa only 0.5% [25]. Although these low levels of condom use reflect both the condom's historical unpopularity and its general unavailability, significant exceptions stand out. The prevalence of condom use among married couples of reproductive age is 15% in Trinidad-Tobago, 12% in Costa Rica, 11% in Mauritius, 8% in Jamaica, and 6% in Mexico. In the developed world, the prevalence is 45% in Japan, 24% in Singapore, 17% in the United Kingdom, and 10% in the United States [25].

These low levels of condom use represent today's sobering reality. U.S.A.I.D.'s data on condoms shipped for AIDS prevention (Table 3), however, show changing trends that are encouraging. Half of the 73 million condoms supplied by U.S. AID in the 2 years ending December, 1988 were shipped in just the last 6 months of 1988. In Tanzania and Uganda (Table 4), each of which has received approximately 7.5 million condoms thus far, 60% were sent in the last half of 1988, and requests for the first semester of 1989 reflect continuing increases in planned distribution. These shipping data do not necessarily reflect increased rates of use, but they are accompanied by numerous anecdotes describing sharp increases in demand, which strongly suggests a change. However, when doubling or tripling of condom use starts from a negligible base, we are still far from achieving the levels necessary to control the pandemic.

If condoms are to fulfill their optimal role in preventing HIV transmission, three challenges must be met: 1) the demand for condoms must be sharply increased, 2) supply needs must be projected so that increased demand can be met, and 3) condoms must be monitored

TABLE 3. Shipments of Condoms for AIDS Prevention by the U.S. Agency for International Development to All Developing Countries and Regions, by 6 Month Time Periods, 1987–1988, and Projected Shipments for First Semester, 1989

	Millions of condoms shipped					
Country	1–6/87	7–12/87	1–6/88	7–12/88	1–6/89[a]	Total
All	2.3	5.3	28.1	37.0	28.7	101.4
Africa	2.3	2.7	13.0	14.9	17.4	50.3
Asia	0	0	5.1	12.3	7.3	24.7
Latin America	0	2.6	10.0	9.8	4.0	26.4

[a]Requested.

TABLE 4. Shipments of Condoms for AIDS Prevention by the U.S. Agency for International Development to Tanzania and Uganda by 6 Month Periods, 1987–1988, and Projected Shipments for First Semester, 1989

	Millions of condoms shipped					
	1–6/87	7–12/87	1–6/88	7–12/88	1–6/89[a]	Total
Tanzania	0	0.5	2.5	4.5	6.0	13.5
Uganda	2.0	1.2	0	4.1	3.9	11.2

[a]Projected.

for quality and improved and research on developing alternatives continued.

INCREASING CONDOM DEMAND

Increasing the demand for condoms is a challenge of highest priority. Resources for education, promotion, marketing, advertising, and distribution must be allocated to stimulate demand for a historically unavailable and unpopular product.

The first priority is to increase condom demand among persons practicing high-risk behaviors, since they are most likely to become infected and transmit infection to others. Persons practicing high-risk behaviors typically include prostitutes, recent and unattached young migrants to towns and cities, young soldiers, students, sea men, and long-haul truck drivers. Because these groups normally are outside the reach of traditional health services, they pose a challenge to AIDS control program managers, who somehow must devise ways to contact and influence them. In many developing countries where HIV is spreading, we are confronted with the question, "Who is going to do the work?'' Governments and health ministries alone cannot do the entire job. Ministries of health often are understaffed and inexperienced in dealing with (and may be disinclined to distribute condoms and information to) persons practicing high-risk behaviors. Likewise, health education departments often are poorly staffed, underfinanced, and unaccustomed to using mass media. Because health ministries are political organizations and health ministers are political appointees, they frequently are constrained from aggressively promoting widespread condom use in what often is regarded as a controversial program.

Because of these limitations in government capacity, the potential contributions of private voluntary organizations (PVOs) increasingly are being recognized. In the past 2 years, established PVOs such as the Red Cross and family planning associations have joined the effort to prevent the spread of AIDS. New organizations also have sprung up, often geared to dealing with people who practice high-risk behaviors. As government and PVO cooperation evolves, new indigenous organizations specifically formed to promote AIDS prevention may need to be created. A historical analogy is the network of country ''chapters'' formed by the Association for Voluntary Surgical Contraception in the 1970s and 1980s, which made male and female sterilization a regular part of international family planning programs.

Discussion is lively about how family planning programs fit into AIDS prevention efforts and whether the relationship will be mutually reinforcing or harmful. The target audiences for contraception (all reproductive-aged couples) are different from the primary audiences of AIDS prevention programs, namely, persons practicing high-risk behaviors. Some administrators are concerned that association with AIDS prevention will damage the reputation of family planning. At the same time, common ground is acknowledged: both programs deal with sexually active people, need counsellors trained and able to talk about sexual behavior, and are involved in condom and spermicide logistics and distribution. In practice, family planning organizations have been leaders in AIDS prevention in a number of countries.

Whether by government, commerical network, or PVO, condoms must be made available wherever and whenever persons at risk congregate. Locations include bars and nightclubs, brothels, lodges and hotels, coffee and tea houses, and truck stops and bus depots. Locations in and near military bases, seaports, colleges, universities, and technical schools also are involved. Ways to supply and resupply condoms include two nongovernmental options. The first is the established private sector commercial distribution system. The companies that distribute pharmaceuticals, beauty products, beer, groceries, and tobacco also can distribute condoms. Likewise, the stores that sell these products can sell condoms too. The second option is social marketing, the use of commercially proved techniques to promote a product of social value. Social marketing has been successfully used in diarrheal disease control and oral rehydration programs and in contraceptive retail sales programs in many developing countries. Programs have marketed condoms successfully in Bangladesh, Ghana, Indonesia, Mexico, and Pakistan [26,27]. Typically, an existing commercial distributor is identified. In an alternative approach, more common some years ago, a not-for-profit organization is created, sometimes affiliated with an existing PVO.

In either case, funds are donated and technical assistance is provided to start the program. Commodities (e.g., condoms) usually are provided free by donors. Consumer surveys help to determine product and packaging design and pricing levels. Promotion and marketing use the channels and means employed by other consumer sales firms. Two strategies that make social marketing work are pricing the commodity below normal cost in the private sector and attracting and keeping top-quality management by paying salaries above traditional civil service scales. Once they are established, social marketing organizations may be able to provide most of a country's condom distribution as well as informational and educational services to persons at risk. However, few such organizations exist. Given the need and the opportunity, social marketing of condoms for AIDS prevention should be promoted as quickly as host government concurrence can be obtained and the technical assistance and financial resources mobilized.

PROJECTING DEMAND

As condom use increases, it will be important to project demand to ensure adequate future supplies. Condom demand today is largely unconnected to demographics (the number of sexually active people), epidemiology (the number of people with AIDS or HIV infection), or previous experience in use (often at too low a level to indicate a trend). Three approaches to the projection of demand are suggested. The first employs sentinel programs, in which a leader in the field, a project activity, or an entire-country program is identified and its progress is observed. The AIDS control programs in Uganda and Zaire are examples; the introductions of condom distribution in the Ghanaian and Tanzanian armed forces are others. Straightforward "pipeline analysis," the second approach, consists of examining the rapidly accumulating record of shipments and reshipments to a large number of countries. Data, such as those shown in Table 3, but broken down by country as in Table 4, provide useful indicators of future demand. Finally, major condom-recipient countries should be visited regularly to monitor supply and demand. Until routine reporting systems exist, this external audit will be necessary, probably twice per year.

QUALITY CONTROL AND PRODUCT IMPROVEMENT

Maintaining continuous quality control of condom manufacturing is essential to keep breakage rates low. In the United States, the FDA has regulated condoms since 1976 to ensure safety and effectiveness as "medical devices." A voluntary standard for condoms developed by the American Society for Testing and Materials (ASTM) and adapted by the FDA states that no more than four condoms per 1,000 should fail a water-leak test. A sampling technique determines if the failure rate is within this limit. If a sample fails to meet the standard, the lot from which the sample was taken is subject to seizure by the FDA. A number of condom recalls have occurred since this action. Both domestically produced and foreign-made condoms are tested and are subject to recall [19,28]. The WHO also is examining condom quality control for AIDS control programs from an international perspective, and progress in deciding international standards is expected in 1989.

Although currently available condoms are effective in preventing HIV transmission, research aimed at product improvement and development of alternatives must continue. New condom materials (e.g., plastics) might prove stronger and cheaper, provide more sensation to the user, and be more impervious to deterioration in hot, humid, and otherwise hazardous storage conditions. Packaging improvements, such as use of foil to reduce exposure to light and ozone, should also be pursued to prolong product quality in storage. New virucides and a female condom can increase a woman's options for protection.

CONCLUSIONS

With the continuing absence of vaccines and curative treatments, condoms are the most promising technology at present to reduce or prevent the transmission of HIV. Emerging data document the effectiveness of condoms in providing direct protection against HIV transmission. Condom use may also indirectly affect HIV transmission by reducing the transmission of the STDs that are cofactors in HIV transmission. Most condom failures result from inconsistent or incorrect use. Breakage rates appear variable but are probably low, and most breakage should be preventable with existing technology and better education of users.

Although condoms can be an effective tool for AIDS prevention, the current prevalence of condom use in the developing world is clearly inadequate to have much of an impact on HIV transmission. Demand has increased of late but is well below the level that is needed. The highest priority for AIDS control programs in developing countries is, therefore, to stimulate demand for condoms, especially among persons practicing high-risk behavior.

Creating this demand will depend on the involvement of nongovernmental providers, including the for-profit and not-for-profit private sectors. Complementing government efforts, commercial distribution using social marketing techniques seems the best way to reach persons at highest risk for HIV infection by making condoms genuinely available. Much can be learned from the experience gained in social marketing of contraceptives and other health-related products. Finally, further research to improve barrier methods and to increase their acceptability and use is required.

REFERENCES

1. **Feldblum PJ, Fortney JA:** Condoms, spermicides, and the transmission of human immunodeficiency virus: A review of the literature. Am J Public Health 78:52–54, 1988.

2. **Rietmeijer CAM, Krebs JW, Feirno PM, Judson FN:** Condoms as physical and chemical barriers against human immunodeficiency virus. JAMA 259:1851–1853, 1988.

3. **Sherris JD, Lewison D, Fox G:** Update on condoms—Products, protection, promotion. Population Rep, pp H122–H156, September, 1982.

4. **Grady WR, Hirsch MB, Keen N, Vaughn B:** Contraceptive failure and continuation among married women in the United States, 1970–75. Stud Family Planning 14:9–19, 1983.

5. **Grady WR, Hayward MD, Yagi J:** Contraceptive failure in the United States: Estimates from the 1982 National Survey of Family Growth. Family Planning Perspect 18:200–209, 1986.

6. **Hatcher RA, Sammon Hughes M:** The truth about condoms. SIECUS Rep 17:1–9, 1988.

7. **Glass R, Vessey MP, Wiggins P:** Use effectiveness of the condom in a selected family planning clinic population in the United Kingdom. Contraception 10:591–598, 1974.

8. **Vessey MP, Mackintosh LV:** Condoms and AIDS prevention. Lancet 1:568, 1987.

9. **Trussell J, Kost K:** Contraceptive failure in the United States: A critical review of the literature. Stud Family Planning 18:257–258, 1987.

10. **Potts M, McDevitt J:** The use effectiveness of spermicidally lubricated condoms. Contraception 11:701–710, 1975.

11. **Gallen ME, Liskin L, Kak N:** Men—New focus in family planning. Population Rep, p J33, 1987.

12. **Simonsen JN, Cameron DW, Gakinya MN, et al.:** Human immunodeficiency virus infection among men with sexually transmitted diseases: Experience from a center in Africa. N Engl J Med 274–278, 1988.

13. **Stamm WE, Handsfield HH, Rompalo AM, Ashley RL, Corey L:** The association between genital ulcer disease and acquisition of HIV infection in homosexual men. JAMA 260:1429–1433, 1988.

14. **Cameron DW, D'Costa LJ, Ndinya-Achola JO, Piot P, Plummer FA:** Incidence and risk factors for female to male transmission of HIV. Abstract 4061: IV International Conference on AIDS, Stockholm, June, 1988.

15. **Cameron DW, Plummer F, Ndinya-Achola JO, Ngugi E, Ronald AR:** The use of condoms by the clients of prostitutes reduce the prevalence of genital ulcer disease. Abstract 6517: IV International Conference on AIDS, Stockholm, June, 1988.

16. **Fischl MA, Dickinson GM, Scott GB, Klimas N, Fletcher MA, Parks W:** Evaluation of heterosexual partners, children, and household contacts of adults with AIDS. JAMA 257:640–644, 1987.

17. **Ngugi EN, Plummer FA, Simonsen JN, et al.:** Prevention of transmission of human immunodeficiency virus in Africa: Effectiveness of condom promotion and health education among prostitutes. Lancet 2:887–890, 1988.

18. **Hatcher RA, Guest F, Stewart F, et al.:** Contraceptive Technology 1988–1989, 14th Ed. Atlanta: Printed Matter, Inc., 1988.

19. **Chapman S, Hodgson J:** Showers in raincoats: attitudinal barriers to condom use in high-risk heterosexuals. Comm Health Stud 12:97–105, 1988.

20. **Richters J, Donavan B, Gerifu J, Watson L:** Low condom breakage rate in commercial sex [letter]. Lancet 2:1487–1488, 1988.

21. **Gotzsche PC, Hording M:** Condoms to prevent HIV transmission do not imply truly safe sex. Scand J Infect Dis 20:233–234, 1988.

22. **Voeller B, Hicks D, Coulson AH, et al.:** Testing HIV leakage through condoms. Abstract 6508: IV International Conference on AIDS, Stockholm, June, 1988.

23. **Rosenberg MJ, Rojanapithayakorn W, Feldblum PJ, Higgins JE:** Effect of contraceptive sponge on chlamydial infection, gonorrhea, and candidiases. JAMA 257:2308–2312, 1987.

24. **Bounds W, Guillebaud J, Stewart L, Steele S:** A female condom (Femshield): A study of its user-acceptability. Br J Family Planning 14:83–87, 1988.

25. **World contraceptive use in 1987:** Chart by Population Division, Department of International Economic and Social Affairs, United Nations Secretariat, New York, 1988.

26. Contraceptive social marketing assessment: Arlington, VA: International Science and Technology Institute, Rpt. No. 87-125-067, 1988.

27. Saunders S, Smith WA, Kilby MA: Contraceptive social marketing and AIDS prevention. Abstract 6519: IV International Conference on AIDS, Stockholm, June, 1988.

28. Centers for Disease Control: Condoms for prevention of sexually transmitted diseases. MMWR 37:133–137, 1988.

DISCUSSION

DR. DODD: On your theme of increasing and meeting demand, is there any information about the current world production of latex condoms and how easily this could be geared up in a very short space of time to meet an increased demand?

DR. HARRIS: Every year about 46 million couples use condoms. I do not know the answer to your question, but I would imagine that it would be difficult to gear up production. It is capital-intensive, but I would ask somebody from the industry to answer.

DR. DODD: I bring up this point because if we suddenly find ourselves facing increasing demand we are really going to be in trouble if we cannot meet it.

MR. SPIELER: And who is going to pay for the increased number of condoms needed to meet the increased demand? Maybe one of the participants from industry can answer the question about worldwide production and capability.

MR. FREED: We (at Ansell, Inc.) have some rough numbers of total worldwide production. In the "free world," probably about 25 million gross are produced worldwide. Now if we multiply 25 million by 144, you will know how many individual condoms there are.

As far as demand continuing and our ability to respond by increasing supply as an industry, we can look at what has happened in the last year or year and a half when the demand that we talked about earlier grew dramatically. All of the condom companies increased their capacity, and, of course, now they have far more capacity than sales. We would be prepared to supply additional quantities as needed.

DR. HARRIS: I think one of the things that we have trouble with, and for which we have not come up with a good answer yet, is how one projects this demand. We complain at the Agency for International Development (U.S.A.I.D.) about the fact that we have only 60 million condoms, but we are meeting the current demand. But we keep thinking that demand is going to increase dramatically and we do not know when that is going to happen.

DR. BIALY: I find this terribly disturbing. The war on AIDS has been declared. The President recommends a considerable sum of money for research on prevention. At the same time, I hear what you are saying, that your budget is only $5,000,000 in 1990 to buy X number of condoms. On one hand we are willing to stimulate excitement for research on AIDS that is going to use billions upon billions of dollars without much of a guarantee that a vaccine or a magic bullet is going to arise, and then we complain that we do not have enough money to buy condoms. There is something weird in this system. I also think a degree of candor on the part of the overall research community is lacking that so fanatically demands, "Give us the billions and we shall conquer; conquer we must, and conquer we shall." But to the need to spend another ten million dollars buying condoms, we say, "The cupboard is bare."

DR. MATA: Dr. Harris, I think you are right about the need to increase demand and production. Taking my country as an example, in 40 years we have seen an 8–20% increase in condom use at the national level by people aged 15–49 years, but the main problem in Costa Rica is that most of the condoms (I think there were 5,000,000 or 6,000,000) are stored at Social Security and the Ministry of Health. I personally put condoms in the car, filling the trunk, bringing them to mechanics, bars, everywhere. When they are available, people use them. Their use was monitored and they were used.

If you have a condom in your pocket, then you may think to use it, but, if you do not have them around, sometimes you cannot buy them. You have to put them in motels. You have to put them everywhere, and have them available almost free.

I want to ask you, is anybody doing this kind of research—systems analysis on the logistics of distribution and models for developing countries—to improve their availability?

DR. HARRIS: Yes. That is precisely on what we are focusing the majority of the efforts through AIDSCOM and AIDSTECH projects.

DR. WILLIAMSON: I am a little disturbed that U.S.A.I.D. distinguishes between two types of condoms: condoms for AIDS prevention and condoms for family planning. The chart you showed in your presentation gives only the number of AIDS condoms. U.S.A.I.D. provided 500 million condoms for family planning last year. What is the difference between the two condoms?

I think we need more coordination. I think we are going to set up two different delivery systems for condoms in some places. In Haiti, there are already two delivery systems, one for condoms through the AIDS program and one for condoms through the family planning program. This does not make sense.

DR. HARRIS: I think that is an excellent point. And, as Paul Cohn, our field officer in Uganda, said, the difference between an AIDS condom and a family planning condom is much clearer in the eyes of the provider than it is in the eyes of the user.

I offered these numbers because I wanted to give you a sense of the demand in AIDS programs. I think what has happened in a couple of countries is that the family planning program people have figured out that they can get "AIDS condoms" for free, whereas they have to use their own resources to obtain "condoms for family planning." There is an official pronouncement from U.S.A.I.D. that programs in the field are not supposed to try to differentiate between AIDS condoms and family planning condoms. It would be foolish to have dual distribution systems, and we are not encouraging that.

DR. ROSENFIELD: Perhaps we need a condom czar. I think that Dr. Bialy's comment about sufficient funds to purchase condoms is very important. There should be no shortage of funds for this particular purpose, and clearly the U.S.A.I.D. Population Office and the Health Office need to plan together in the distribution of condoms.

DR. HARRIS: I would like to reiterate my point that we are currently meeting the demand for condoms. We need to work on more effective national distribution systems, but the demand must increase before we can honestly make a very strong case for increasing supply.

MR. SPIELER: You indicated that we are saved by the fact that, right now, there is a small demand for condoms. You also pointed out that, if only 10% of the eligible men in Nigeria were to start using condoms, U.S.A.I.D. would have to provide four times more condoms than are currently being provided under the AIDS program.

Now, let us assume that demand is increased tremendously and that the private sector can produce more condoms to meet the demand, who is going to provide the additional funds to purchase the condoms? Is it your belief that, in the presence of increased demand, there will be no problem obtaining an increased allocation from Congress to purchase the number of condoms that U.S.A.I.D. could deliver?

DR. HARRIS: No, I do not think that is true. We build cost participation into social marketing programs. The cost participation usually goes for subsidizing the distribution system, but we also should think about building in some cost participation that pays for the basic product. I think you are absolutely right that we must be concerned about how condoms are going to be financed. Through social marketing, hopefully, we can get government out of the picture altogether in some places.

33

HIV and Contraception: Research Priorities

Gary D. Hodgen

At first glance, the association between human immunodeficiency virus (HIV) infection and contraception is not obvious. In retrospect, perhaps those of us committed to contraceptive development were slow to recognize this relationship, in part because so much of the initial publicity and research focused on homosexual relations or intravenous drug use as the main modes of viral transmission. However, early in 1987 shortly after the CONRAD Program began, we did develop in collaboration with the Office of Population, Agency for International Development (U.S.A.I.D.) an initial plan to pursue research related to the linkage between heterosexual HIV transmission and contraception.

This research priority was encouraged because it filled an investigational niche not yet developed aggressively by other public or private agencies concerned either with the spread of HIV or with development and evaluation of contraceptive methods. Significant momentum was added by the Contraceptive Development Branch, NICHD, through both scientific collaboration and additional funding via an interagency agreement with U.S.A.I.D. Together, this impetus led the CONRAD Program to initiate both extramural and intramural subprojects addressing, inter alia, fundamental questions about the factors influencing heterosexual HIV transmission from men to women and vice versa. For example, we became interested in understanding the routes and vectors of HIV transmissions; the relative efficiency of HIV infectivity by stage of disease; if the tissues coming in contact with the virus must have lesions to permit HIV entry; if transmissibility was a function of endocrine status at different times in the menstrual cycle; if HIV is borne on or within somatic

Heterosexual Transmission of AIDS, pages 415–418

cells, germ cells, or reproductive tract fluids. Moreover, we believe that the impact of various contraceptive methods on heterosexual HIV transmission requires an in-depth understanding of transmission modes. Accordingly, we have sought to develop an appropriate laboratory animal model to investigate heterosexual transmission of HIV. Because physical and chemical barriers are thought to provide some degree of first-line defense to coitally transmitted HIV, the CONRAD Program has, simultaneously, established programs to evaluate spermicidal agents that may also be effective virucides; two screening programs have been set up for this purpose. Thus the linkage of contraceptive technology to prevention of heterosexual HIV infection was inevitably an investigational priority for the CONRAD Program.

During the evolution of the research efforts summarized above, we recognized that an international workshop could provide a significant scientific forum to elaborate and define further research priorities aimed toward understanding the mechanisms of, and developing methods to prevent, heterosexual HIV transmission. Also, the potential for interactions of contraceptive use on the factors affecting transmission deserved consideration.

Throughout this workshop, many points of controversy arose, however; several issues generated heated discussion, including whether HIV is transmitted heterosexually as free virus or in a cell-associated form or both; if the virus can be found on the sperm membrane, within the sperm, or only in the nonsperm portion of the semen; whether spermicides alone offer sufficient protection against transmission or whether they should be used only in combination with condoms; if oral contraceptives actually promote the rate of infectivity or if the studies showing this association suffer from methodological biases; and what is the specific nature of an appropriate animal model to investigate the mechanism and prevention of the heterosexual transmission of HIV. Research priorities related to these questions identified during the workshop included, but were not limited to, the following six.

1 The elucidation of the routes and vectors of the heterosexual HIV transmission. This was discussed at length regarding the male. We have a great deal to learn about the constituents of semen responsible for transmission and whether the epididymis and/or the sex accessory glands play a role and what role the blood testes barrier plays. A considerable amount of basic physiology research still needs to be undertaken. For the female, we need to look at infectivity rates

during different phases of the menstrual cycle. How important is it to say that a person shedding virus can shed it at any time in the menstrual cycle? Is the risk of transmission quantitatively different at one time or another? It may be that during menses, or during the midcycle events when the cervical mucus is abundant and very thin, there is easier passage of virus in the vagina and the uterus.

2 Testing of the feasibility of contraceptive methods that directly or indirectly limit the heterosexual transmission of HIV. Directly, of course, would be the barrier methods, such as condoms and spermicides. An example of an indirect method would be something like progesterone or progestins, which make the cervical mucus very thick. The steroid milieu has a direct impact on the immunologic state of the reproductive tract; this has been known for 30 years. What parts of that knowledge are relevant to the risk factors in HIV transmission?

3 Determining the reliability of the virucidal activity of nonoxynol-9-containing spermicides. Spermicides assist in reducing the transmission rate of sexually transmitted diseases (STDs). Their in vivo effectiveness in preventing heterosexual HIV transmission is not known. Do the formulation, frequency of application, and duration of action have an impact on efficacy? The public needs from us answers to these questions.

4 Evaluating alternative spermicidal agents that have high virucidal efficacy. This, again, is one of the key activities in which the CONRAD Program is involved, and I come out of this meeting thinking that it deserves to remain at the top of our priority list. Perhaps we can find compounds that will be better tolerated than nonoxynol-9; we want compounds that are more effective virucides, without forfeiting spermicidal activity. On the other hand, perhaps we should be looking at overlapping methods; i.e., one method provides effective contraception and the other provides an effective virucide. Is it necessary to have both activities in one product?

5 Development of one or more animal models to study heterosexual HIV transmission. This, again, is a key priority of the CONRAD Program, and this meeting reaffirmed our belief that we should have begun earlier and perhaps worked more industriously. We particularly need a model with an efficient virus transmission rate from the coital act

(from the male of that animal species to the female and from the female to the male). If we had such an animal model, we would have a system to test such things as spermicidal and virucidal activity and the efficacy and duration of action, and we would, certainly, also hope that that model would teach us about the issues related to infectivity.

6 Understanding the risk factors associated with contraceptive methods as they affect transmission. Here we need to look at primary vector systems of male-to-female and female-to-male transmission, and, certainly, secondary vectors, where the mother may pass the virus to the fetus or child, primarily through the placenta and, to a lesser degree, through breast milk.

If we are advocating certain contraceptive methods, we have to take into account whether the methods have a high contraceptive failure (pregnancy) rate, especially in a population with a high rate of heterosexual HIV transmission. A 5–10% unplanned pregnancy rate would certainly be exposing people to HIV infection. Furthermore, we would then expect that 80% or 85% of the fetuses may contract the virus from their mothers, so we would see a cascade of negative events occurring from ineffective contraceptive methods, which is really why all of this basic research has to be done.

On behalf of all of the CONRAD staff and U.S.A.I.D., let me express our sincere appreciation to all the contributors to these proceedings in the hope and expectation that these proceedings will serve to guide our efforts in understanding the factors influencing heterosexual transmission of HIV as well as assisting in the development of contraceptive methods that prevent or reduce the spread of HIV.

ACKNOWLEDGMENTS

Financial support was received from U.S.A.I.D. and the National Institute for Child Health and Human Development (NICHD). The views expressed in this chapter do not necessarily reflect those of U.S.A.I.D. and NICHD.

Summary Discussion

Jeffrey M. Spieler, Moderator

MR. SPIELER: In this closing session, we would like to give everyone who has something to say a chance to speak. A few people have asked for an opportunity to address the group, and I am pleased to call on them first.

DR. POTTS: First, on the evidence available today, should we recommend the use of spermicides to prostitutes who have refused to use a condom? Second, in the absence of additional data, should we still prescribe oral contraceptives to prostitutes?

MR. SPIELER: You have asked two important questions, and I do not know many people who are more qualified than you to venture an answer. Then, we will seek the opinions of others.

DR. POTTS: I would not prescribe the pill to a prostitute. I would give it, enthusiastically, to every other woman, as I always have. I think I would give her a spermicide in the 100 mg dose range if she was going to have several partners, but I would do that knowing that I may be doing her a disservice because of the problem with monilial infection and things like that. However I am uncomfortable about the use of spermicides alone, based on the present data.

DR. LAMPTEY: I would like to comment on the question about spermicides. We have actually used spermicides in two programs in Ghana and Cameroon. We told the women that, first, they should get the man to use a condom. If he refuses, she should use a spermicide. What eventually happened was that most women found it easier to use a spermicide than to convince the man to use a condom. We discontinued the use of spermicides because of some of the data, especially from Nairobi, that have not been presented here but that have been available to us. In Cameroon, on the other hand, a policy decision was made to continue to recommend both condoms and spermicides, but we should bear in mind the danger that women would find it easier to use spermicides than a combination of the two or condoms alone.

DR. HARRIS: I would like to comment on Dr. Lamptey's point. We are kidding ourselves if we think that we can give women the infor-

Heterosexual Transmission of AIDS, pages 419–426

mation needed to allow them to make an informed choice in that situation.

DR. POTTS: What we cannot do is present to the world's prostitutes the excellent information and discussion from this Workshop, and let them decide what they are going to use. I acknowledge the problem that if you offer a simple thing, such as spermicides alone, people will use it. I am still uncomfortable with not offering spermicides.

DR. PHANUPHAK: I would just give the example that our Minister of Health, who is not a doctor, decided to provide spermicides to prostitutes because it was something they could do for themselves irrespective of whether they were more or less effective than condoms.

MR. SPIELER: Do any of our colleagues from Africa wish to comment on this?

DR. CHIKAMATA: Unfortunately, our country is not very well organized in terms of prostitutes, who are scattered all over the city. And we have no experience in organizing them, or with prostitutes organizing themselves. So I am not comfortable commenting on this point.

DR. BURNHILL: I must confess that I am a little put off by Malcolm Potts' statement that he would recommend that prostitutes stop using oral contraception. Knowing Malcolm, I am not quite sure whether that was a serious statement or not. Nevertheless, there are two considerations that would lead me to continue to recommend oral contraceptives (OCs). First, they are very effective in preventing pregnancy, and this would result in a reduction in perinatal transmission. There is a vast difference in the contraceptive effectiveness of OCs vs. spermicides and condoms. Second is the fairly well recognized prevention of upper genital tract infection with OCs. In fact, if we use OCs with slightly more potent progestational agents, we would get an even thicker cervical mucus, which might be more protective. I cannot imagine making a recommendation that we should not be prescribing oral contraceptives for prostitutes. If *Candida* infection is the problem, I would submit that most *Candida* infection in prostitutes is the result of repeated doses of tetracycline that are giving them a persistent fecal carriage of the infection. They are reinfecting themselves perpetually because no efforts have been made to eliminate that source of *Candida*.

DR. SHELTON: I am puzzled by Malcolm's position on oral contraceptives. He is making a public health decision on the basis of one study, which I would characterize as only a fair study. My general rule of thumb is to make an important decision like that on the basis of at least two good studies or the equivalent. Of course, the choice really depends on what the alternatives are. But, in the case of the prostitute, the alternatives to oral contraception for preventing pregnancy are not great, assuming sterilization is not acceptable. I also think that, although the Kenya study showed an association with oral contraceptives, we ought to remember that a number of other groups have not been able to find a relationship between human immunodeficiency virus (HIV) and OCs.

DR. POTTS: The last point is comforting. What we heard about Nairobi prostitutes is that these women are getting gonorrhea every 10 days, so they probably are not very fertile. It looks like OCs increase the relative risk of HIV infection, and I do not accept totally some of the arguments made by Dr. Meirik. I think that there are plausible biological reasons for this association, and they have to do with cervical erosion.

DR. SHELTON: I think you have to differentiate among prostitutes. Not all prostitutes are like the Nairobi prostitutes. Many of them are mothers and will be mothers again, without question.

DR. ROSENFIELD: I think one thing we cannot say for certain is that a prostitute using a condom faithfully will not enjoy almost the same contraceptive effectiveness as pills, which she may not be using as well. Also, it may be very difficult to convince people that they ought to be using two methods, one to prevent AIDS and one for contraception. Also, it may well be that if we really want to focus on condoms, we have to go all out with condoms and double the message that they are effective if used correctly. In practice, I think it is highly unlikely that people will use two methods.

DR. FATHALLA: Let me add a piece of information. In the World Health Organization (WHO) consultation examining the relationship of contraceptive methods to HIV, Dr. Francis Plummer was one of the participants, and he presented his data. I asked him whether, based on his findings in Nairobi, he has recommended that prostitutes change their contraceptive behavior? He said no, he did not feel that the data justified the change.

MR. SPIELER: I asked Dr. Olaf Meirik the same question. In his paper, he made this point even more strongly. He certainly found fault in a study that should be of some concern to all of us. He said that in the unpublished papers given to him to prepare for his presentation there was no information that would lead him to conclude that the OCs themselves are causing the increase in HIV transmission.

DR. HODGEN: We saw some data this morning that showed that a rule of thumb would be that the prostitute may have five customers per day. If she takes no holidays, that is 1,825 coital acts per year. If half of the customers are clients who are HIV-shedding individuals, then she has over 900 exposures per year. It would not take very many condom failures, or many acts when condoms were not used, to lead to real exposure. The use of a condom would have to be almost absolute, with no failures, or the woman is likely to get the disease.

DR. HARRIS: I hesitate to ask this question, because it may sound terribly naive, but is there any justification for conducting studies in animals to obtain information on the ease of transmission between the cervical epithelium and vaginal epithelium? One could study the effects on transmission using a barrier with or without spermicide. Most of the data that we have seen did not address whether HIV transmission requires the virus to reach the reproductive tract beyond the cervix.

DR. BERNSTEIN: There is one concern I have about mechanical barriers such as the diaphragm. The rate of trauma they cause is higher than people think. In the study we completed comparing diaphragms with cervical caps, we were able to detect abrasions in 3% of diaphragm users, so I think, if we are contemplating developing a device that is atraumatic, if it covers the cervix, we may be opening a new portal of viral entry.

DR. ALEXANDER: Based on the Simian immunodeficiency virus (SIV) model we have developed with Dr. Preston Marx, we showed that you could transmit the virus by placing it into the vagina without any evidence that virus has reached the uterus. If this holds true for humans, it would indicate that diaphragms might not be very useful in preventing HIV transmission.

DR. ROSENFIELD: If prostitutes work long hours, potentially they would have continuous diaphragm use and all the problems that would entail. Spermicides alone may be a more practical recommendation than the diaphragm.

DR. WITKIN: It seems to me that there are two kinds of people in the world, the rational and the irrational. The rational we can educate to use condoms or spermicides, but a large number of people at high risk for AIDS are not rational and will not be educated. We have heard almost nothing about what to do with this large population of people.

MR. SPIELER: I do not think it is fair to say people are either rational or irrational, and that the irrational cannot be educated. Uneducated people can be very rational. Uneducated is not the same as irrational.

DR. WILLIAMSON: I would want to respond to Malcolm Potts'

question about spermicides. I think we still are unclear about what our position should be on spermicides. When you are working with high-risk prostitutes, the first thing you should tell them is to get out of that field. If they cannot do that, the second thing to tell them is to get their partners to use condoms. If the partner will not do that, they should refuse sex with that partner. If they will not do that, then the use of spermicides is the fourth line of defense. It seems to me we should not deny that fourth line of defense because it may not be as effective as other lines. It may be that the female condom will be another fourth line of defense. We are doing a small clinical trial of the female condom involving 20 prostitutes in Chunchon, Thailand. I am very uncomfortable with the idea that prostitutes should not be given spermicides because we have some misgivings, when there are so many in vitro and in vivo studies showing that spermicides have some impact on sexually transmitted diseases (STDs).

DR. ANDERSON: I noticed a summary statement in the newspaper yesterday that free HIV in semen was not a problem; rather, infected cells were the transmitters of HIV. I would like to emphasize that yesterday's session on HIV in semen pointed out, in my opinion, that we know nothing about the mechanisms of transmission. We do not know if free virus or cell-associated virus is responsible for transmission.

DR. ADA: I think this meeting has properly emphasized the role of spermicides and condoms as measures we have at hand for controlling HIV. As Gary Hodgen pointed out, the use of condoms is not going to stop AIDS, it is only going to slow down the spread of HIV. I think we would all agree with what Dr. Bialy said: If more money for condoms is needed, we have to provide those funds even at the expense of some of the research. However, in the long run, we have to develop a vaccine. An encouraging thing about this meeting was the discussion on mechanisms of transmission of this infection. Unquestionably, sexual transmission is one of the most important routes, if not the most important route, in the world today. We have to find out more about the properties of the virus present in semen, whether the infected cells transmit the infection. There is no experiment of which I am aware that shows that infected cells can transmit the infection. There is some work at Johns Hopkins University showing that, among a cohort of homosexuals, three or four people who were seropositive at one stage have seroreverted. They have no virus nor antibody present that we can detect, but they are positive by the polyerase chain reaction (PCR), so we have to think that there are probably latent infections. I believe we must keep working on the development of an effective vaccine because, in the long run, I think that is the only way we are going to defeat this affliction.

DR. BURNHILL: I want to comment on Dr. Witkin's statement about rationality. There is no rationality connected with sexuality. What is needed are reasonably effective tools; e.g., barriers and spermicides. What we need is to have, say, one-tenth of the marketing knowledge that is put into underarm deodorant TV advertising. Somehow we have to find appropriate messages that will make users of nonusers and regular users of sporadic users. At the moment, that is all we have.

MR. SPIELER: I want to make sure that everybody has had an opportunity to say something. And, having said that, the comment that I want to make deals with condom testing. For 2 years I have been recommending something that I have not yet taken action on myself, although I actually could. I think there is one way to get some hard data on how well condoms perform in use that could be compared to the results we get from in vitro tests. Without putting anybody at risk of disease, we could go to family planning clinics where condoms are widely distributed, or find cohorts of people who receive condoms from a social marketing program, or who buy them in a pharmacy. These people could be brought into a study where we have couples who are both HIV-negative and who do not appear to have any risk factors for HIV. What we would do is provide condoms and request the couples to keep coital logs, and record condom use and breakage. We would obtain their actual experience with condoms in a prospective study. The statisticians could tell us the number of couples needed to make some conclusions about how frequently, and where, condoms actually break. A similar study could also be conducted on a gay population in monogamous relationships who have no other risk factors, who are seronegative, and who practice anal intercourse.

DR. RESNICK: I want to come back to a point that Dr. Hodgen mentioned about animal models. It is quite intriguing to me that we have arrived at this point, including studies with humans, before we actually discovered an analogous virus in an animal model. I believe that there is an opportunity for trying to develop a small animal model with natural infection. I think the mouse model or rabbit model may be applicable, and we could use large numbers of animals to get statistically significant data. I would caution, again, about the results that one gets from experimental systems such as putting large quantities of virus in vaginal areas or other mucus membranes of subhuman primates, because it is extremely debatable whether this really has any applicability to what occurs naturally.

MR. SPIELER: Under an interagency agreement between the Agency for International Development and the National Institutes of Health, the CONRAD program has funds to support research on animal models. If there is anybody in this room, or anybody who reads the proceedings, who thinks that he or she can develop a better or more appropriate animal model, we would certainly appreciate receiving your proposal.

DR. VOELLER: In 1984 I testified before Ted Wise's subcommittee on the importance of providing money for animal models and was told by the Public Health Service that there was no need in molecular biology for such things, and that was when the budget for AIDS was $10,000,000. The points I want to make are simple ones, and one of them basically is endorsing what Deborah Anderson said. When we do not even know what the infectious unit is, since financial support is as limited as it is, I think that animal models should be given high priority. There is another side to the problem as well, which really needs some concentrated thinking, and that is, what are the mechanisms at the physiological and cellular level by which the infection takes place? Perhaps Virginia Scofield and Deborah Anderson would be key people to organize a small group to think about this. There has been precious little analysis of this, and I think it is as essential as looking at possible drug and vaccine solutions. Also, I think there are mechanisms that have been proposed for rectal infection that do not involve abrasions or the like as the route. This needs to be explored. A final point relates to what Bill Masters and I have talked about for quite some time and which no one has picked up. I think it is worth looking at the effect of vaginal pH on virus inactivation. Steve McDougall and colleagues at the Centers for Disease Control (CDC) a number of years ago showed a very striking inactivation curve around pH 7 falling in both directions by log units. The striking effect was at the acid end and well within lower physiological vaginal pH values.

DR. LAUFER: We have heard a lot about factors that may influence the acceptability of condom use, including things such as packaging, marketing, distribution, availability, cost (particularly in developing countries, as well as in this country), and physical characteristics of the condom itself such as texture, color, etc. We have not heard very much about things like peer values, peer pressure, peer worries. And we know that, for the very people who are at increased risk for STDs, pregnancy, and HIV, particularly in the younger age groups, peer pressure is particularly important. We also know that it is easier to instill a new habit than it is to change established behavior. Given these two factors, I am very interested in what is taking place in the school system. Dr. Harris talked about a window of opportunity as a vehicle for influencing people's behavior and communication about condoms. I wonder if any studies are going on in school systems? Could other people comment on this?

DR. PADIAN: I know of a study in San Francisco that actually was not conducted in the school system but was conducted among adolescents. The investigators were looking at factors that predicted when adolescents would and would not use condoms, and it had nothing to do with health behavior. I think the main factor that predicted that they would not use condoms was that they thought they would look silly. Therefore, marketing is a key factor. I think that, especially with young people, we need to think about eroticizing the use of condoms and associating them with pleasure rather than making them a caveat for health. It really amazes me that this has not been done. There is some good precedence for that in safe-sex advertizing in the gay community, but we have not seen that among heterosexuals.

MR. SPIELER: In family planning we have seen a tremendous swing in the promotion and use of condoms. Not so many years ago, condoms were promoted strictly for disease prophylaxsis purposes. Then we tried to take the stigma of STDs away from condom use and promote condoms as romantic. Now, with AIDS, we have gone in the other direction again.

DR. MARX: I will close with the KISS principle, which applies to what we do with animal models, and that is, "keep it simple, stupid." What we are able to do with the animal models is the simple application of feline immunodeficiency virus (FIV) or SIV to genital surfaces to model and predict what vaccines will do and whether or not they will be effective. No amount of molecular biology study will replace that at this time. In the future, perhaps it will, but there is nothing that mimics the intact animal, and this has been known for many years. What we try to do is keep the model simple and deal with one variable at a time. We do not usually have social problems to deal with in the animal. We do not have income to think about. We can look at one variable at a time, and that is the contribution we can make. The value of animal models can be argued back and forth, but they are really only as good as the experimenters who use them. Therefore, we try to keep our models and questions simple, and we think we can make a contribution.

Workshop Participants

Anibal Acosta
The Jones Institute for Reproductive Medicine
Norfolk, Virginia

Gordon Ada
The John Hopkins University School of Hygiene and Public Health
Baltimore, Maryland

Biran Affandi
University of Indonesia School of Medicine
Jakarta Pusat, Indonesia

Nancy J. Alexander
The Jones Institute for Reproductive Medicine
Norfolk, Virginia

Kate Altman
Agency for International Development
Washington, D.C.

Cindy Anderson
The Jones Institute for Reproductive Medicine
Norfolk, Virginia

Deborah J. Anderson
Harvard Medical School
Boston, Massachusetts

Amaury Andrade
Family Health International
Durham, North Carolina

David Archer
The Jones Institute for Reproductive Medicine
Norfolk, Virginia

Subhash Arya
Centre for Logistical Research and Innovation
New Delhi, India

Rebecca Bacon
The Jones Institute for Reproductive Medicine
Norfolk, Virginia

Terri Bauer
Eastern Virginia Medical School
Norfolk, Virginia

Stephen Beebe
Eastern Virginia Medical School
Norfolk, Virginia

Kathy Berghorn
Eastern Virginia Medical School
Norfolk, Virginia

Gerald S. Bernstein
Women's Hospital
LA County USC
Los Angeles, California

Gabriel Bialy
NIH/Contraceptive Development Branch
NICHD/GDB
Rockville, Maryland

Benjamin Brackett
College of Veterinary Medicine
Athens, Georgia

Cosima Brucker
Eastern Virginia Medical School
Norfolk, Virginia

Michael Burnhill
University of Medicine and Dentistry of New Jersey
New Brunswick, New Jersey

Virginia Cain
National Institute of Child Health and Human Development
Bethesda, Maryland

Bill Cameron
Ottawa General Hospital
Ottawa, Ontario, Canada

Robert Caspari
GynoPharma Inc.
Somerville, New Jersey

Christopher Castle
American Red Cross
Washington, D.C.

Willard Cates
Centers for Disease Control
Atlanta, Georgia

Agnaldo Cedenho
Eastern Virginia Medical School
Norfolk, Virginia

Eric N. Chantler
University Hospital of South Manchester,
Manchester, England

Davy Chikamata
The Population Council
New York, New York

Richard A. Cone
The Johns Hopkins University
Baltimore, Maryland

Kathleen Cooper
The Jones Institute for Reproductive Medicine
Norfolk, Virginia

Russell Culp
Ansell-Americas
Eatontown, New Jersey

Maryanne Danello
Department of Health and Human Services
Washington, D.C.

Isabelle De Vincenzi
WHO Collaborating Centre on AIDS–Europe
Paris, France

Nicholas Dodd
World Health Organization
Geneva, Switzerland

Laneta Dorflinger
Office of Population
Agency for International Development
Washington, D.C.

William Droegemueller
University of North Carolina School of Medicine
Chapel Hill, North Carolina

Martin Dym
Georgetown University School of Medicine
Washington, D.C.

Robert Endias
State University of New York Health Science Center
Brooklyn, New York

M.F. Fathalla
World Health Organization
Geneva, Switzerland

Lisa Feingold
Brown University
Providence, Rhode Island

Paul J. Feldblum
Family Health International
Durham, North Carolina

Patricia Flemings
National Institutes of Health
Bethesda, Maryland

Jill Flood
The Jones Institute for Reproductive Medicine
Norfolk, Virginia

Robin G. Foldesy
Family Health International
Durham, North Carolina

Jacqueline Forrest
The Alan Guttmacher Institute
New York, New York

Jean Fourcroy-Behr
6310 Swords Way
Bethesda, Maryland

Michael J. Free
Program for Appropriate Technology in Health
Seattle, Washington

Eugene Freed
Ansell-Americas
Eatontown, New Jersey

Matthew Freund
New Jersey School of Osteophathic Medicine
Camden, New Jersey

Patrick Friel
World Health Organization
Geneva, Switzerland

David Fulgham
The Jones Institute for Reproductive Medicine
Norfolk, Virginia

Henry L. Gabelnick
CONRAD Extramural Programs
Arlington, Virginia

Murray B. Gardner
University of California
Davis, California

Keith Gordon
Eastern Virginia Medical School
Norfolk, Virginia

Forrest Greenslade
Population Council
New York, New York

A.T. Gregoire
National Institutes of Health
Bethesda, Maryland

Mary Guinan
Centers for Disease Control
Atlanta, Georgia

E.S.E. Hafez
Reproductive Health Center
Kiawah Island, South Carolina

Jeffrey R. Harris
Agency for International Development
Washington, D.C.

Cindy Hastings
Eastern Virginia Medical School
Norfolk, Virginia

Evelyn Hess
University of California Medical Science Center
Davis, California

David L. Heymann
World Health Organization
Geneva, Switzerland

Joseph Hill
Harvard Medical School
Boston, Massachusetts

Gary D. Hodgen
The Jones Institute for Reproductive Medicine
Norfolk, Virginia

Scott Holmberg
Atlanta, Georgia

Marlene Horowitz
Ansell-Americas
Eatontown, New Jersey

E. Howett
University of Cincinnati Medical Science Center
Cincinnati, Ohio

Mohamed Isahakia
Institute of Primate Research
Karen, Nairobi, Kenya

Morgan Jackson
Department of Health and Human Services
Washington, D.C.

Mary Jenkins
Eastern Virginia Medical School
Norfolk, Virginia

Jacob John
Christian Medical College and Hospital
Vellore Tamilnadu, India

Anne M. Johnson
University College and Middlesex School of Medicine
London, England

Deborah Johnson
Eastern Virginia Medical School
Norfolk, Virginia

Jeanette Johnson
The Alan Guttmacher Institute
New York, New York

Jeffrey Johnson
Eastern Virginia Medical School
Norfolk, Virginia

Georgeanna Jones
The Jones Institute for Reproductive Medicine
Norfolk, Vitginia

Howard Jones
The Jones Institute for Reproductive Medicine
Norfolk, Virginia

Michael Kafrissen
Johnson Pharmaceutical Research Institute
Raritan, New Jersey

Inonge Kamungoma
University of Zambia School of Medicine
Lusaka, Zambia

Lenni W. Kangas
Consultant, Agency for International Development
Washington, D.C.

Leonard Kaplan
Ortho Pharmaceutical Corporation
Raritan, New Jersey

Joseph Kelaghan
National Institute of Child Health and Human Development
Bethesda, Maryland

David Kleinbaum
Centers for Disease Control
Atlanta, Georgia

Maciej Kurpisz
Eastern Virginia Medical School
Norfolk, Virginia

Peter Lamptey
Family Health International
Durham, North Carolina

Brad Langmaid
Bureau for Science and Technology
Washington, D.C.

Deborah Laufer
Memorial Hospital
Pawtucket, Rhode Island

Dale N. Lawrence
Centers for Disease Control
Atlanta, Georgia

Allan Leftwick
London International Group
Cambridge, England

Leonard Levin
American Eagle Insurance Agency
Trevose, Pennsylvania

Laurie Liskin
The Johns Hopkins University School of Hygiene and Public Health
Baltimore, Maryland

Martha Lynch
Agency for International Development
Washington, D.C.

Catherine Lyons
University of California
Davis, California

Andria Maestello
Old Dominion University
Norfolk, Virginia

Mary Mahony
Eastern Virginia Medical School
Norfolk, Virginia

Bohdan Malyk
Ortho Pharmaceutical Corporation
Raritan, New Jersey

Preston Marx
University of California
Davis, California

Leonardo Mata
Ciudad Universitaria "Rodrigo Facio"
San Jose, Costa Rica

Kenneth Mayer
Memorial Hospital
Pawtucket, Rhode Island

Erin McDavid
Agency for International Development
Washington, D.C.

Olav Meirik
World Health Organization
Geneva, Switzerland

Marilyn Mendelson
Eastern Virginia Medical School
Norfolk, Virginia

Kelly Metcalf
Office of Technology Assessment
U.S. Congress
Washington, D.C.

Veronica E. Miller
UCLA School of Medicine
Los Angeles, California

Kamenga Munkolenkole
CDC/Project Sida
U.S. Embassy
Kinshasa, Zaire

Barbara B. North
Healthworks Medical Group
Laguna Niguel, California

Viveca Odlind
Uppsala University
Uppsala, Sweden

James Overstreet
University of California
Davis, California

Thomas O'Brien
Centers for Disease Control
Atlanta, Georgia

Nancy Padian
San Francisco General Hospital
San Francisco, California

Jerri Perkins
Perkins and Perkins, Inc.
Potomac, Maryland

Elisabeth Persson
Karolinska Institutet
Stockholm, Sweden

Thomas A. Peterman
Centers for Disease Control
Atlanta, Georgia

Heidi Peterson
University of California
Davis, California

Herbert Peterson
Centers for Disease Control
Atlanta, Georgia

Praphan Phanuphak
Chulalongkorn Hospital
School of Medicine
Bangkok, Thailand

Joseph Politch
Harvard Medical School
Boston, Massachusetts

John L. Portis
Public Health Service
NIAID
Hamilton, Montana

Malcolm Potts
Family Health International
Durham, North Carolina

Jeffrey Pudney
Harvard Medical School
Boston, Massachusetts

Vanaja Ragavan
Food and Drug Administration
McLain, Virginia

Lionel Resnick
Mount Sinai Medical Center
Miami Beach, Florida

Roselyn Rice
Virginia State Health Department
Virginia Beach, Virginia

Margaret Richman
American Red Cross
Washington, D.C.

Cornelis A.M. Rictmeijer
Dijkzigt University Hospital
Rotterdam, The Netherlands

Allan Rosenfield
Columbia University School of Public
Health
New York, New York

Barbara Ross
The Jones Institute for Reproductive
Medicine
Norfolk, Virginia

Patrick Rowe
World Health Organization
Geneva, Switzerland

Virginia L. Scofield
UCLA School of Medicine
Los Angeles, California

Ruby Senie
Centers for Disease Control
Atlanta, Georgia

James D. Shelton
Office of Population
Agency for International Development
Washington, D.C.

Joyce Sigaloff
Embryonics, Inc.
New York, New York

Jill Silverman
Old Dominion University
Norfolk, Virginia

Joseph Sodroski
Dana-Farber Cancer Institute
Boston, Massachusetts

Kenneth D. Somers
Eastern Virginia Medical School
Norfolk, Virginia

Jeffrey M. Spieler
Office of Population
Agency for International Development
Washington, D.C.

Robert Staab
Schmid Laboratories, Inc.
Little Falls, New Jersey

Ralph Stevens
Old Dominion University
Norfolk, Virginia

A. Charles Tanquary
Family Health International
Durham, North Carolina

Sabita Tejuja
81 Pontiac Way
Gaithersburg, Maryland

Nina Tumosa
Office of Population
Agency for International Development
Washington, D.C.

Linda Valleroy
Office of Population
Agency for International Development
Washington, D.C.

William Vander Haar
Carter-Wallace, Inc.
Cranbury, New Jersey

Bruce Voeller
The Mariposa Foundation
Topanga, California

Mary Vogler
Bellevue Hospital Center
New York, New York

Brendan Waddell
Eastern Virginia Medical School
Norfolk, Virginia

Kevin J. Whaley
The Johns Hopkins University
Baltimore, Maryland

Robert Williams
The Jones Institute for Reproductive Medicine
Norfolk, Virginia

Nancy Williamson
Family Health International
Durham, North Carolina

Steven S. Witkin
Cornell University Medical College/The New York Hospital
New York, New York

Dale Wurster
University of Iowa College of Pharmacy
Iowa City, Iowa

Margan Zajdowicz
Portsmouth Naval Hospital
Norfolk, Virginia

Thaddeus Zajdowicz
Portsmouth Naval Hospital
Norfolk, Virginia

Index